HANDBOOK OF PHARMACY HEALTH EDUCATION

HANDBOOK OF PHARMACY HEALTH EDUCATION

Editor
John Martin

Editorial Staff
Gail C. Neathercoat
Sunayana A. Shah
Prakash Gotecha

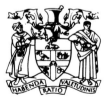

London
THE PHARMACEUTICAL PRESS
1991

 # 24850103

CONTENTS

PREFACE

The *Handbook of Pharmacy Health Education* is produced by direction of the Council of the Royal Pharmaceutical Society of Great Britain, and is one of a series of books to replace the *Pharmaceutical Handbook* (19th Edition, 1980) and *The Pharmaceutical Codex* (11th Edition, 1979). The first replacement volume, *Handbook of Pharmacy Health-care: Diseases and patient advice*, was published in 1990. This latest *Handbook* comprises completely new material and is intended to provide the pharmacist with background information to the aims of health education. It provides comprehensive accounts of areas in which pharmacists may choose to become actively involved and about which they will almost certainly be required to provide advice.

Although the pharmacist is regarded as a specialist in the knowledge of medicines, the future development of the profession and its place within the overall framework of the health-care team requires that this knowledge should be supplemented by a proficiency in other related areas. The public expect pharmacists to possess a broad knowledge of many aspects of health-care. In the course of their work, pharmacists have the opportunity to raise the individual's awareness and understanding about health and illness. In order to fulfil this role, the pharmacist should seek greater collaboration with other health-care professionals and increased personal involvement with the public in giving advice on matters relating to health-care.

Health education is essentially a branch of preventive medicine. In conjunction with effective screening measures (e.g. cervical cytology and plasma-cholesterol concentration monitoring), it seeks to reduce the individual's ultimate needs and demands for health-care resources. Health education involves every aspect of the health—illness continuum and contributes to primary prevention, before the illness starts; secondary prevention, after the illness has started; and tertiary prevention, after the disease has occurred. Patients are demanding to know more about their illnesses, and are showing a greater willingness to take more responsibility for their health.

The main responsibility of the pharmacist in educating the public is helping them to understand their medicines — what they are for, and how and when they should be taken. While giving this advice pharmacists have the opportunity to educate patients on other matters. Pharmacists should be prepared to discuss all issues of concern that patients may raise about their health when such opportunities arise. The purpose of health education is to make health a valuable community asset, to give individuals and communities knowledge and skills so that they can solve their own health problems, and to promote the proper use and development of health-care resources.

The public needs an accessible source of health education to enable and encourage the adoption of healthier life-styles and subsequent avoidance of disease. The pharmacist is the health-care professional who will potentially have the greatest contact with both sick and healthy people, and should take the opportunity to fulfil the role of health educator. Campaigns to increase public recognition of the pharmacist's role in community health-care have generally been directed at the symptomatic treatment of minor illnesses. There is now a need to promote the role of the pharmacist and the pharmacy premises as a first-line source of general health-care advice. In the past, individuals most in need of health-care services have sometimes been the least likely to seek it or receive it. It is important that any improvements in the choice and accessibility of health-care services should benefit those in greatest need. The *Pharmacy Healthcare* scheme has demonstrated the value of community pharmacies as a source of material on such topics as contraception, giving up smoking, dental health-care, and the benefits of a healthy diet. The provision of health education, both verbal and written, is of undoubted value to any community and can only serve to enhance the value and professional image of the pharmacist. However, while pharmacists should develop further their role as health educators, it is imperative that they are also capable of maintaining high standards in the traditional disciplines such as dispensing and advising on drug use.

In *The Health of the Nation* (1991), a Green Paper discussion document, the Government describes Britain's failure to reduce heart disease at the same rate as other countries, its high infant mortality rates, a recent rise in breast cancer deaths and lung cancer deaths among women, and an increase in obesity. The Government recognises that many people are dying prematurely or suffering from preventable conditions, and there are significant ethnic, social, and occupational variations in health. In addition, the report concedes that there are considerable differences in the provision of NHS services across the UK. The Green Paper sets out the Government's targets for improvements to health and ways of achieving them. The Government recognises that community pharmacists have a central role to play in promoting better health and preventing sickness.

The issues involved in health education and the subject matter central to many health promotion activities are both detailed and frequently outside the accepted expertise of pharmacists and their traditional training. The primary aim of the *Handbook of Pharmacy Health Education* is to provide practising pharmacists with the background information that will enable them to raise the awareness and knowledge of their customers or patients about health and illness; the ultimate aim is to discourage participation in essentially 'unhealthy' activities and encourage healthy eating and exercise.

By using the *Handbook*, pharmacists can react to health-related enquiries from members of the public and provide information to help put into perspective the often emotive reports in the media. The coverage of health-related topics in the media may generate frank and open discussion on health topics. This can increase people's awareness of health and subsequently the need for readily available information and advice. However, sensationalised and biased reports on health matters have considerable potential for harm. In order to respond constructively and effectively in such situations, pharmacists must possess a sound and broad scientific and medical knowledge base.

The *Handbook of Pharmacy Health Education* comprises ten chapters on a range of health matters, which frequently present in overt or hidden fashion in the modern pharmacy. The opening chapter considers some of the broader aspects of health and disease, and the issues associated with health education and health promotion.

Nutritional deficiency diseases are still prevalent in many countries, and are an important cause of ill-health and premature death. Nutrient-associated disease due to an incorrect balance or an excess of nutrients is now a problem in virtually all countries, developing and developed alike. The chapter on **Dietary Management** provides an account of dietary constituents, the complex issue of nutritional requirements necessary to maintain health and prevent disease, and examines the dietary needs of specific groups of people. It also considers the risks associated with food additives and other chemicals used by the food industry and in agriculture, and the importance of careful food production and hygiene.

The **Dental Health-care** chapter describes many of the diseases associated with the teeth and gingivae and provides information on plaque control, prevention of dental caries including the protective effect of fluoride, and the care of dentures. The chapter highlights the insidious and often painless nature of dental disease and the importance of daily dental health-care and regular check-ups.

The pharmacist's contribution towards reproductive health and knowledge within the community is vital, particularly with regard to the prevention of HIV infection and other sexually transmitted diseases. The **Contraception** chapter describes the events of the menstrual and ovarian cycles and considers the methods available to prevent conception. The mode of action, reliability, and the beneficial and adverse effects of each method are considered.

Smoking is probably the single most harmful activity affecting the population and giving up is the most beneficial step towards better health that smokers can take. Community pharmacists have supported national 'No Smoking' campaigns for many years now. The success of such campaigns may be enhanced by a more persistent approach and long-term support for the individual. The chapter on **Smoking** looks at the behavioural aspects of the habit and its prevalence. The diseases that occur as a direct effect of smoking are described and the consequences of passive smoking are considered. The chapter also deals with the prevention of smoking and the methods used in trying to give up.

There can be little doubt that there exists a positive correlation between excessive alcohol consumption and morbidity and mortality trends. The **Excessive Alcohol Consumption** chapter gives an account of the social problems and diseases associated with alcohol consumption, and identifies specific groups such as children, the elderly, and pregnant and breast-feeding women, who may be at increased risk from alcohol-related problems. The measurement of alcohol intake and the promotion by the pharmacist of sensible limits of consumption are discussed.

Misuse of both prescribed and illicit drugs is a major national problem. The need to prevent or control drug misuse in view of the spread of HIV infection, hepatitis B, and other infectious diseases is now a priority among health-care professionals. The **Drug Misuse** chapter describes some of the commonly misused drugs and their patterns of use, and considers ways in which a pharmaceutical service can be provided to drug misusers.

Regular exercise promotes good health whereas lack of activity has a deleterious effect. The **Sport and Exercise** chapter describes the physiology of exercise and the benefits and risks associated with sport and exercise. Sports injuries, their management, and the principles of treatment are explained, and the restrictions on the use of drugs in sport are described.

It has been suggested that as many as one in ten travellers abroad becomes ill, and one in twenty ends up in hospital because of failure to take elementary precautions. The chapter on **Health and Travel** gives an account of the measures necessary before travelling, the prevention and management of conditions associated with travel and staying in an unfamiliar environment, and advice for travellers on return. The chapter includes sections on chemoprophylaxis and immunisation, infectious diseases, and sunburn.

The pharmacist is in an ideal position to provide advice to contact lens wearers on effective care regimens and suitability of available preparations for particular types of lenses. The **Contact Lens Care** chapter provides an introduction to the types of lenses currently in use, and describes the different solutions and regimens that are used in the care of contact lenses. The chapter also details some of the complications associated with contact lens wear and includes the adverse effects of some systemically and topically administered drugs.

The further reading section included at the end of most chapters provides a selected list of reading matter that will enable the pharmacist to study the background details relevant to the subject area. General references to health education have been included at the end of chapter one. Useful addresses are included at the end of most chapters. These sections include addresses of professional organisations, which may be able to provide the practising pharmacist with information additional to that included in the chapter. The pharmacist is often asked by patients for information about self-help groups and addresses of these have therefore been included. Important functions of self-help groups are the provision of literature for patients, which should reinforce the information given by health-care professionals, and the provision of contact with other individuals with similar health problems. Addresses relevant to health education and health-care in general have been included at the end of chapter one.

In providing detailed information on these important issues, the *Handbook of Pharmacy Health Education* examines the role of the pharmacist in health education alongside other health-care professionals. This · book should assist the pharmacist to maintain and develop the advisory role confidently and effectively. The *Handbook* is intended to help the pharmacist to achieve a recognised role as a health educator within the community.

Acknowledgements

It is a pleasure to acknowledge the advice and assistance of the experts who have reviewed certain chapters of the *Handbook*. Particular thanks are due to Toni Belfield, Family Planning Association, for her assistance with Chapter 4 and also to Professor M.N. Naylor, Department of Periodontology and Preventive Medicine, Guy's Hospital, for his invaluable contribution to Chapter 3. I am also grateful to Dr Elizabeth Clubb, Catholic Marriage Advisory Council, for her advice and assistance with the illustration of Section 4.4. Appreciation is also due to many organisations including LRC Products Ltd, Organon Laboratories Ltd, The Sports Council, and Wyeth Laboratories for their help and cooperation in the provision of information and illustrations. I also wish to acknowledge *The Sourcebook of Medical Illustrations*, P. Cull (ed.) London: Pantheon Publishing, 1989, from which some of the figures have been taken.

The planning and initial work on this volume were carried out by Robin J. Harman, BPharm, PhD, MRPharmS and I am glad to have this opportunity to record my gratitude and appreciation of the diligent services and enthusiasm of the editorial staff, Gail Neathercoat, BSc, MRPharmS, Sunayana Shah, BPharm, MRPharmS and Prakash Gotecha, BSc, MRPharmS.

The support provided by Pamela North and the staff of the library and information department has also been much valued. I am grateful to have been able to call freely on the expertise of many of the Society's staff, particularly A. Wade, General Editor of Scientific Publications, and W.G. Thomas, Director of the Department of Pharmaceutical Sciences. The secretarial assistance provided by Thelma M. Roberts has been greatly appreciated.

Comments and constructive criticism will be welcome, and should be sent to the Editor, Handbook of Pharmacy Practice series, Royal Pharmaceutical Society of Great Britain, 1 Lambeth High Street, London SE1 7JN.

John Martin, BPharm, PhD, MRPharmS
September 1991

Chapter 1

HEALTH, DISEASE, AND HEALTH EDUCATION

1.1 HEALTH AND ILL-HEALTH

The profession of pharmacy has always been intimately involved with ill-health and its treatment, the drug management of major and minor disease, and the promotion of health. A fundamental role of the pharmacist has been, and will increasingly be, as an adviser on all aspects of drug treatment to the medical and paramedical professions, and to the public.

However, recently, there has been a greater awareness of the problems created by the increasing burden of ill-health on national resources, and the seemingly infinite demands placed upon the health-care systems of many developed nations. In the UK, this has led to a gradual change in government policy, leading to the recognition of the value of enhancing disease prevention and health promotion.

A consultative document on prevention and health (*Prevention and health: everybody's business. A reassessment of public and personal health*, 1976) was distributed that stressed the need for 'the preventive approach to permeate and inform all aspects of health services'. Since that time, further policy statements from government have emphasised the importance of health promotion (*Primary health care. An agenda for discussion*, 1986; *Promoting better health. The government's programme for improving primary health care*, 1987). This emphasis on greater personal responsibility for health has coincided with a trend to increase services within the community, as outlined in the *Griffiths Report* (1988) and extended by a follow-up

report *Caring for people: community care in the next decade and beyond* (1989).

It is important to consider the concept of health and perceptions of ill-health, in order to understand the value of the pharmacist's input towards health education.

Health is an imprecise and elusive concept. One of the most quoted definitions of health is that first proposed by the World Health Organization (WHO) in 1946 and reiterated in 1978. It states that 'health is a state of complete physical, mental, and social well-being, and not simply the absence of disease or infirmity'. This confirms the derivation of the word 'health', which is Anglo-Saxon for 'wholeness'. The WHO definition of health can be succinctly summarised as 'health is being able to cope successfully'. In addition, definitions of health must reflect the changing meaning that we, as individuals, give to life.

Despite, or possibly as a reflection of, these imprecise definitions, many people are unable to express clearly what health means to them (except in terms of the absence of disease, illness, or sickness). People fortunate enough to be in good health tend to take it for granted. Many individuals consider that worrying about health, particularly when there are no apparent health problems, is counter-productive and a waste of time and energy. Many people consider that health is a state of equilibrium and this èquilibrium is perceived as something that comes from within; it is thought to be influenced by temperament and heredity. Perception of a stable equilibrium is commonly related to happiness, relaxation, feeling strong, and having good relations with others; being cheerful and enthusiastic are other positive traits. All of these characteristics enhance the quality of life.

It is often only when individuals, or someone close to them, suffer from ill-health that the positive aspects of good health become appreciated. Most people accept that their everyday life will be occasionally punctuated by minor illness; but there is considerably less willingness to accept those conditions that seriously affect normal activities (e.g. work or social contacts) within the community. Examples of those diseases that are therefore considered more serious and warrant medical attention include cancer, heart disease, and tuberculosis. Such considerations of the relative severity of disease are obviously important when attempts to promote health are proposed.

A further important point to consider in determining health and the value of health education is the wide divergence in the interpretation of health and ill-health by health-care professionals on the one hand and by members of the public on the other. When individuals seek advice from health-care professionals, the application of a disease label by the professional is the result of considering the symptoms reported by the patient and signs noted by the doctor, pharmacist, or nurse. Often, the term used to describe the diagnosed disease is incomprehensible to the patient suffering from it. Nevertheless, the patient's condition can be conveniently and neatly categorised; and this labelling commonly suggests appropriate measures to be taken by the health-care professional.

Conversely, the symptoms experienced by the patient can be termed an illness. The willingness on the part of the sufferer to take action to relieve the illness is determined partly by their ability to cope; and the severity of the illness is subjectively related by the sufferer to past experiences. People may report symptoms and have an illness (e.g. general malaise) but not suffer from a disease; equally, they may be diagnosed as having a disease (e.g. hypertension) but not perceive any symptoms that they would consider indicates the presence of an illness.

Another facet of ill-health sometimes used to indicate levels of morbidity (*see below*) in a population is sickness; this describes an action taken by a patient that may be taken to indicate ill-health. Individuals may seek medical advice, take time off work, or curtail their social activities of their own accord. Sickness may occur in the absence of disease or illness; conversely, the presence of disease or illness does not necessarily imply that any action suggestive of sickness will be taken.

Measurements of health and disease

Valid measurements of health and disease, and application of the data in determining priorities and establishing effective programmes of health promotion and health education, can only be based upon assessment of large populations, not individuals. The study of disease in relation to populations is termed epidemiology, and mortality data (*see below*) that have contributed to the development of this science have been collected in the UK since 1838.

It is not usually possible to monitor an entire population in specific studies of health and disease. Normally, the population under study is a defined group and includes both those that are healthy and those that are unwell. The possible causes of a disease may be determined by comparison of disease rates in different population groups; further comparisons may identify those members of the population at a higher risk of developing a disease than the general population.

More importantly for health promotion and health education, epidemiology permits trends in health and disease to be monitored. Determination of trends identifies those diseases that are declining in importance, and highlights those that may require special attention in the future. One problem, however, in identifying trends, and in particular associated with disease monitoring over several decades, is that the criteria for reporting a particular disease may change with time. This can lead to false optimism (e.g. about the success of a particular form of treatment) when in fact the disease is currently being recorded under a new or different name.

Similarly, as awareness of certain disease states increases (e.g. AIDS), so too does the incidence of diagnosis. The most commonly quoted statistics to identify trends are morbidity and mortality data. These and other terms commonly used in epidemiology are defined in Table 1.1. Mortality statistics are produced by extracting and coding the causes recorded on the death certificate.

In the UK, measurements of morbidity are assessed by the *General Household Survey*, published annually. This survey determines ill-health by seeking information on people's own opinion of their health, details of consultations with general practitioners, attendance at hospital out-patient clinics, and in-patient data. In assessing chronic ill-health, people are asked to indicate whether they have a long-standing illness, infirmity, or disability.

All epidemiological measurements of disease incorporate certain disadvantages. Measurements of the prevalence of a disease are only valid if the condition is chronic, persistent, and stable. However, some chronic

TABLE 1.1
Definition of terms used in epidemiology

Term	Definition
Birth rate	number of live births expressed as a proportion of the population
Fertility rate	number of live births expressed as a proportion of the number of women aged between 15 and 44 years of age
Incidence rate	proportion of a defined group developing a condition within a stated period of time
Infant mortality rate	number of infant deaths (under one year of age) expressed as a proportion of the number of live births
Mortality	frequency of death
Morbidity	frequency of illness and disability
Perinatal mortality rate	number of stillbirths and deaths in the first week of life expressed as a proportion of the total births
Prevalence rate	proportion of a defined group having a condition at one point in time
Standardised mortality rate	number of deaths actually occurring in a given year expressed as a proportion of the number of deaths that would have been expected in that year had the conditions of a period of reference years prevailed
Stillbirth rate	number of intra-uterine deaths after 28 weeks expressed as a proportion of the total births

sufferers will be omitted from the count if the condition is chronic but intermittent, because the prevalence indicates people that actually have the disease at any one point in time. Similarly, prevalence of acute conditions will be underestimated.

The incidence of a disease is often assumed to reflect the actual number of cases, whereas in epidemiology it is the number of new cases expressed as a proportion of the defined population at a stated point in time. As the incidence only counts the number of new cases, it does not take into account those cases that already exist, and therefore underestimates the number of chronic sufferers.

Historical perspectives and trends in disease

Perhaps as a result of the ready availability of comprehensive health services in the UK for more than a generation, many people have come to accept without question that the apparent improvements in general health, and the increased numbers of people living to old age, are a direct consequence of developments in health-care. The public observes a wide range of hospital

services that can be readily and freely used in the event of acute emergencies; a bewildering array of medicines that promote the image of 'a pill for every ill'; and a high profile in the media for 'high technology' medicine that promotes an image of successful management of many formerly untreatable conditions.

However, careful analysis of mortality and morbidity statistics collected throughout this and the last century has led many health-care professionals to the conclusion that the greater proportion of the improvements in life expectancy, and the decreased mortality, can be attributed to:

• improved standards of living
• developments in standards of hygiene
• control of the physical environment
• measures to limit population growth
• introduction of preventive and therapeutic measures.

The early improvements in health in the second half of the nineteenth century were primarily a consequence of:

• public health measures to cover open sewers
• provision of better quality drinking water
• long-term changes in agricultural production and distribution of food supplies.

These social developments led to a significant decline in the mortality from infectious diseases.

The single largest cause of death in the mid-nineteenth century was tuberculosis. Although the tubercle bacillus was identified by Koch in 1882, the first effective drug treatment with streptomycin did not become available until 1947, and widespread BCG vaccination did not commence until 1954. Although the introduction of additional antituberculous drugs has further reduced the mortality, 57% of the initial reduction occurred before 1900.

A similar pattern of decreased mortality before the introduction of effective therapeutic measures can be observed with other airborne infectious diseases (e.g. pertussis, measles, and scarlet fever) and in infections carried by food and water (e.g. cholera and dysentery).

The reduced incidence of infectious diseases generated the greatest impact on the health of the population by significantly increasing the life expectancy of people under 45 years of age. In 1850, the life expectancy at birth was 40 years for men and 42 years for women; by 1984, this had risen to 72 and 78 years respectively.

Although these trends reflect reduced infant mortality rates, even today the death rate during the first year of life still remains higher than at any time below 55 years of age in males and 60 years of age in females. The

TABLE 1.2
Main causes of death in the first year of life

Neonatal period (under 4 weeks)	Post-neonatal period (4 to 52 weeks)
Complications of childbirth	Accidents
Complications of pregnancy	Congenital malformations
Congenital malformations	Infections
Low birth-weight	Respiratory diseases Sudden infant death syndrome

predominant causes of death in the first four weeks of life, and in the remaining period up to the end of the first year of life, are summarised in Table 1.2. The measurement of infant mortality rate is important because it is generally taken as an indicator of a country's quality of health-care and standard of living.

Unfortunately, the advances in the prevention and management of infectious diseases of the past have not produced continued improvements in the overall health of the population (as shown by mortality and morbidity statistics). Epidemics of the past have been replaced by epidemics of the 'industrial' or 'modern' present. Among the most common causes of mortality and morbidity in the 1980s (which will presumably continue to be so in the 1990s) are:

- arthritis
- cancer, and especially lung cancer
- cerebrovascular disease (e.g. stroke)
- chronic bronchitis and emphysema
- diabetes mellitus
- ischaemic heart disease (coronary heart disease)
- mental disorders.

In data collected between 1946 and 1948, circulatory diseases (incorporating ischaemic heart disease and cerebrovascular disease) and cancer accounted for approximately 50% of all deaths in people over 35 years of age; between 1980 and 1982, the proportion had increased to 73%. The dramatic increase in numbers of deaths from cancer and circulatory diseases in people above 35 years of age during the past 40 years has resulted in little overall change in the mortality rate, particularly for men. Most of the 'modern' diseases can be attributed to life-style changes rather than social or environmental changes. Many diseases are caused by behaviour that is entirely voluntary; by far the most important for morbidity and mortality statistics are smoking, poor dietary intake, and alcohol consumption. It has been estimated that as many as 100 000 of the annual 600 000 deaths, can be attributed to smoking.

The most important factors predisposing to ischaemic heart disease are smoking, raised plasma-cholesterol concentrations and a high-fat diet, and hypertension; other contributory factors are obesity and lack of exercise. Many of these factors are interrelated: obesity is commonly associated with a lack of exercise; raised plasma-cholesterol levels, obesity, and high blood pressure can be related to poor diet; and a high dietary salt intake, excessive alcohol consumption, and obesity can all cause hypertension. Each of the contributory factors in the predominant causes of morbidity and mortality is discussed in subsequent chapters.

Highlighting specific important facts serves to illustrate the scale of the health problems facing the population in the 1990s:

- 180 000 deaths occurred and an estimated 38 million working days were lost in 1987 as a result of ischaemic heart disease
- 25% of young people are overweight
- 2.25 million teeth are extracted and 6.5 million fillings are inserted each year in children under 16 years of age
- more than 30% of attendances at hospital accident and emergency departments by men are related to excessive alcohol consumption
- almost 18 000 drug addicts were registered in 1990; a 20% increase compared to the previous year.

1.2 Disease prevention, health education, and health promotion

Misunderstanding sometimes exists concerning the terminology used to describe the methods employed to facilitate disease prevention, and to improve the health of individuals and of the population. Interchange can occur between the use of terms, leading to confusion.

Disease prevention may be classed as primary, secondary, or tertiary. Primary prevention is intended to stop people from developing ill-health or a disease. Primary prevention can be carried out collectively within a population by changing social or environmental conditions, or by providing protection against certain hazards by measures directed at the whole population (e.g. seat-belt legislation or mass immunisation).

Secondary prevention takes place once symptoms are reported by an individual, or a disease has been diagnosed. Initial treatment may help the patient overcome the acute episode of the illness, but prevention of subsequent recurrences or relapses are promoted by careful monitoring of the patient.

At the tertiary level, after a disease has occurred, the pharmacist is able to offer advice on the manner in which a patient's life-style may influence the progression of the condition, and on the appropriate use of their medicines.

Health promotion is the term used to describe a broad and all-embracing concept. Health promotion recognises the need and provides the opportunities for the changes necessary for individuals and communities to improve their health. The breadth of the definition implies that a comprehensive approach is necessary, and not one limited strictly to health matters. Successful health promotion also requires action to improve the communal environment, legislation from central government, economic measures, and social improvements.

Health education is a much more specific concept, directed primarily, but not exclusively, at individuals. It aims to raise the awareness of individuals' knowledge about health and illness, and thereby reduce their participation in essentially 'unhealthy' activities. Health education also facilitates the effective use of the available health-care resources, and attempts to modify individual or collective beliefs, producing a reduction in morbidity and mortality.

Health education is essentially a branch of preventive medicine. When used in conjunction with effective screening measures (e.g. cervical cytology, and plasma-cholesterol concentration monitoring), it seeks to reduce the individual's needs and demands for health-care resources.

The primary aims of health education are not only to increase the length of an individual's life but to reduce morbidity and improve the quality of life. Ageing is inevitable but need not be associated with increased ill-health. Ideally, health education should establish good habits in childhood and early adulthood; early establishment of good habits is more likely to last throughout life, and can lead to compression of the period of morbidity that almost inevitably occurs towards the end of life.

Pharmacists are primarily involved in health education and not health promotion.

Factors influencing the effectiveness of health education

One of the major problems in achieving effective health education is the apparent unwillingness of many sectors of the population to understand or recognise the risks of some of their activities. Most people find it extremely difficult to accept that their behaviour at the time they are between 20 and 30 years of age will have a bearing on their health in 20 or 30 years time. Social and peer pressures demand that they conform (e.g. in excessive alcohol consumption or in smoking); advertising aims to create and emphasise the close association between some activities (e.g. drinking alcohol and acceptance by friends and associates). Fatalism, illustrated by statements such as 'It won't happen to me', and 'Bill drank and smoked all the time − and he lived to be 90', is a potent force counteracting the effectiveness of health education.

Prevention is also sometimes perceived as a negative concept, seen as stopping people from doing something that they enjoy and from which little or no immediate or foreseeable benefit can be determined.

Conversely, on the positive side, there is an increased determination in certain sectors of the population to ensure that they do as much as is possible to remain healthy, and to lead as fulfilling and active a life as possible. There is a growing trend for people to try and positively influence their own health, possibly in recognition that individual efforts can have a bearing on the quality of life.

The age of those receiving health education can also influence the success of its uptake. People up to about 40 years of age have little interest in their own health, particularly if they have been in predominantly good health. It is only when 40 and more years of age is reached that a greater concern with health matters tends to develop. However, the value of adopting preventive measures after this age, both to society and to the individual, is difficult to assess, but measures can still be useful. For example, if measures are taken to stop smoking early enough in life, the risks of ischaemic heart disease will be reduced and the length of the productive working life of the individual will be increased, producing a benefit to society as a whole. By comparison, smoking in later life may be associated with a greater burden on society. This can be attributed to: increased demands for proportionally more expensive health services in old age; and possible social costs of care for the individual.

On a positive note, however, all human beings are inherently valuable and attempts should be made to dissuade them from doing things that are potentially harmful. Pharmacists should encourage all members of the population to adopt a healthier life-style, so producing a healthier society.

Methods of disseminating health education

A wide variety of methods are used to transmit information used for educating people about health. The methods vary in the size of their target audience, the level of involvement between educators and their audience, and the degree of feedback that can be obtained to monitor the effectiveness of the process.

The mass media reaches a significant proportion of a target population but, by definition, its messages are largely impersonal. Information will be relayed to all members within a defined population, not just those who may be at high risk of developing a particular condition. Posters, television, radio, and books are the most commonly used channels of the mass media, and these can be extremely influential in drawing attention to particular issues; appropriate sales promotion, advertising, and sponsorship can highlight a link with a healthy activity. To be effective, messages conveyed by the mass media must be simple and non-stressful; they should also be enjoyable and interesting. Because of their potential audience and effect, it is vital that the message conveyed is accurate and responsibly portrayed. Endorsement by an authoritative personality (e.g. a well-known doctor or a government minister) may reinforce the positive nature of the message. However, the effectiveness of mass media techniques in actually influencing and changing people's behaviour in the desired direction is extremely difficult to quantify.

More personal measures adopted in health education can be carried out in specific environments and targeted towards specific groups. The importance of providing health education at as young an age as possible has been recognised by the inclusion of health topics in the curricula of schools and colleges, and in activities at other centres where young people gather socially. It has been found that the most effective means of influencing attitudes can be produced by participation in small discussion groups (inter-personal approaches). Individuals may be pressurised by their peers to adopt a change in attitude, emphasising the perceived importance of conformity with the general consensus of the group. Similar educational activities can take place in the workplace, although the adoption of specific policies (e.g. introduction of no-smoking policies) can have a more immediate impact.

The greatest level of involvement and the maximum degree of feedback can be obtained with discussions between health educators and clients on a one to one basis. Ideally, the opportunities for education should be grasped by adopting an interactive approach. A much greater response will be obtained from clients if they actively participate in the discussions, rather than merely being told what is good for them and what they should do. By adopting such a stance, clients can be guided to develop a much greater responsibility for their own health.

The most important setting for pharmacists to carry out health education is in the pharmacy, although pharmacists can and do extend their health education role by talking to small meetings outside normal working hours. In the pharmacy, pharmacists work face to face with patients and can tailor the information and responses to the specific needs of the individual. The role of the pharmacist in providing health education is discussed in more detail in Section 1.3.

No one method of imparting information about health is appropriate for all situations. The most effective health education measures are usually a combination of impersonal mass media messages reinforced by inter-personal or personal information.

Ethical issues in health education

Ethical issues in health education have mainly concentrated upon the concerns about the balance between trying to persuade people to change their attitudes and life-style, and allowing people the right of self-determination. Ideally, education in its broadest sense aims to provide people with the information they need to make informed decisions. Health education attempts to provide details of the likely effects of particular activities on health; it is then up to individuals to decide whether to continue that activity in the light of that knowledge.

Ethical discussions also centre upon the degree to which people should be told what to do when it comes to their own bodies, and how much intervention can be justified on the grounds of the common good. Smoking in some public places has been prohibited; but individuals cannot be forced to stop smoking altogether, they can only be advised of the health risks that ensue from the habit.

In providing people with the information they require to assess the risks to themselves, they must also be informed of the potential consequences of their activities on others. Passive smoking has become a recognised health hazard to non-smokers, and this should be borne in mind by smokers when they smoke in the presence of others. Certain potentially harmful activities require community action to prevent the risks to others. Legislation exists in an attempt to protect people from those who would drink excessive quantities of alcohol and subsequently drive. Other measures enforced by legislation for the overall benefit of the community also exist (e.g. fluoridation of water supplies to prevent dental caries, and seat-belt legislation). Restriction of personal liberties may be claimed but accusations of authoritarianism can only be justified when the measures taken are against the wishes of the majority of the population.

1.3 THE ROLE OF THE PHARMACIST

Integration within the primary health-care team

There appears to be an encouraging trend in the general population that is leading to the gradual recognition of the importance of preventive medicine, as opposed to the traditional emphasis on curative procedures. Demands for the introduction of policies to ban smoking in public places, of increased health education in schools, and the banning of the advertising of tobacco products, appears to be gaining momentum. These trends are reflected by an increased desire among all health-care professionals to take an active part in health education, not only relating to smoking but also to many of the closely related topics of nutrition, ischaemic heart disease, and excessive alcohol consumption.

It has been estimated that about 90% of all contacts that people have with the health-care professionals are through the primary health-care services. These include the family practitioner services (general practitioners, dentists, community pharmacists, and opticians) and the community health services (community nurses, midwives, health visitors, and other professions allied to medicine, including chiropodists and physiotherapists). Community pharmacists have a prominent position within the primary health-care services because of their free and ready accessibility to the public.

However, there is the danger that involvement of increasingly large numbers of health-care professionals in health education can lead to a fragmented approach. All members of the primary health-care team should attempt to provide an integrated and coordinated approach that emphasises those activities whose modification could lead to improvements in the health of the population. In the UK, attempts to provide an integrated approach involving all health-care professionals are overseen by the Health Education Authority (HEA), the successor to the Health Education Council. The HEA published a five-year strategic plan in 1990, operational from 1990 to 1995, which it believes identifies those areas of health that warrant particular attention. The list of preventive health measures given priority by the HEA are listed in Table 1.3.

Great emphasis in many aspects of pharmacy practice research is placed upon the estimated numbers of daily visitors to community pharmacies. The six million visits which are made to pharmacies each day in the UK represents the maximum potential pool of those to whom health counselling could be given; but perhaps a more realistic estimate of those who enter pharmacies

TABLE 1.3

HEA strategic plan 1990–1995

Programme	Aims include
HIV/AIDS and sexual health	guidance on drug injection practices by addicts, and sexual health (e.g. use of condoms)
Look after your heart!	prevention of ischaemic heart disease, and promotion of a physically active way of life
Cancer education	integration of Look after your heart!, smoking, and alcohol programmes, and prevention by screening of breast and cervical cancer
Smoking education	encouraging teenagers not to smoke; provision of information on harmful effects of smoking; and support for the introduction of smoke-free workplaces
Alcohol education	helping people to make informed choices about alcohol use, and reducing the number of people drinking above sensible limits
Nutrition education	provision of a consistent, authoritative source of advice and information on all aspects of nutrition, and encouragement to food providers to make available a wider choice of healthy foods
Family and child health	provision of information on pregnancy, parenthood, and the care of young children, and information on immunisation

and approach the pharmacist is closer to the 650 000 people who visit pharmacies each day to have prescriptions dispensed. Irrespective of the actual figure, it is clear that the potential for advising on health matters is enormous. One important point to consider is that many of the visitors to pharmacies are healthy, and it is to this group that health education activities should be directed.

Health education activities can also take place within the hospital pharmacy. However, by virtue of the nature of the secondary referral procedure to hospitals, these activities tend to be related more to specific problem areas (e.g. drug misuse and needle exchange schemes), with less emphasis on opportunities for general health advice.

It has been suggested that whereas many people are happy to consult their doctor when they are ill, they are less willing to request time for general health education and advice when they are healthy. In many cases, health education has been delegated within group practices to the practice nurse, who can devote a greater length of time to counselling and advising visitors to the surgery. More importantly, practice nurses will commonly be able to tailor the discussion to the particular needs of the patient as a result of knowledge of the relevant medical history. The government in the UK aims to recognise the contribution that doctors and practice nurses can make by encouraging the development of scheduled health education sessions for their patients.

Pharmacists should be prepared to offer their expertise to assist in these sessions (e.g. to advise on health when travelling and on the prevention of drug misuse). Clearly, any offers of participation will be much more readily received if pharmacists already have good working relationships and regular contacts (e.g. collaborative meetings) with staff working in group practices.

Pharmacy Healthcare scheme

Pharmacists are ideally placed through their direct personal contact with the public to fully develop their advisory role on all health matters. In the UK, more formal promotion of this role was facilitated by the launch in February 1986 of the *Family Health Care* or *Health Care in the High Street* scheme. This was launched by the Pharmaceutical Society of Great

Britain in conjunction with the Family Planning Association, the HEA, the Scottish Health Education Group, the National Pharmaceutical Association, and Boots the Chemists Ltd. To reflect the position of pharmacies as primary distribution outlets for the leaflets, the scheme has subsequently been renamed *Pharmacy Healthcare*.

The *Pharmacy Healthcare* scheme highlights the importance of pharmacists as a source of information on a wide range of health topics through the display of leaflets produced and distributed by a diverse group of health organisations (Table 1.4). New leaflets, which are produced by participating organisations, are supplied every 4 to 6 weeks. Guidance for pharmacists on the information contained in new leaflets is given before the time of distribution by articles in the pharmaceutical press.

It is vital to the success of the scheme that all pharmacists play as full a part as possible. Display stands, supplied as part of the scheme, should be prominently positioned within the pharmacy. Pharmacy staff should familiarise themselves with the content of the leaflets at the time of distribution so that questions raised by members of the public can be confidently answered. Opportunities for discussing the content of

TABLE 1.4

Leaflets and organisations involved in the Pharmacy Healthcare *campaign, 1990 to 1991*

1990		
Jan	Healthy teeth and fresh breath	Warner Lambert
Feb	Warmth in winter	HEA
Mar	National no smoking day	HEA
Apr	Thrush	HEA/PHC
May	Emergency contraception	PHC/FPA
Jun	NHS breast screening: the facts	HEA/PHC
Jul	Are you dying to get a suntan	HEA/PHC
Aug	Solvent abuse	ReSolv/PHC
Sep	Headlice	PHC/NPA
Oct	Herpes	HEA/PHC
Nov	European Cancer Week	
Dec	HIV/AIDS and you	HEA/PHC
1991		
Jan	Alzheimer's disease	Alzheimer's Disease Society/PHC
Mar	National no smoking day	HEA
Apr	Medic-Alert	Medic-Alert Foundation
May	Oral hygiene	Gibbs
Jul	Skincare: Are you dying for a suntan	HEA/PHC
Aug	Better communicating with your doctor and pharmacist	Medical Advisory Service/PHC
Sep	Diet and exercise for people	Arthritis Care/PHC
Oct	Migraine	Glaxo
Nov	Cystitis	
Dec	11 Methods of contraception	FPA/PHC

Abbreviations used:
FPA	Family Planning Association
HEA	Health Education Authority
NPA	National Pharmaceutical Association
PHC	Pharmacy Healthcare Campaign

the leaflets may commonly arise at periods when patients are waiting to collect dispensed medicines.

Evaluation of the widespread uptake, reading, and use of leaflets by the public has been recorded by reports from participating organisations of the return rate of tear-off responses. Recognition of the importance of the *Pharmacy Healthcare* scheme in promoting a greater awareness on health topics within the community has come by continued financial backing from the UK government to consolidate and expand the scheme.

1.4   USEFUL ADDRESSES

AGE CONCERN ENGLAND
National Council on Ageing
Astral House
1268 London Road
London SW16 4EJ
Tel: 081-679 8000

Age Well is Age Concern England's health promotion project for older people, which aims to raise public and professional awareness, and to encourage the adoption of healthier lifestyles after the age of 60 or around retirement.

BRITISH ASSOCIATION FOR COUNSELLING (BAC)
37a Sheep Street
Rugby CV21 3BX
Tel: (0788) 578328
Promotes the understanding and awareness of counselling throughout society.

BRITISH HEART FOUNDATION
14 Fitzhardinge Street
London W1H 4DH
Tel: 071-935 0185

THE CHEST, HEART AND STROKE ASSOCIATION
CHSA House
Whitecross Street
London EC1Y 8JJ
Tel: 071-490 7999

THE CORONARY PREVENTION GROUP
60 Great Ormond Street
London WC1N 3HR
Tel: 071-833 3687

DEPARTMENT OF HEALTH (DoH)
Hannibal House
London SE1 6TE
Tel: 071-972 2000

DEPARTMENT OF HEALTH AND SOCIAL SERVICES
Dundonald House
Upper Newtownards Road
Belfast BT4 3FS
Tel: (0232) 63939

HEALTH EDUCATION AUTHORITY
Hamilton House
Mabledon Place
London WC1H 9TX
Tel: 071-383 3833

THE HEALTH PROMOTION AGENCY FOR NORTHERN IRELAND
The Beeches
12 Hampton Manor Drive
Belfast BT7 3EN
Tel: (0232) 644811

HEALTH PROMOTION AUTHORITY FOR WALES
Brunel House (8th Floor)
2 Fitzalan Road
Cardiff CF2 1EB
Tel: (0222) 472472

THE HEALTH PROMOTION RESEARCH TRUST
49–53 Regent Street
Cambridge CB2 1AB
Tel: (0223) 69636

THE LOOK AFTER YOURSELF PROJECT CENTRE
Christ Church College
Canterbury
Kent CT1 1QU
Tel: (0227) 455564

NATIONAL PHARMACEUTICAL ASSOCIATION
Mallinson House
38–42 St Peter's Street
St Albans
Herts AL1 3NP
Tel: (0727) 832161

PHARMACEUTICAL SERVICES NEGOTIATING COMMITTEE (PSNC)
59 Buckingham Street
Aylesbury
Bucks HP20 2PJ
Tel: (0296) 432823

PHARMACY HEALTHCARE SCHEME
1 Lambeth High Street
London SE1 7JN
Tel: 071-735 9141

THE ROYAL SOCIETY OF HEALTH (RSH)
RSH House
38A St George's Drive
London SW1V 4BH
Tel: 071-630 0121

THE SCOTTISH HEALTH EDUCATION GROUP
Woodburn House
Canaan Lane
Edinburgh EH10 4SG
Tel: 031-447 8044

SCOTTISH HOME AND HEALTH DEPARTMENT
St Andrew's House
Edinburgh EH1 3DE
Tel: 031-556 8400

WELSH OFFICE
Cathays Park
Cardiff CF1 3NQ
Tel: (0222) 825111

1.5   FURTHER READING

Black D, *et al. Inequalities in health. The Black report*. Harmondsworth: Penguin, 1982.

Black N, *et al.*, eds. *Health and disease: a reader*. Milton Keynes: Open University Press, 1984.

Calnan M, *Health and illness. The lay perspective*. London: Tavistock Publications, 1987.

DHSS. *Prevention and health: everybody's business. A reassessment of public and personal health*. London: HMSO, 1976.

DoH. *On the state of the public health*. London: HMSO, 1989.

Griffin T, ed. *Social Trends 21*. London: HMSO, 1991.

Griffiths R. *Community care: agenda for action*. London: HMSO, 1988.

Rose G, Barker DJP. *Epidemiology for the uninitiated*. 2nd ed. London: British Medical Journal, 1986.

Secretaries of State for Health, Social Security, Wales and Scotland. *Caring for people. Community care in the next decade and beyond*. Cm 849. London: HMSO, 1989.

Secretaries of State for Social Services, Wales, Northern Ireland, and Scotland. *Primary health care. An agenda for discussion*. Cmnd 9771. London: HMSO, 1986.

Secretaries of State for Social Services, Wales, Northern Ireland, and Scotland. *Promoting better health. The government's programme for improving primary health care*. London: HMSO, 1987.

Smith A, Jacobson B, eds. *The nation's health. A strategy for the 1990s*. London: King Edward's Hospital Fund for London, 1988.

Smith GT, ed. *Measuring health: a practical approach*. Chichester: John Wiley & Sons, 1988.

Chapter 2

DIETARY MANAGEMENT

2.1 DIET AND HEALTH

Food is essential to ensure growth, maintenance and repair of tissues, correct functioning of metabolic processes, and to provide energy to enable all these functions to be carried out. In addition, food has a social function and is a means of getting people together, whether it be a family, a group of friends, or business people entertaining clients. Food is also used as a means of comfort or reward.

A great deal is written and spoken about modern diets by the lay press, professional bodies, government departments, and the food industry itself. The result is a plethora of conflicting information from all quarters, which can, at times, be highly controversial. It is not surprising that there is a lot of confusion over what constitutes a good, well balanced, nutritious diet. Some people take an extreme standpoint and indulge in faddish diets in an effort to eliminate totally certain components. In doing so, their diet becomes unbalanced and they run the risk of both excesses and deficiencies. Others attempt a more rational approach but quickly run into trouble because they do not have the background knowledge to objectively assess the contradictory information presented to them. They either struggle on, labouring under a variety of misconceptions, or revert to their original habits in the belief that 'nobody knows what they are talking about anyway'. At the other extreme, there are those who refuse to give any thought to dietary matters at all and continue to indulge in dietary excesses, possibly at the expense of other, more nutritious, alternatives.

People in the western world are as much at risk of malnutrition as those in developing countries but for different reasons. Diets in affluent societies contain a high proportion of fats and sugars, and it has been recommended by many authorities that both of these should be reduced, and a greater emphasis placed on starchy foods as a means of providing food energy. Conversely, people in developing countries are likely to be undernourished and should increase their intake of proteins and fats, and aim for consumption of a greater variety of foods.

The modern diet has changed drastically in other respects too. Busy life-styles and a steady reduction in the time spent in planning, shopping, and preparation of food has led to reliance on a vast array of 'convenience' foods. Products with a long shelf-life coupled with minimal preparation and cooking are now expected in addition to certain standards of appearance (e.g. good colour and texture). Consequently, a whole multitude of substances are added as preservatives, stabilisers, emulsifiers, binders, colouring and flavouring agents, and flavour enhancers. Salt and sugar are also added in large amounts (sometimes to the most unlikely products) to improve flavour. Modern food processing methods and prolonged storage also reduce the levels of valuable vitamins, although it is not often appreciated that losses also occur from fresh foods on storage and preparation.

Fresh foods are not without risks of contamination, and the skins of fruit and vegetables may be coated with chemicals (e.g. insecticides and herbicides). Ready-to-eat salads are widely available and, if improperly prepared, have proved to be a source of *Listeria monocytogenes*. Cook-chill foods provide a fertile growing medium for bacteria, notably *Salmonella* spp. and *Listeria monocytogenes*, and may cause food poisoning if not reheated thoroughly. Modern intensive farming methods have also increased the level of bacteria in food (e.g. *Salmonella* spp. in poultry and eggs), and meat may contain residues of veterinary drugs.

Pharmacists have an important role as providers of health-care, and are in an effective position to advise on nutrition. Counselling may be required in a variety of cases including:

- advice about basic nutritious diets to maintain health and prevent diet-related diseases
- objective interpretation of the information available from different sources
- recommendations about vitamin and mineral supplements
- consideration of the needs of specific groups (e.g. vegetarians, infants and children, pregnant and lactating women, the elderly, and the sick and convalescent)
- assessment of the potential risks associated with food additives and other chemicals used by the food industry and in agriculture
- counselling on food preparation and hygiene to reduce the risks of food-borne infections.

Diet-related diseases

Some diseases can be directly related to food or its lack and these are well documented. Such disorders were common in the UK until comparatively recently, and still are in developing countries. Undernourishment results in poor growth and repair of tissues, and specific deficiency syndromes are caused by lack of some vitamins (*see* Section 2.2.4).

Fungal contamination may occur during growth of crops or on subsequent storage: ergotism (St. Anthony's fire) is caused by ingestion of rye contaminated with *Claviceps purpurea*, and formerly occurred as epidemics but is now rarely seen; and aflatoxins, which have been implicated in the development of liver cancer, are potent toxins produced by *Aspergillus flavus*, which grows on many vegetables, particularly peanuts. Helminthic infections have always been a problem, and still are in areas where raw or undercooked meat or fish form part of the traditional diet. Bacterial or protozoal contamination of food is responsible for cholera, dysentery, giardiasis, and salmonellal infections in areas where poor sanitation results in contamination of the water supply or human excrement is used as a fertiliser. Brucellosis is caused by the ingestion of unpasteurised milk and milk products obtained from cows infected with *Brucella* spp.

Improvements in agricultural yields, hygiene, health education, and the increased availability of a wide range of foods to all income-levels of society have eliminated most of these diseases in industrial nations. However, the incidence of other diseases has increased, and this has been linked to the increase in consumption of sugars, fats, and salt. It may be that, in some cases, poor diet is not the sole aetiological factor; other factors that must be taken into consideration include smoking (*see* Chapter 5), excessive alcohol consumption (*see* Chapter 6), lack of exercise (*see* Chapter 8), and emotional stress. The diet-related disorders referred to in this Chapter are those considered to be caused or precipitated by the long-term consumption of the traditional diet of industrial nations. It is felt by many authorities that the incidence of these diseases would be significantly reduced if overall dietary adjustments were made. The role of diet in the development of dental caries is discussed in Chapter 3.

Obesity is common in the western world and is caused by consumption of fats and sugars in excess of an individual's energy requirements. Being overweight may affect a person psychologically because obesity is not considered attractive. Obese people are also at a physical disadvantage because they do not possess the suppleness or stamina of a person of desirable body-weight. Obesity also predisposes an individual to disease (e.g. cardiovascular disease, diabetes mellitus, and joint disorders). Cardiovascular disease and gallstones are directly attributed to a high fat intake, and hypertension may be associated with excessive salt consumption. Insufficient non-starch polysaccharides (*see* Section 2.2.1) in the diet has been linked to the development of several gastro-intestinal and related disorders (e.g. appendicitis, colorectal cancer, constipation, diverticulitis, and irritable bowel syndrome). Poor diet may also cause or precipitate diabetes mellitus, and diet has been linked with some forms of cancer.

Symptoms of some disorders are produced as a direct reaction to certain components in the diet, but the underlying aetiology may involve immunological mechanisms or inappropriate biochemical reactions. Such conditions include food allergies and food intolerance, malabsorption syndromes, and inborn errors of metabolism. Treatment usually involves removal of the offending food, and may require substitution with some other component. For more detailed information on dietary products for specific disorders the reader is referred to Dietary Products in Harman RJ, *Patient care in community practice: A handbook of non-medicinal health-care*, 1989.

Energy requirements

Energy values

The unit of energy in the International System of Units (SI) is the joule (J). This is the work done when a force of 1 newton is displaced through a distance of 1 metre in the direction of the force. In nutrition, the kilojoule (1 kJ = 1000 J) and megajoule (1 MJ = 10^6 J) are used as more convenient units. Energy values were formerly expressed in units of heat, employing the calorie. One calorie is the amount of heat required to raise the temperature of 1 g of water by 1°C at a specified temperature (i.e. from 14.5 to 15.5°C). This was formerly known as the 'small calorie' (cal) and distinguished from the 'large Calorie' (Cal) used in nutrition, which is equivalent to 1000 calories or 1 kilocalorie (kcal). Although, it is preferable to use the SI unit, the kilocalorie is widely used in nutrition.

In food, fats form the most concentrated source of energy, and 1 g provides 0.037 MJ (8.8 kcal), whereas carbohydrates (expressed as monosaccharides) provide 0.016 MJ (3.8 kcal), and proteins 0.017 MJ (4 kcal). Energy values can therefore be calculated when the proportion of these constituents in food is known. Alcohol is also a source of energy, and 1 g provides 0.029 MJ (7.0 kcal). Vitamins and minerals do not contribute any energy. Additional heat is provided by hot food cooling to the body's temperature of 37°C, and although this amount of energy is very small compared to the overall contribution, the effects are felt immediately and may be of considerable psychological benefit in producing feelings of comfort and warmth. There is, however, no nutritional advantage of hot food compared to cold food.

Individual requirements

Human energy requirements are variable and depend upon a number of different factors (e.g. age, sex, and body composition and size). Climate, environment, and the state of a person's health must also be considered, but it is the amount of physical activity that has the greatest effect on individual energy requirements.

The basal metabolic rate (BMR) is the rate at which the body uses energy when the body is at complete rest. Values depend on age, sex, and body-weight. Examples of BMRs are:

- 7.56 MJ/day (1800 kcal/day) for a 65 kg man
- 5.98 MJ/day (1424 kcal/day) for a 55 kg woman.

The proportion of lean tissue (i.e. the fat-free mass or FFM) dictates the energy needed, and the BMR is therefore lower in the elderly or during starvation.

Extra energy above the BMR is required when food is eaten and for any sort of activity. More energy is required for strenuous activity than light exercise, and heavier people need more energy than light people to carry out the same amount of activity. The Estimated Average Requirement (EAR) for energy is an estimate of the average requirement or need, and is equivalent to the BMR multiplied by the Physical Activity Level (PAL). PAL is the ratio of overall daily energy expenditure to BMR, and values range from 1.4 to 1.9. Most people in the UK have a PAL of 1.4, which represents very little physical activity.

Dietary reference values and food tables

The control of dietary energy intake is dictated by appetite whereas nutrient consumption is not. However, a good, regular, mixed diet should provide all the nutrients required and, in theory, in-depth nutritional knowledge is not necessary. However, in practice, the correct balance of nutrients may not be achieved. In many parts of the world, deficiencies occur because there may be a general shortage of food or a lack of variety. In developed nations, where these problems do not exist, clinical deficiencies are uncommon. However, there may still be a poor balance of nutrients in the diet as a result of over-consumption of fats and refined carbohydrates (especially sugars) at the expense of other foods.

The diets of adults are largely determined by what was eaten during childhood and reflects the nutritional knowledge of their parents, which in turn would have been based on the level of general health education available at the time. In addition, restrictions may have been imposed by culture, ethics, or religion. In order for individuals to assess the adequacy of their diets and to make any appropriate adjustments, an awareness of nutritional needs is necessary.

Dietary reference values

A knowledge of the disease states produced by deficiencies of some nutrients has enabled the compilation of a list of nutrients that are essential to maintain health and activity. Furthermore, controlled scientific studies have been able to assess the minimum amounts of some nutrients required to prevent clinical deficiency syndromes (e.g. 10 mg per day of ascorbic acid prevents scurvy). However, solely preventing a clinical condition does not necessarily guarantee health because the actual amount needed to maintain health may be in excess of that required to prevent disease. There are other nutrients for which clinical deficiency states are unknown, presumably because they are required in such small amounts, or are widely distributed throughout foods, or both. Nevertheless, research has highlighted essential roles of such nutrients in metabolic pathways and, consequently, they too are considered necessary to maintain health. Various authorities have made recommendations regarding the amounts of essential nutrients necessary to maintain health. However, the amounts suggested may differ because different criteria are used as the basis for the recommendations.

In 1979, the DHSS set Recommended Daily Amounts (RDAs) of food energy and nutrients for groups of people in the United Kingdom. The definition of the RDA for a nutrient was 'the average amount of the nutrient which should be provided per head in a group of people if the needs of practically all members of the group are to be met'. Therefore, to ensure that everyone received adequate amounts, RDAs were higher than the average amount required by the group. This was widely misinterpreted as the minimum amount required by individuals to maintain health. Individuals vary in their needs and some may consume less than the RDA without any apparent ill effects and problems may not arise until the intake falls significantly below the RDA. RDAs were intended to be used when planning food supplies for groups of people, or when interpreting data obtained from surveys of food supplies or dietary intake.

The DoH has issued a new set of guidelines in Dietary reference values for food energy and nutrients for the United Kingdom, *Report on Health and Social Subjects No. 41*, 1991. It has been recognised that nutritional reference values are required in a variety of applications, including assessment of the adequacy of individual diets. Consequently, four standards have been defined to replace the former RDAs. All four standards are covered by the term Dietary Reference Values (DRVs).

- EAR

    Estimated Average Requirement of a group of people for energy or a nutrient. About half will usually need more than the EAR, and half less.

- LRNI

  Lower Reference Nutrient Intake for a nutrient. An amount of the nutrient that is enough for only the few people in a group who have low needs. Most people will need more than the LRNI if they are to eat enough, and if individuals are habitually eating less than the LRNI they will almost certainly be deficient.

- RNI

  Reference Nutrient Intake for a nutrient. An amount of the nutrient that is enough, or more than enough, for about 97% of people in a group. This level of intake is, therefore, considerably higher than most people need. If individuals are consuming the RNI of a nutrient, they are most unlikely to be deficient in that nutrient.

- Safe intake

  A term used to indicate intake or range of intakes of a nutrient for which there is not enough information to estimate EAR, LRNI, or RNI. It is an amount that is enough for almost everyone but is not so large as to cause undesirable effects.

EARs of energy are the average values of energy required by various groups and, consequently, some people within a group will require more, and others less, than this amount. The exact amount of energy required by an individual is equal to the amount of energy expended, and therefore varies with the level of physical activity. Energy requirements are controlled quite accurately by appetite, which should maintain a constant body-weight.

Fats, sugars, and starches are major contributors to energy intake, and an inadequate intake results in weight loss. There are, however, no deficiency signs or symptoms specifically associated with a low intake of these nutrients, and there is no EAR, LRNI, or RNI. Research has shown that health is affected by the proportions in the diet of fats, starches, and sugars, and it was deemed by the DoH (1991) that some guidance was required on the desirable intakes of these nutrients. DRVs are quoted as representing the average contribution that fats, sugars, and starches should make to dietary energy for groups of people.

The DoH (1991) has emphasised that all DRVs for proteins, vitamins, and minerals should be treated cautiously because they are only indications of the ranges of requirements likely to be found within the UK populations, and the values for energy, fats, sugars, and

TABLE 2.1

Daily EARs for energy and daily RNIs for nutrients for adults of 19 years of age and over

	Men	Women[a]
Energy (PAL = 1.4)	8.77 to 10.60 MJ[b]	7.61 to 8.10 MJ[b]
Protein[c]		
19 to 50 years of age	55.5 g	45.0 g
over 50 years of age	53.3 g	46.5 g
Ascorbic acid	40 mg	40 mg
Vitamin A (retinol equivalents)	700 mg	600 mg
Vitamin B group		
total folate	200 mg	200 mg
nicotinic acid equivalent	16 to 17 mg [b]	12 to 13 mg[b]
pyridoxine [d]	1.4 mg	1.2 mg
riboflavine	1.3 mg	1.1 mg
thiamine	0.9 to 1.0 mg[b]	0.8 mg[b]
vitamin B_{12}	1.5 mg	1.5 mg
Vitamin D	(e)	(e)
Calcium	700 mg	700 mg
Chloride	2.5 g	2.5 g
Copper	1.2 mg	1.2 mg
Iron	8.7 mg	8.7 to 14.8 mg[f]
Magnesium	300 mg	270 mg
Phosphorus	550 mg	550 mg
Potassium	3.5 g	3.5 g
Iodine	140 mg	140 mg
Selenium	75 mg	60 mg
Sodium	1.6 g	1.6 g
Zinc	9.5 mg	7.0 mg

(a) The requirement for many nutrients increases during pregnancy and lactation and, where appropriate, these are discussed in Section 2.3.

(b) The actual value depends on age, the level of physical activity, or both.

(c) Milk or egg protein. These figures assume complete digestibility. For diets based on high intakes of vegetable proteins, correction may need to be applied.

(d) Based on protein providing 14.7% of EAR for energy.

(e) No dietary sources may be necessary for people who are sufficiently exposed to sunlight, but the DoH recommends that the RNI after 65 years of age is 10 μg/day for men and women; supplements may be required by children and adolescents during the winter (*see* Section 2.3), and housebound adults.

(f) This intake may not be sufficient for women with large menstrual losses and iron supplements may be required.

The figures for this table are derived from DoH, Dietary reference values for food energy and nutrients for the United Kingdom, *Report on Health and Social Subjects No. 41*, London: HMSO, 1991.

starches are just intended to be indications of appropriate intakes.

DRVs have been assessed for healthy groups, including those with extra needs (e.g. infants, children, and pregnant and breast-feeding women), but have not taken into account the increased demands made by illness and convalescence (*see* Section 2.3). Specific deficiency syndromes or disorders requiring specialised dietary management are clinical problems and should be treated by specialists. Table 2.1 lists EARs for energy and RNIs for nutrients for adults aged 19 years and over.

Food tables

Tables listing the composition of nutrients and energy provided by various foods are available, and may help to assess the adequacy of a diet. They may also be useful in highlighting those foods that contain a specific nutrient needed by an individual (e.g. the requirement for calcium dramatically increases during pregnancy and lactation and may not be met by the individual's regular diet, *see* Section 2.3). Tables may be arranged as a list of foods under each nutrient, or as an alphabetical list of foods with analysis of composition. Publications listing food tables are included in Section 2.7.

The actual values quoted are based upon the laboratory analysis of several samples. Tables from different laboratories, particularly in different countries, will not necessarily show the same figures because there are many factors that may influence the nutrient levels. These include the variety of plant or animal used for analysis, the season or climate, the level of minerals in the soil, and other growing and feeding conditions. The level of nutrients also falls after harvesting. For example, some vitamins are destroyed by heat, light, or prolonged storage (especially if allowed to dry out), or if the flesh of fruits and vegetables is bruised. Losses during cooking must be taken into account if the tables quote values for raw food only, and nutrients may be lost in preparation because the skins of many fruit and vegetables are discarded.

Food tables are not intended to be used to calculate the exact amount of nutrients ingested because this is time-consuming and the final result would be very inaccurate. However, they are useful as a means of comparing the composition of foods, and they may help to introduce new foods into the diet when attempting to increase the variety. Food tables are also useful in assessing the energy provided in the diet and will be familiar to those attempting to reduce weight. Tables may also be used to estimate the contributions to total dietary energy made by carbohydrates, fats, and proteins, and to assess the extent of adjustment required to comply with the recommendations made by the DoH (*see* Section 2.2).

2.2 DIETARY CONSTITUENTS

2.2.1 Carbohydrates

Carbohydrates contain carbon, hydrogen, and oxygen, and are based upon a chemical structure consisting of sugar units (usually glucose) linked together in a variety of ways. They may be classified as monosaccharides or disaccharides (sugars) and polysaccharides. Dietary sugars are further classified as 'intrinsic', which comprises sugars contained within the cell walls of fruits and vegetables, and 'extrinsic', which are not found in the cell walls of food. Extrinsic sugars include lactose, honey, and sucrose used in baking or added at the table.

Monosaccharides

Monosaccharides are the simplest sugars. Glucose (dextrose) occurs naturally in some foods (e.g. fruit and vegetable juices) as free glucose, or is obtained from other carbohydrates following digestion. Fructose (laevulose) occurs in honey and also in some fruits and vegetables, and is the sweetest sugar. Galactose does not occur freely but is a constituent of lactose.

Disaccharides

Disaccharides may be hydrolysed to yield two monosaccharide units.

Sucrose is a combination of glucose and fructose, and occurs naturally in sugar cane, sugar beet, and some fruits and root vegetables (e.g. carrots). Lactose is less sweet than sucrose, and is a combination of glucose and galactose; it occurs in the milk of all animals. Maltose is a combination of two molecules of glucose and is formed during digestion of starch.

Polysaccharides

Polysaccharides (complex carbohydrates) ultimately yield a number of monosaccharide units on hydrolysis. Those that can be digested by man are starches, which are broken down in the body to the simplest sugar unit, glucose. Any glucose not immediately required by the body is converted into glycogen, which acts as a reserve supply (*see* Section 8.5). Further excesses are converted into fat and deposited in adipose tissue. Starch is the form in which energy is stored in the seeds and roots of many plants. It is enclosed within granules and cannot easily be digested until treated with moist heat, which allows the granules to swell, burst, and release the starch. Good food sources of starch include baked beans, bread, cereals, potatoes, and yams.

Non-starch polysaccharides (NSP) were formerly

called roughage and then dietary fibre. NSP is present in food that has undergone minimal processing, and includes plant polysaccharides that are water insoluble (e.g. cellulose) and water-soluble polysaccharides (e.g. pectins, gums, mucilages, and other hemicelluloses). The latter are abundant in barley, oats, fruits, and legumes, although most sources contain both types of NSP. Good sources of NSP include whole grain cereals, nuts, and fruits and vegetables (especially legumes). The NSP content of fruits is increased if the skins are consumed, although the beneficial effects are diminished if the fruit is pulped or puréed.

The role of carbohydrates in the diet

Sugars

When the general term 'sugar' is used, it usually means sucrose, which is the most common sugar consumed in the modern diet. Sucrose is a relatively recent addition to man's diet and has only been widely used in the last 150 years. Before that, it was only available in small quantities for the wealthy, and the only sugars ingested in the general diet were those occurring naturally in foods. Sugars are purely a source of energy and are often referred to as 'empty calories' because they do not contain proteins, vitamins, minerals, or NSP. A high sugar consumption removes the need for more nutritious foods as a source of dietary energy.

Increased use of sugar has been linked to many diseases (e.g. behaviour disorders, cancer, cardio-vascular disease, diabetes mellitus, and gallstones), although there are many conflicting reports. Excessive consumption of sugar does, however, cause obesity which, in turn, is associated with many of these diseases.

All authorities are agreed on the need to reduce the intake of non-milk extrinsic sugars, which are not an essential form of dietary energy and could be eliminated from the diet completely. However, this is probably impractical in a western diet. The DRV for non-milk extrinsic sugars is about 60 g/day, representing 10% of total energy intake. This is an average figure for the UK population, and is based on a contribution by protein of 15% to dietary energy (which is above the RNI, see Section 2.2.3) and by alcohol of 5%. If alcohol is excluded from the diet, then the DRV increases to 11% of total energy. A substantial proportion (about 66%) of the sugars consumed are present in processed foods, including savouries (e.g. tomato soup, tomato sauce, and baked beans). In some cases the sugars could be removed or reduced, as their function is merely one of flavouring. A re-educated palate would soon adapt to less sweet alternatives. However, in many cases the sugar in a recipe has a specific function (e.g. as a preservative in jams, to lower the freezing point in ice-creams, or in influencing the texture of biscuits and cakes). The only alternative in such cases would be to select more nutritious alternatives.

Foods or drinks rich in sugars are used by many people as an immediate source of energy in the belief that the feelings of fatigue commonly attributed to 'low blood sugar levels' will be relieved. In healthy, well-nourished individuals the plasma-glucose concentration is maintained within very narrow limits, relying on the body's own stores of glycogen and fat to make up any deficit. This does not, however, alter the fact that there are some people who report hypoglycaemic symptoms that are immediately relieved by consumption of food. The condition has been labelled 'functional hypoglycaemia' because blood testing produces no evidence of chemical hypoglycaemia. Such individuals, once diabetes mellitus has been excluded, should be advised to substitute NSP-rich complex carbohydrates, and fruits and vegetables for sugar-rich foods. Frequent small meals and snacks may help prevent the symptoms, although the intake of total dietary energy must be carefully controlled to avoid weight gain.

There is nothing to be gained by substituting white sugar with any of the other forms available (e.g. brown sugar, raw cane sugar, glucose syrups, honey, and molasses). There is no difference between them, apart from flavour and appearance, and all have the same effects on metabolism. There are alternative methods of sweetening available (see below), but it should be borne in mind that substitutes do not play a part in reducing the basic desire for sweet foods.

Sugar substitutes

These may be derived from sugars, which have been chemically altered so that they can no longer be classified as sugars or they may be totally unrelated to sugars (artificial sweeteners) and are many times sweeter than sucrose. Artificial sweeteners possess no nutrient value at all.

Sorbitol   Sorbitol is half as sweet as glucose, from which it is prepared by reduction, and has the same energy value. It also occurs naturally in some fruit and vegetables. It is used as a bulk sweetener (i.e. when a large quantity is required for cooking or sprinkling on foods) and a carbohydrate source. It is converted in the liver to fructose by the enzyme sorbitol dehydrogenase or to glucose by aldose reductase. It is absorbed slowly and incompletely from the gastro-intestinal tract and does not directly need insulin for metabolism. It is, therefore, a useful sweetener in diabetic products. Mannitol is an isomer of sorbitol used as a bulk sweetener, and has no energy value because most of it is eliminated from the body unmetabolised.

Aspartame   Aspartame is 200 times as sweet as sucrose. It is derived from the amino acid phenylalanine and therefore should not be used by patients with phenylketonuria. Aspartame is mainly used as a table-top sweetener because its sweetness is lost at high temperatures; this restricts its use in cooking. It is also present in soft drinks although poor stability in solution may limit the shelf-life of products sweetened with this agent alone. It is consequently often mixed with saccharin.

Acesulfame potassium   Acesulfame potassium is 130 to 200 times as sweet as sucrose, and may be used in cooking. There may be a slight after-taste when used alone.

Cyclamates   Cyclamates (usually sodium cyclamate) are 30 times as sweet as sucrose, stable at high temperatures, and have a good shelf-life. They are used in some European countries, but are not permitted at present in the UK.

Saccharin   Saccharin is 200 to 500 times as sweet as sucrose. It has on rare occasions caused allergic or photosensitivity reactions. It has a characteristic bitter after-taste and some of the salts (e.g. saccharin sodium) are considered more palatable.

Thaumatin   Thaumatin is 2000 to 3000 times as sweet as sucrose, and is the sweetest natural substance known, although it has a liquorice-like after-taste. It is a polypeptide obtained from a West African fruit, Katemfe (*Thaumatococcus daniellii*). It is not used as a table-top sweetener but is usually found in combination with other sweetening agents in processed food and drinks. It is also used in very small amounts as a flavour enhancer.

Starch

Foods with a high starch content have, in the past, been considered 'fattening' and were often avoided in weight-reducing diets. In fact, weight for weight, starch provides about the same amount of energy as proteins, and less than half the amount provided by fats. It is only fattening if quantities in excess of individual energy requirements are consumed. In the UK, the DoH has made recommendations to reduce the contribution to dietary energy made by fats (*see* Section 2.2.2), and this may be effected by a simultaneous increase in the starch contribution. The DRV for starch, intrinsic sugars, and

lactose in milk and milk products is 37% of total energy; there are not separate values for each of these components. This figure is based on a contribution by protein of 15% to dietary energy, and by alcohol of 5%. If alcohol is excluded from the diet, the DRV increases to 39% of total energy.

Non-starch polysaccharides

Epidemiological studies show that populations in rural Africa and other non-industrialised communities consuming a diet rich in NSP are less likely to develop certain gastro-intestinal diseases (e.g. appendicitis, constipation, diverticular disease, haemorrhoids, and irritable bowel syndrome) than those in industrialised nations where the NSP intake is substantially lower. Absence of disease has been related to large stool size and epidemiological studies show that stool weights below 150 g/day are associated with increased risks of bowel cancer and diverticular disease. In the UK, the average stool weight is about 100 g/day. Stool consistency is equally important, and colonic disorders may be related to the increased difficulty experienced in passing small, hard stools. This is a well accepted cause of constipation and diverticular disease, and treatment of both conditions involves an increase in NSP. Diet appears to be an important aetiological factor in the development of appendicitis, although the exact mechanism is unknown. NSP reduces colonic transit time, which may reduce contact time of potential carcinogens with the mucosal surface. Increased intestinal bulk may have the effect of diluting the effect of any carcinogenic elements or there may be an anticarcinogenic component present in the NSP.

Many trials have shown a correlation between an increase in NSP and a reduction in plasma-LDL-cholesterol concentrations, although some workers claim that it is only those foods rich in soluble NSP that have this effect. Other trials have, however, shown that there is no difference between oat bran (which contains soluble fractions) and wheat bran (which contains partly soluble fractions) in their cholesterol-lowering effect. The actual mechanism is not clear, and the reduction in concentrations may simply be a result of the replacement of saturated fats in the diet by NSP-rich foods. In general, insoluble NSP (e.g. cellulose) decrease colonic transit time and also absorb water, resulting in the production of soft stools with an increase in volume and frequency; they have little effect on plasma-cholesterol concentrations. Conversely, soluble NSP (e.g. guar gum and pectins) appear to lower plasma-cholesterol concentrations but have little effect on bowel function. There are, however, exceptions and ispaghula and xanthan gum (both soluble NSP) have a good laxative action as well as a beneficial effect on plasma-cholesterol levels whereas sterculia (karaya gum) has no effect on either.

The DoH (1991) proposes an average intake of NSP of 18 g/day for adults (range 12 to 24 g/day) from a variety of foods whose constituents contain it as a naturally integrated component. Young children should eat proportionately less because there is a small risk that, if eaten to excess, high-bulk NSP-rich foods may prevent sufficient energy-rich foods being eaten to ensure adequate growth. No increase in stool weight occurs with intakes of NSP above 32 g/day and, although there is no evidence of adverse effects above this level, the DoH sees no virtue in exceeding this value. Too rapid an increase in NSP intake can cause abdominal pain, flatulence, and diarrhoea, and the increase should be made gradually with plenty of fluid taken at the same time.

Phytic acid, present in all grains, reduces the absorption of some important minerals (e.g. calcium, magnesium, manganese, phosphorus, and zinc), and this may need to be taken into consideration when increasing the NSP intake in diets low in mineral content. There is eight times as much phytic acid in wholemeal flour as white flour, although when flour is used to make bread, phytase present in yeast destroys up to one-third of the phytic acid content of wholemeal flour and nearly all that in white flour. Yeast phytase also occurs in the gastro-intestinal tract, and there is some evidence to suggest that the body can adapt to a large intake of phytic acid. However, vegetarians (*see* Section 2.3) may experience deficiencies of those minerals bound by phytic acid for which the best dietary source is animal products (e.g. iron and zinc).

2.2.2 Fats and cholesterol

Fats, like carbohydrates, are composed of carbon and hydrogen, but contain less oxygen. Chemically, they are esters of glycerol (glycerin) and fatty acids. Most are triglycerides (i.e. one molecule of glycerol is combined with three fatty acid molecules), and this is the form of most dietary fats. The essential fatty acids (formerly called vitamin F) are the unsaturated linoleic acid and alpha linolenic acid; they cannot be synthesised in the body and must be obtained in the diet. Fatty acids are classified as saturated (no double bonds), mono-unsaturated (one double bond), or polyunsaturated (two or more double bonds). Myristic acid, palmitic acid, and stearic acid are saturated fatty acids; oleic acid is a monounsaturated fatty acid that occurs in all fats. Polyunsaturated fatty acids are derived from two sources: linoleic acid (the omega-6 series) from plants,

meat, and poultry; or linolenic acid (the omega-3 series) from marine mammals and fish, and some plants (e.g. evening primrose oil obtained from *Oenothera biennis*). The main source in western diets is the omega-6 series. Arachidonic acid is a polyunsaturated fatty acid present in animal fats and synthesised in the body from linoleic acid.

All natural fats contain both saturated and polyunsaturated fatty acids, but the nature and proportion of the constituent fatty acids dictate the properties of the fat. Polyunsaturated fatty acids are less stable than saturated fatty acids and react gradually with air, turning the fat rancid. Products made with poly-unsaturated fats therefore have a short shelf-life. A high polyunsaturated content renders a fat liquid at room temperature, although it will generally solidify at low temperatures (e.g. in a refrigerator). In everyday terms, fats that are solid at room temperature are referred to as 'fats', whereas those that are liquid at room temperature are termed 'oils'; however, in reality, they are all fats. Polyunsaturated fatty acids can be converted by hydrogenation (reduction) into saturated fatty acids and *cis* and *trans* monounsaturated fatty acids. This process is used during the manufacture of some products to increase the shelf-life or alter the physical properties (e.g. to make hard margarines). Animal fats generally contain a higher proportion of saturated fatty acids than plant oils, although there are some exceptions (e.g. the semisolids, coconut oil, palm kernel oil, and palm oil contain a high proportion of saturated fatty acids).

Dietary fat occurs in two forms: visible fat, which includes butter, margarine, lard, vegetable oils, and the fat that can be seen on meat; or invisible fat, which includes that contained in lean meat, milk, and nuts.

Cholesterol is a fat-like steroid alcohol. It is involved in the formation of bile acids and some steroid hormones, and is a component of cytoplasmic membranes. Cholesterol is present in many animal products, especially in saturated fats, and particularly high levels are found in egg yolk, shellfish, and offal (e.g. brain, liver, and kidney). About half of the dietary cholesterol is absorbed. Eggs provide the main dietary source of cholesterol in the UK, of which an average of 3 to 4 are consumed per person each week.

The role of fats in the diet

The amount of energy derived from all fats is roughly equivalent; some animal fats may contain vitamins A and D, and cholesterol whereas vegetable fats may contain carotene (a precursor of vitamin A) and vitamin E. Fats are a more concentrated source of dietary energy than carbohydrates or proteins and are the form in which most of the energy reserve is stored in animals and some plant seeds. Fats are the slowest of the food types to pass through the stomach (carbohydrates are the fastest), and as a consequence are said to have a 'high satiety value'.

Essential fatty acids have a variety of functions including maintaining the function and integrity of cellular and sub-cellular membranes, the regulation of cholesterol metabolism, and as precursors of prostaglandins and arachidonic, eicosapentaenoic, and docosahexaenoic acids.

A high intake of saturated fatty acids raises plasma-cholesterol concentrations, which in turn is linked to an increased risk of cardiovascular disease. Mono-unsaturated fatty acids probably have no effect on plasma-cholesterol concentrations whereas linoleic acid and its derivatives lower cholesterol levels. Linolenic acid and its derivatives inhibit clot formation. A high-fat diet has also been implicated as a risk factor for cancer (e.g. breast cancer and colorectal cancer), although there is insufficient evidence to support this. However, on the evidence that is available, it would seem prudent to moderate intake of saturated fatty acids and total fat.

Epidemiological studies show that populations consuming diets with a high ratio of dietary polyunsaturated to saturated fatty acids (P:S ratio) do not have a high rate of cardiovascular disease, breast cancer, or

colorectal cancer. Reports that diets high in poly-unsaturated fatty acids increase the risk of gallstones and pancreatic cancer have not been substantiated, and there is no evidence of association with any human disease. The effects of *cis* and *trans* isomers of fatty acids on the body remain to be elucidated. However, it would be prudent not to exceed the current estimated average level. DRVs for adults for fatty acids and total fat are given in Fig. 2.1.

To achieve the proposed dietary modifications, the following changes are suggested:

- avoid cream
- use semi-skimmed or skimmed milk
- reduce consumption of fatty meat (e.g. red meat) and replace with poultry or white fish*
- replace butter and lard with soft margarine and cooking oils low in saturated fatty acids.

These recommendations are not intended for children under five years of age. When a household elects to change from whole milk to low-fat forms, whole milk should still be provided for the under-fives (*see also* Section 2.3).

One problem in achieving these goals is that not all nutrition labels on foods state the content or composition of fats. As a general guide, however, butter contains 59 to 63% saturated fatty acids (including *trans* fatty acids), and lard up to 48%. The amount in margarine varies according to the type of oil used and the method of production. Hard margarines can contain 39 to 57% saturated fatty acids and soft margarines between 21 and 49%. Vegetable oils vary widely in their composition, and by no means are they all low in saturated fatty acids. Tropical oils have very high levels of saturated fatty acids, and some of them (e.g. coconut oil and palm kernel oil) contain even more than butter. The lowest levels are found in corn oil, olive oil, peanut oil, rapeseed oil, safflower oil, soyabean oil, and sunflower oil. Rapeseed oil and olive oil are the best sources of monounsaturated fatty acids (62 and 72% respectively). Total fat intake will also be reduced if food is grilled, poached, steamed, or baked rather than fried.

The role of cholesterol in the body

The link between high plasma-cholesterol concentrations and ischaemic heart disease is now well established. A reduction in plasma-cholesterol concentrations by dietary modification (*see below*)

saturated fatty acids	10 (11)
cis-monounsaturated fatty acids	12 (13)
cis-polyunsaturated fatty acids [a] including: linoleic acid 1.0% linolenic acid 0.2%	6 (6.5)
trans-fatty acids	2 (2)
total fatty acids	30 (32.5)
total fat (i.e. the sum of fatty acid intake and glycerol)	33 (35)

These figures are the average intake for the population and assume that the contribution by protein to food energy is 15% and that of alcohol is 5%. Figures in parentheses indicate DRVs as a percentage of food energy excluding alcohol.

(*a*) *Cis*-polyunsaturated fatty acids should provide an average of 6% of total dietary energy for the population but individual intake should not exceed 10%.

Fig. 2.1
Dietary Reference Values for fatty acids and total fat for adults as a percentage of daily total energy intake.

* Consumption of fatty fish will increase the amount of polyunsaturated fatty acids in the diet but will not aid in the reduction of total fat intake.

appears to reduce the risk for developing atherosclerosis. In established disease, there is evidence that reducing plasma- cholesterol concentrations decreases the rate of progression of atheromas and stimulates regression. High plasma-cholesterol concentrations may also contribute to the formation of gallstones. The British Hyperlipidaemia Association has recommended that adults with a plasma-cholesterol concentration between 5.2 and 6.5 mmol/litre should receive advice on diet (*see below*) and other risk factors (e.g. smoking, *see* Chapter 5, and lack of exercise, *see* Chapter 8), and those with higher levels may, in addition, require drug therapy.

Fats are water insoluble and are carried in the circulation by various fractions of lipoproteins to muscles for utilisation as an energy source, or to adipose tissue for storage. Very low-density lipoproteins (VLDLs) are produced in the liver, and transport endogenous triglycerides and cholesterol. Hydrolysis of VLDLs produces low-density lipoproteins (LDLs), which transport about 70% of the cholesterol in the circulation.

Most of the cholesterol utilised for various functions in the body is synthesised in the liver. When sufficient cholesterol is stored to meet these requirements further synthesis is inhibited. There is also a mechanism that can alter the number of active LDL receptors (the uptake site) on cell membranes, so that cholesterol taken into the cells from the bloodstream is regulated. LDLs are catabolised in the liver, but if the LDL receptors are suppressed, cholesterol remains in the circulation. This process contributes to the deposition of cholesterol on the arterial walls and the formation of atheromas.

High-density lipoproteins (HDLs) are synthesised in the liver, and carry about 25% of the circulating cholesterol. They take cholesterol away from the tissues, including the arterial walls, and transport it to the liver for catabolism. Thus, a high plasma-concentration of LDL-cholesterol is harmful whereas a high concentration of HDL-cholesterol may be beneficial. A low plasma-concentration of HDL-cholesterol may be harmful independent of the LDL-cholesterol concentration. Measurement of the total plasma-cholesterol concentration may not be a useful indicator of risk because total cholesterol includes the HDL fraction, which is protective. It is thought by some that the ratio of LDL-cholesterol to HDL-cholesterol is a more important determinant of risk for ischaemic heart disease.

Age and sex have an effect on plasma-cholesterol concentrations. In men, the plasma concentration of LDL-cholesterol increases steadily until it peaks between 40 and 50 years of age. Women have lower plasma concentrations of LDL-cholesterol initially, but these rise after the menopause until about 60 years of age, and the final plasma concentration in women is higher than in men. This is reflected in the difference in ages between men and women at which ischaemic heart disease may occur.

Plasma-cholesterol concentrations are influenced by saturated fatty acid intake rather than dietary cholesterol, which has only a small effect. Adoption of a low-fat, high-NSP diet, increasing the polyunsaturated fatty acid content should not necessitate any further reduction in dietary cholesterol, and the DoH (1991) does not give any specific recommendations about the dietary intake of cholesterol. The average daily intake in adults is 350 to 450 mg, which would fall without any further dietary adjustment if the above guidelines were followed.

Saturated fatty acids increase plasma-cholesterol concentrations, particularly the LDL fraction, whereas polyunsaturated fatty acids lower plasma concentrations when substituted for saturated fatty acids. However, the exact mechanism of action and role in the diet of polyunsaturated fatty acids is not clear. Plasma concentrations are lowered to a greater degree by reducing saturated fatty acid intake than by increasing polyunsaturated fatty acid intake. There are insufficient data available on long-term use of large quantities of polyunsaturated fatty acids to justify any recommendations about excessive increases in consumption.

Marine fish oils form a high proportion of the diet of Eskimos and appear to protect them from developing ischaemic heart disease. There are two omega-3 polyunsaturated fatty acids implicated, eicosapentaenoic acid (EPA) and docosahexaenoic acid (DHA). They reduce platelet numbers and aggregation, and have also been shown in some studies to lower the plasma concentrations of fats and LDLs, although others dispute this. They may also slightly raise the plasma concentrations of HDLs. The presence of EPA and DHA is rare in the average British diet, which has a greater bias towards meat than fish. Trials in which western men were given regular supplements of fatty fish or fish oil have shown a beneficial effect on plasma-cholesterol concentrations. Oily fish (e.g. herring, mackerel, and salmon) are good sources of these fatty acids, although those reared on fish farms are not because they do not feed on plankton, which is the original source in the food chain. Not all fish represent good sources, and the fatty acids are not found in freshwater fish and only in very small amounts in white fish. However, a regular diet of lean fish has been shown to be protective, although the mechanism of action is not clear. It has been suggested that eating fish twice a week may reduce the risk of ischaemic heart disease.

Fish oil supplements should not be recommended without supervision because there are insufficient data available on long-term use. Their antiplatelet action may cause an interaction with aspirin or anticoagulants. There may also be potential adverse effects from the long-term ingestion of excessive quantities of fatty fish, particularly those derived from areas associated with problems of marine pollution, because lipophilic toxins may concentrate in the fish oils. Increase in fish-oil consumption is only of benefit if there is a concomitant decrease in total fat intake. It should also be borne in mind that the overall life-style of Eskimos is somewhat different from that of western people, and this may also be a significant factor in their relative freedom from ischaemic heart disease.

2.2.3 Proteins

Proteins are made up of carbon, hydrogen, oxygen, and nitrogen; some also contain sulphur. Proteins are made up of chains of amino acids, some of which may be synthesised by the body using any excess of other amino acids available. These are the non- essential amino acids:

- alanine
- arginine*
- aspartic acid
- cysteine
- glutamic acid
- glycine
- histidine*
- proline
- serine
- tyrosine.

The eight amino acids that must be provided in the diet and are classified as essential are:

- isoleucine
- leucine
- lysine
- methionine
- phenylalanine
- threonine
- tryptophan
- valine.

Amino acids are found in both animal and plant foods, but the types and proportion vary widely. The quality of

* Arginine and histidine are required in infant growth and therefore considered essential amino acids for infants. Histidine may also be essential in adults.

a protein is dependent on the content of essential amino acids. Animal proteins are rich in the essential amino acids and are therefore described as having a high biological value. Plant foods have a low biological value because each individual source does not provide all the essential amino acids in sufficient quantities. However, mixing several plant foods together provides the total complement required, a fact that must be borne in mind by vegetarians (see Section 2.3).

The role of proteins in the diet

Proteins are required for growth and repair of tissues, and any excess is used as a source of energy. However, if the diet is deficient in other energy-producing foods, proteins will be used instead, and this function supersedes their main function of tissue regeneration. It is therefore essential that sufficient carbohydrates and fats are provided with proteins.

In the average UK diet, one-third of the proteins ingested are derived from plant sources and the remainder from animal foods. Animal products (and some plant sources) also contain saturated fats, and this should be borne in mind when selecting foods. Proteins from vegetable sources are commonly associated with NSP.

The DoH (1991) estimates that the protein RNI for all adults of 19 years of age and over is 0.75 g/kg/day. Additional requirements are necessary during pregnancy and lactation, and for children (see Section 2.3). The RNI for the elderly is the same as for younger adults, but because of the small amount of lean body mass per kg body weight in the elderly, the resultant figure per unit lean body mass is higher than in younger adults. There is some evidence that very high protein intakes may aggravate poor or failing kidney function, and because there is no proven benefit of protein intakes in excess of the RNI, the DoH concludes that intakes should not exceed twice the RNI.

2.2.4 Vitamins

Most vitamins cannot be synthesised in the body but must be provided in the diet. They are organic compounds required by the body in small amounts for a variety of metabolic functions. They do not, however, provide any energy. They are often grouped together with minerals (see Section 2.2.5), which are inorganic elements also essential in small amounts.

Vitamins are classified as water soluble or fat soluble. This property is important in consideration of their food source, stability (especially during cooking), and storage in the body. Fat-soluble vitamins (A, D, E, and K) may be found in foods with a high fat content (e.g. vitamins A and D in oily fish). They are stored in the body, and ingestion of excessive quantities over a long period may be toxic. Water-soluble vitamins (B complex and ascorbic acid) are less stable than fat-soluble vitamins, particularly in boiling water. They do not accumulate in the body and so must be provided in the diet on a regular basis. Most are less toxic in large doses than fat-soluble vitamins because they are rapidly excreted in urine; nevertheless adverse effects can occur following ingestion of large quantities over a prolonged period (see Section 2.2.6).

Ascorbic acid

Ascorbic acid (vitamin C) is a water-soluble vitamin essential for the formation of collagen and intercellular material. It is therefore required for the development of bone, cartilage, and teeth, and for wound healing. Ascorbic acid is important in the maintenance of capillaries and is also involved in the regulation of intracellular oxidation-reduction potentials. Ascorbic acid is an antioxidant and is one of several dietary antioxidants that is being investigated for a protective role against tumour formation involving free radicals. Man cannot synthesise ascorbic acid and must provide it in the diet.

Ascorbic acid occurs mainly in fruits and vegetables, but exists in only small amounts in milk and other animal products. It is readily absorbed from the gastro-intestinal tract. Valuable food sources include black currants, Brussels sprouts, citrus fruits, green peppers, and mangoes. Potatoes (especially new potatoes) contain relatively little ascorbic acid, but nevertheless represent a good source in the diet because of the amount commonly eaten. There is no ascorbic acid in whole grain cereals. The amount present in food can vary considerably depending upon the season, and large amounts are lost during cooking, storage, and on exposure to light. Cutting or bruising fruits and vegetables activates the destructive ascorbic acid oxidase enzyme. The minimum amount of ascorbic acid necessary to prevent clinical scurvy is 10 mg/day, and the RNI is 40 mg/day for adults, 50 mg/day for pregnant women, and 70 mg/day during lactation. High costs of seasonal foods in the winter may price foods rich in ascorbic acid out of the reach of low-income households. Supplements may be required, particularly during the winter, for vulnerable groups (e.g. the very young and the elderly, those with chronic illnesses, cigarette smokers, and pregnant and breast-feeding women).

Vitamin A

Vitamin A is a fat-soluble vitamin obtained from animal and plant sources. It is essential for growth, vision (especially night vision), and for maintenance of epithelial tissue. Deficiency of vitamin A causes xerophthalmia, a progressive disorder characterised by night blindness, corneal drying, corneal ulceration, and keratomalacia. Vitamin A is an antioxidant and is one of several dietary antioxidants that is being investigated for a protective role against tumour formation involving free radicals. Retinol is the form found in animal foods (e.g. liver, kidney, eggs, and dairy products) and accounts for two-thirds of the vitamin A intake. The remainder is supplied by carotenoids such as beta-carotene, which are found in plants (e.g. carrots and other green or yellow vegetables). These are converted in the body to retinol, although they are less effectively utilised than animal sources. There is a legal requirement in the UK to fortify all margarine with vitamin A to provide the same amount as butter. Vitamin A is readily absorbed from the gastro-intestinal tract, although absorption may be impaired if fat or protein intake is low and in the presence of fat malabsorption. There is little lost from food during cooking, except when high temperatures are used (e.g. in frying), but vitamin A is unstable in the presence of light and oxidising agents. The RNI of vitamin A for adult males is 700 μg/day and for females 600 μg/day. Requirements increase during pregnancy and lactation although it is important not to consume excessive amounts during pregnancy (see Section 2.3). Excessive doses of vitamin A over a long period are toxic; acute toxicity may also occur with ingestion of high doses.

Vitamin-B group

There are several water-soluble vitamins in this group which, although chemically unrelated, all act as cofactors in various enzyme reactions. They occur together in similar foods and can lead to multiple deficiency disorders in cases of low dietary intake.

Biotin

Biotin (vitamin H) is an essential coenzyme in fat metabolism, and may be supplied in sufficient quantities by bacterial synthesis in the colon. Good dietary sources of biotin are egg yolk and offal; other sources include cereals, dairy products, fish, fruits, and vegetables. Deficiency is unlikely except in the unusual circumstance of excessive consumption of raw egg-white. Egg-white contains a protein, avidin, which binds with biotin and prevents its absorption. Deficiency may also occur in long-term parenteral nutrition. No RNI has been set in the UK, although 10 to 200 μg/day has been assessed as a safe intake for adults.

Folic acid

Folic acid is a coenzyme in several metabolic processes, including nucleic acid synthesis (see also Vitamin B_{12} below). Deficiency causes megaloblastic anaemia, and may arise as a result of low dietary intake, malabsorption, or in pregnancy. Folic acid is present in liver, nuts, pulses, fresh green leafy vegetables, and yeast, and is well absorbed from the gastro-intestinal tract. It is, however, readily destroyed by cooking. The RNI is 200 μg/day total folate for adults, increasing to 300 μg/day during pregnancy and 260 μg/day during lactation. A Medical Research Council vitamin study has demonstrated that taking folic acid supplements before and during pregnancy reduces the incidence of neural tube birth defects.

Nicotinic acid and nicotinamide

Nicotinic acid and nicotinamide are both called niacin (vitamin B_3). They are converted in the body to coenzymes that are involved in electron transfer reactions in the respiratory chain, and thus play a part in the utilisation of energy from food. Deficiency causes pellagra. Nicotinic acid is formed in the body from tryptophan (an essential amino acid); food that contains tryptophan but little nicotinic acid (e.g. eggs and milk) does therefore provide the body with nicotinic acid. The RNI is calculated as nicotinic acid equivalents, and is 6.6 mg/1000 kcal for all ages, increasing to 8.9 mg/1000 kcal during lactation. RNIs in mg/day based on DRVs for energy are given in Table 2.1. Good dietary sources (including tryptophan-containing foods) are Cheddar cheese, eggs, fish, meat, milk, pulses, and potatoes; absorption from the gastro-intestinal tract is good. Nicotinic acid and nicotinamide are heat-stable and little is lost during cooking.

Pantothenic acid

Pantothenic acid (vitamin B_5) is a component of coenzyme A, which is involved in the metabolism of carbohydrates, fats, and proteins, and thus in the release of energy from foods. Pantothenic acid is also involved in the synthesis of sterols (including cholesterol) and acetylcholine in the body. It is widely distributed in foods, including egg yolk, fresh vegetables, liver, kidney, milk, whole grain cereals, and yeast, and is readily absorbed from the gastro-intestinal tract. Some may be lost during cooking. There is no RNI in the UK as deficiency is unlikely but the current dietary intake of 3 to 7 mg/day has been assessed as a safe intake for adults.

Pyridoxine

Pyridoxine is 1 of 3 similar compounds that may be referred to as vitamin B_6; the other two are pyridoxal and pyridoxamine. These compounds are converted in the body to the active forms, pyridoxal phosphate and pyridoxamine phosphate. The main function of pyridoxine is in amino acid metabolism, although it also plays a part in carbohydrate and fat metabolism. Two metabolic functions of particular note are the conversion of tryptophan to nicotinic acid, and the formation of haemoglobin. Pyridoxine is also involved in enzyme reactions that control the synthesis and metabolism of most neurotransmitters (e.g. dopamine and nor-adrenaline). Good sources include fruits, eggs, fish, meat, potatoes and other vegetables, and whole grain cereals although there may be some losses during cooking. Pyridoxine is readily absorbed from the gastro-intestinal tract. The dietary requirement depends on protein intake and the RNI is 15 μg/g protein per day. Absolute RNIs are given in Table 2.1 and are based upon protein providing 14.7% of dietary energy. Certain people may, however, need supplements (e.g. people who consume excessive amounts of alcohol and those taking some drugs including isoniazid). Excessive supplementation for long periods can cause peripheral neuropathies.

Riboflavine

Riboflavine (vitamin B_2) is involved in oxidation-reduction reactions in tissues, and therefore in the utilisation of energy from food. Deficiency results in ariboflavinosis, a disorder characterised by angular stomatitis, cheilosis, glossitis, and seborrhoeic keratosis. Good sources of riboflavine include Cheddar cheese, eggs, green leafy vegetables, kidney, liver, milk, and yeast extract; riboflavine is well absorbed from the gastro-intestinal tract. In Britain, about one-third of the average intake of riboflavine is derived from milk. There is some loss of riboflavine during cooking but exposure to light causes greater losses, which is an important consideration in Britain where many households have milk delivered to the home and bottles may be left on doorsteps for long periods during the day. The RNIs for riboflavine are 1.3 mg/day for men and 1.1 mg/day for women, increasing to 1.4 mg/day during pregnancy and 1.6 mg/day during lactation. It is considered that a good mixed diet will provide the required amounts, and deficiency of this vitamin is rare in the western world.

Thiamine

Thiamine (vitamin B_1) is principally involved in the metabolism of carbohydrate, and the dietary requirements are consequently related to the carbohydrate intake and metabolic rate of an individual. Deficiency of thiamine causes beri-beri. Thiamine is also involved in the metabolism of alcohol, which puts people with chronic alcohol dependence at risk of developing a deficiency syndrome (see Chapter 6). Valuable sources include cereals, peanuts, peas, pork, potatoes, soya beans, and rice. In the UK, all flour (except wholemeal) is fortified with thiamine because so much is lost during processing. Thiamine is well absorbed from the gastro-intestinal tract. An average of 20% is lost during cooking; this percentage is even greater if the medium is alkaline. The RNI for thiamine is 0.4 mg/1000 kcal for most groups of people. Absolute RNIs for adults are given in Table 2.1.

Vitamin B$_{12}$

Vitamin B$_{12}$ refers to a group of cobalt-containing compounds called cobalamins, and includes cyanocobalamin and hydroxocobalamin. Together with folic acid, vitamin B$_{12}$ is involved in nucleic acid synthesis and is required by rapidly dividing cells, particularly those involved in erythropoiesis. It is also involved in the metabolism of amino acids and fats. Deficiency causes megaloblastic anaemias and nerve cell degeneration. The best source is liver, although vitamin B$_{12}$ is also present in other forms of meat, dairy products, fish, fortified cereals, and in yeast extract. The RNI is 1.5 μg/day for adults, increasing to 2.0 μg/day during lactation. It is not found in any plant products, which puts vegetarians (see Section 2.3), particularly strict vegans, at risk of deficiency. Other people at risk are those who do not secrete intrinsic factor in gastric juice and are therefore unable to absorb vitamin B$_{12}$.

Vitamin D

Vitamin D refers to several related fat-soluble sterols that possess the common property of preventing or curing rickets. The natural form is cholecalciferol (activated 7-dehydrocholesterol or vitamin D$_3$), which is produced by the action of ultraviolet light on 7-dehydrocholesterol present in the oily secretions of the skin. The main commercial form is ergocalciferol (calciferol or vitamin D$_2$). Active metabolites of vitamin D, produced in the liver and kidneys, regulate calcium and phosphorus homoeostasis by action in the bones, gastro-intestinal tract, and kidneys.

Vitamin D is not widely distributed in foods but is readily absorbed from the gastro-intestinal tract. Oily fish are a good source (especially fish liver), and other sources, which contain much smaller amounts, include dairy products, eggs, and liver. There is a legal requirement in the UK to fortify all margarine with vitamin D. Vitamin D is not destroyed by cooking. The form present in animal products is cholecalciferol, which was formed in the living animal by the action of sunlight on its skin or obtained from its food. There are therefore seasonal variations in the quantity present. In the UK, exposure of the skin to the sun's ultraviolet radiation during the summer months builds up liver stores of vitamin D to last through the winter months, and no dietary source is necessary. However, a dietary supply is required by people who cover up their skin during the summer, or by the housebound. This is particularly important for the elderly, and the RNI for people over 65 years of age is 10 μg/day. The RNI for pregnant and breast-feeding women is also 10 μg/day (see Section 2.3). Vitamin D is the most toxic of all the vitamins in excessive doses, and results in more calcium being absorbed than excreted. The excess is deposited in the kidneys, which consequently become damaged.

Vitamin E

Vitamin E (alpha tocopherols) refers to fat-soluble compounds, of which alpha tocopheryl acetate has the highest vitamin E activity. Vitamin E acts as an antioxidant and may protect cytoplasmic membranes from damage by free radicals; it is one of several dietary antioxidants that is being investigated for a protective role against tumour formation involving free radicals; it also assists the absorption of fatty acids. It is essential in the diet, and neurological deficiency syndromes can occur in patients with malabsorption syndromes, genetic blood disorders, or in malnourished premature infants. Good sources are cereals, eggs, peanut butter, and vegetable oils (e.g. cottonseed oil, safflower oil, sunflower seed oil, and wheat-germ oil). Absorption requires the presence of bile. Vitamin E is not destroyed by cooking, although it may be subject to oxidation reactions, and may be destroyed by freezing. Vitamin E requirements are largely determined by the polyunsaturated fatty acid content of the diet, which varies widely, and so it is not possible to set DRVs. However, safe intakes have been assessed as above 4 mg/day for men and above 3 mg/day for women.

Vitamin K

Vitamin K refers to fat-soluble compounds essential for the formation of prothrombin and other clotting factors, and for the maintenance of a normal prothrombin concentration in the plasma. The clotting time of the blood is prolonged and spontaneous haemorrhage may occur in vitamin-K deficiency. Phytomenadione (vitamin K$_1$) is the naturally occurring form and is found in cauliflower, cereals, egg yolk, green leafy vegetables (e.g. cabbage and spinach), peas, and vegetable oils. A series of compounds called menaquinones (vitamin K_2) are synthesised by bacteria in the colon and can provide sufficient vitamin K. Absorption of vitamin K depends on the presence of bile. Losses may occur on exposure to light but little is lost during cooking. Too little information exists to establish accurate DRVs for vitamin K but intakes of 1 μg/kg/day appear to be safe and adequate for adults. Deficiency may occur in obstructive jaundice, severe liver disease, or as a result of inadequate absorption. Oral anti-coagulants (e.g. warfarin) act by antagonising the actions of vitamin K.

2.2.5 Minerals

There are a number of minerals that are essential for life and must all be obtained from the diet. The major minerals are needed in relatively large amounts whereas the trace elements, although still essential, are only required in small amounts and may be toxic in excess.

Major minerals

Calcium

The greatest proportion (99%) of calcium in the body is in the bones and teeth where it provides strength and support. It also acts as a reserve supply that may be drawn on to fulfil its other functions, which include roles in blood clotting, enzyme activity, muscle contraction (e.g. in the heart), and nerve function. Deficiency causes rickets in children and osteomalacia in adults. Calcium is present in bread, dairy products, dried figs, eggs, peanuts, sardines, and some vegetables (e.g. aubergines, cabbage, onions, and watercress). The amount of calcium absorbed from dietary sources is generally between 20 and 30%, although this varies with requirements. Absorption may be impaired by phytic acid present in NSP (see Section 2.2.1). The RNI of calcium is 700 mg/day for adults, with increased requirements during infancy, childhood, and lactation (see Section 2.3). Vitamin D is essential for calcium absorption, and in British diets, calcium deficiency is more likely to be caused by vitamin-D deficiency rather than dietary deficiency of calcium.

Iron

Most of the iron in the body is present in haemoglobin; the rest is in myoglobin and the cytochrome enzymes, or stored as ferritin and haemosiderin. Iron in haemoglobin is principally involved in the transport of oxygen from the lungs to the tissues. A lack of iron eventually causes iron-deficiency anaemia because the body's stores become depleted. Dietary sources include meat (especially kidney and liver), eggs, figs, dried apricots, and cocoa. Small amounts may also be found in some vegetables (e.g. aubergines, cabbage, potatoes, and watercress). Only about 5 to 15% of the iron in the diet is absorbed, although this increases when body stores are low or when needs are greatest (e.g. in children, or in pregnant and breast-feeding women). It is absorbed most readily from meat, which accounts for 20% of the total dietary intake. The overall absorption is increased in the presence of ascorbic acid but decreased in the presence of tannins (e.g. in tea). The RNI is 8.7 mg/day for men and postmenopausal women and 14.8 mg/day for premenopausal women. Women suffering regular heavy menstrual losses may require even more.

Magnesium

More than half the magnesium content of the body is in the skeleton. It is also present in all cells and acts as a cofactor in many enzyme systems. Magnesium is involved in muscle contractility, neuronal transmission, and phosphate transfer. It is an essential constituent of chlorophyll and is found in green vegetables. Other sources include bread, eggs, meat, milk, and peanuts. The average amounts ingested in the diet are 237 mg/day (women) and 323 mg/day (men). Deficiency is rare, although it may occur in chronic alcoholic dependence or in severe diarrhoea. The RNIs for magnesium are 270 mg/day for women and 300 mg/day for men, and for breast-feeding women, 320 mg/day.

Phosphorus

Phosphorus (as phosphates) has many functions in the body, ranging from provision of strength and support in bones and teeth (calcium phosphate) to liberation and utilisation of energy from nutrients. Phosphates are constituents of cells, nucleic acids, carbohydrates, some fats, and proteins, and are essential in activating some of the B-group vitamins. The RNI for phosphorus is 550 mg/day for adults and increases to 990 mg/day during lactation. Phosphorus is present in many foods and deficiency is not known.

Potassium

Potassium is the principal cation of intracellular fluid, and is involved in carbohydrate metabolism, enzyme reactions, muscle contraction, and nerve conduction. Potassium is present in a wide range of foods (e.g. bread, cauliflower, cheese, eggs, meat, milk, oranges, potatoes, raisins, and tomatoes). The average amounts ingested in the diet are 2.43 g/day (women) and 3.19 g/day (men), of which most is absorbed. Dietary deficiency of potassium is unlikely to occur, but losses may arise during diuretic therapy or in chronic diarrhoea, and must be corrected clinically rather than nutritionally. The RNI for potassium is 3.5 g/day for adults.

Sodium

Sodium is the principal cation of extracellular fluid, and is involved in maintaining the fluid and electrolyte balance, and in muscle and nerve activity. The sodium content is low in unprocessed foods but high in many processed foods, especially smoked foods. Particularly high levels are found in bacon, baked beans, cornflakes, Marmite, smoked fish, and soy sauce; sodium is even present in instant coffee. The main dietary intake is in the form of sodium chloride (salt), although other food additives (e.g. sodium bicarbonate present in baking powder, sodium alginate, sodium ascorbate, sodium benzoate, and sodium citrate) also contribute sodium to the diet. Sodium is readily absorbed from the gastro-intestinal tract. Average intakes of sodium in the British diet are 2.35 g/day (women) and 3.38 g/day (men), with individual intakes ranging from 2 to 10 g/day. The amount required in a temperate climate is considerably less than this. The amount of sodium lost in the urine is homoeostatically regulated by the kidneys to maintain the plasma concentration within narrow limits. The amount lost in sweat is less readily controlled, and extra sodium may be required in the diet during periods of strenuous work, particularly in high temperatures, to prevent muscular cramps (see Section 8.4). However, adaptation does occur so that the sodium concentration in sweat decreases and sodium requirements return to normal. The RNI for sodium is 1.6 g/day for adults.

Some epidemiological studies across different populations have shown a correlation between high sodium intake and hypertension. Populations with a low sodium intake do not show as marked an increase in blood pressure with age as seen in western nations. These results have been difficult to reproduce within populations, which may be a result of the difficulty in obtaining consistent blood pressure readings from individuals since these can be subject to considerable personal variation. There may also be certain inherent factors that make some people susceptible to developing hypertension in the presence of a high sodium intake. Other factors (e.g. excessive alcohol intake, lack of exercise, obesity, smoking, and stress) influence the development of hypertension and need to be considered when interpreting data. People moving into areas with a high average intake of sodium do show an increase in blood pressure, although other factors may also be responsible since a change in culture inevitably results in overall social and nutritional changes. In some studies, restriction of sodium intake has not shown significant changes in blood pressure in normotensive individuals and only a marginal improvement in mildly hypertensive subjects.

Although quantitative information on high sodium intakes is lacking, the DoH (1991) advises that intakes of more than 3.2 g/day may lead to raised blood pressure in susceptible adults.

The functions of salt in industrial food processing are similar to those of sugars (i.e. it is used as a preservative, to influence texture, or to enhance flavour). Salt from this source can only be reduced if processed foods are largely avoided. There is no justification for adding salt to food during home cooking or at the table other than one of personal taste, and this source can be reduced immediately. Salt substitutes (usually potassium salts) may be used to flavour food after cooking, although these are contra-indicated in renal disease because of the risk of hyperkalaemia. Alternative means of flavouring foods are varied and include herbs, spices, garlic, onion, pepper, vinegar, lemon juice, and yoghurt. Increasing carbohydrate and NSP consumption (see Section 2.2.1) may cause a slight increase in salt consumption because it is added to bread and some breakfast cereals. However, provided that the recommendations to reduce overall consumption are followed, this should not represent a major source. For those who have to follow a low-salt diet as part of the management of a clinical condition, it is suggested that they regularly scan nutrition labels and select only those products claimed to be salt-free (although initially, professional advice from a dietician may be necessary).

Trace elements

Trace elements are widely distributed in foods and deficiency is rare because minute quantities are required. They have only recently been recognised as essential.

Cobalt

Cobalt forms part of the vitamin B_{12} molecule, and can only be utilised by man in this form.

Copper

Copper is a component of many enzyme systems, including cytochrome oxidase. It is involved in haemoglobin synthesis, nerve function, bone growth, and connective tissue metabolism. The principal sources in the diet are bread, cereals, meat, and vegetables. Shellfish and offal (e.g. heart, kidney, and liver) are particularly rich in copper. An adequate diet provides sufficient copper and deficiency is rare, although premature infants may be at risk (see Section 2.3). The

RNI for copper is 1.2 mg/day, increasing to 1.5 mg/day during lactation.

Chromium

Chromium is involved in carbohydrate metabolism and the utilisation of glucose, and acts as a cofactor for insulin. It is widely distributed and good food sources include liver, milk, and vegetables, although the best source is brewers' yeast. A little is also present in chicken, fish, fruits, and cereals. Deficiencies may arise in those consuming large quantities of sugars, fats, and refined cereals. There is no RNI in the UK for chromium, but more than 25 μg/day has been assessed as a safe intake.

Fluorine

Fluorine is present in bones and teeth, and contributes to the prevention of tooth decay (see Section 3.4). The principal food sources are salt-water fish (especially those eaten whole) and tea. Small amounts may be found in cereal, meat, fruits, and vegetables. Drinking water contains the ionised form, fluoride, but in variable amounts, and may be below the optimum level for temperate climates of 1 mg per litre (1 ppm). In warmer climates, where more water is likely to be consumed, the optimum level is lower. Some authorities undertake fluoridation of the water supply, and this should be borne in mind before recommending fluoride supplements for children because excessive ingestion of fluoride can cause mottling of the teeth. No supplementation is required if the level of fluoride in the water exceeds 700 μg/litre. For levels below this, see the guidelines in Section 3.4. There is no RNI in the UK for fluoride, but 0.05 mg/kg/day has been assessed as a safe upper limit for infants and young children; there is no figure for adults.

Iodine

Iodine is essential for the formation of the thyroid hormones, thyroxine (T_4) and liothyronine (T_3 or tri-iodothyronine), and a deficiency may cause hypothyroidism. The best dietary source is seafood, but iodine is also found in cereals and vegetables grown in iodine-rich soil. Animal products are a source of iodine but the amount depends on their dietary intake. In Britain, iodides are widely used in animal feeds, and thus milk and milk products are the main source; other important sources are meat and eggs. Absorption may be reduced by goitre-producing compounds present in some members of the cabbage family. Deficiency is generally rare, although it may occur in isolated parts of the world where the soil is iodine-deficient and the population relies totally on locally produced food. Iodised salt may be used as a supplement if necessary. The RNI for iodine is 140 μg/day for adults. An upper intake of 17 μg/kg/day, or no more than 1000 μg/day, has been set.

Manganese

Manganese is a cofactor for the enzymes arginase and the phosphotransferases. Good sources include leafy vegetables, nuts, pulses, spices, and whole grain cereals; tea is a particularly rich source. There is no RNI in the UK for manganese, but more than 1.4 mg/day has been assessed as a safe intake for adults.

Selenium

Selenium is a component of the enzyme glutathione peroxidase, and is involved in the removal of harmful peroxides. Sites of action include the blood vessels (endothelium), eye (lens), kidney, liver, and erythrocytes. There is also an association with vitamin E, although the exact relationship is unclear. Selenium is an antioxidant and is one of several dietary antioxidants that is being investigated for a protective role against tumour formation involving free radicals. Good dietary sources include seafood and meat (particularly liver and kidney). Cereals also contain selenium but the content depends on the level of selenium in the soil. No deficiency disorders have been recognised in man, although a form of cardiomyopathy has been observed in children living in an area of China where the selenium content of grains and beans in the diet is low. The RNI for selenium is 75 μg/day for men and 60 μg/day for women. In high doses, selenium is toxic and a maximum safe intake from all sources has been set at 450 μg/day for adult males.

Zinc

Zinc is an essential component of many enzyme systems involved in a variety of pathways, including insulin synthesis, nucleic acid metabolism, and spermatogenesis. It also has a role in wound healing and may be involved in taste sensation. Deficiency results in retarded growth in children. Most of the zinc in the body is in the bones, but this does not act as a reserve and zinc must be provided in the diet on a regular basis. Zinc is associated with proteins in foods and the best source is meat (especially liver). Other sources include cereals, cheese, eggs, milk, legumes, and nuts. Absorption is poor (less than 50%), and this is further reduced in the presence of whole grain cereals and other foods with a high-NSP content because of the presence of phytic acid. The RNI for zinc is 9.5 mg/day for men and 7 mg/day for women. In the UK the average daily intake has been assessed as 9 to 12 mg, although vegetarians and vegans may ingest less because of the lack of meat in their diet coupled with a high-NSP intake.

2.2.6 Vitamin and mineral supplements

A very popular question for pharmacists concerns the value of vitamin and mineral supplements, and their ability to boost energy. It must be stressed that vitamins and minerals contribute absolutely nothing to dietary energy. The only way they could possibly be of benefit is if fatigue is a symptom of a deficiency disorder, which is unlikely in a well balanced diet. Similarly, emotional disturbances would benefit more from relaxation therapy than vitamin supplementation. However, in many instances, counselling alone may not be enough and the value of a placebo effect should not be overlooked. For some groups, however, regular vitamin supplements are essential, and these are discussed in Section 2.3. People who consume excessive quantities of alcohol may also need vitamin supplements because alcohol provides energy and may therefore preclude the intake of more nutritious alternatives. Moreover, thiamine is required in the metabolism of alcohol, and excessive alcohol consumption causes thiamine deficiency. For a more detailed discussion on nutritional deficiency associated with excessive alcohol consumption *see* Chapter 6.

It should, of course, be made clear to many of those requesting vitamin and mineral supplements that their best source is in a good diet. Pharmacists may offer guidance on food sources, and could also offer the following advice as to how vitamin losses from foods may be reduced:

- eat raw fruits and vegetables whenever possible
- use the minimum amount of water for cooking and avoid overcooking
- eat food as soon as possible after cooking and avoid reheating
- store fruits and vegetables in a cool dark place and use as soon as possible after purchasing
- do not use sodium bicarbonate when cooking vegetables
- cook frozen vegetables without prior thawing and for as little time as possible
- use vegetable water in stocks or gravies.

Clinical deficiency syndromes should not be treated by self-medication with vitamin supplements or by diet alone. These pathological states must be referred to medical practitioners.

There is absolutely no justification for dosage in excess of RNIs or for megadoses of dietary supplements for which no RNI has been set. In some cases this can even prove harmful. Fat-soluble vitamins in excess of requirements are stored in the body and may produce toxic effects. Although water-soluble vitamins are not stored, megadoses may still cause adverse effects by exacerbating existing conditions, or interacting with some drugs. Ascorbic acid in large doses reduces the absorption of vitamin B_{12} and may aggravate megaloblastic anaemia. It has also been shown to exacerbate diarrhoea. Large doses of nicotinic acid may precipitate asthmatic attacks, aggravate peptic ulceration, or produce hepatotoxicity. Nicotinic acid also raises the plasma-urate concentration and may therefore aggravate gout. Folic acid supplementation is not advised except under medical supervision because this could mask the clinical symptoms of megaloblastic anaemia caused by vitamin-B_{12} deficiency. Patients treated with levodopa for Parkinson's disease should not be given pyridoxine supplements, even at low doses, because of an interaction with the drug unless a dopa decarboxylase inhibitor is also given. Long-term supplementation with high doses of pyridoxine has been shown to cause peripheral neuropathies.

Some water-soluble vitamins have been shown to induce a state of dependency and produce withdrawal symptoms. Megadoses increase the efficiency of the elimination pathways and, consequently, if the supplementation is stopped abruptly, the vitamin obtained naturally from dietary sources may be eliminated too quickly. For example, clinical scurvy may follow abrupt withdrawal of megadoses of ascorbic acid, and convulsions have been seen in some infants born to mothers who ingested large doses of pyridoxine during pregnancy.

2.2.7 Non-nutritive constituents

There are some substances present in foods and drinks that have no nutritional value at all and, indeed, may actually have adverse effects.

Caffeine   One example of a non-nutritive constituent that has been the subject of many studies is caffeine. It has been proposed as an aetiological agent for many conditions, including benign mammary dysplasias, cancers, ischaemic heart disease, spontaneous abortion, and teratogenic effects. The evidence to support these claims is, in many cases, inconclusive or conflicting, and moderate consumption is not a significant risk to health. However, caffeine is known to be a central nervous system stimulant and in moderate doses (200 to 300 mg) it elevates mood. In larger doses, caffeine produces anxiety, diarrhoea, insomnia, irritability, headache, nausea, and tremor. Tolerance and physical dependence occur, and withdrawal may cause symptoms of anxiety, irritability, headache, lethargy, poor concentration, and restlessness.

Caffeine is automatically associated with coffee but it is in fact contained in other beverages and also in chocolate; some analgesic preparations, particularly headache tablets, contain caffeine. The amount of caffeine present in plants varies according to species, and the final amount contained in drinks depends on the method and length of time of brewing. Average amounts of caffeine present in a mug (about 300 mL) of some drinks are:

- ground coffee   230 mg*
- instant coffee   130 mg
- tea   80 mg
- cocoa or drinking chocolate   8 mg
- decaffeinated coffee or tea   6 mg
- cola   36 mg

Chocolate bars contain some caffeine, although the amount is well below that likely to cause stimulation. Dark chocolate contains about 80 mg of caffeine per 100 g bar whereas milk chocolate contains only about 20 mg per 100 g bar; white chocolate contains almost none.

No firm conclusions have been reached to suggest that caffeine should be avoided by the general population, although in view of its stimulant properties, the recommendations are to moderate intake. Caffeine in tea and coffee has been shown to reduce the absorption of iron from food. Decaffeinated coffee may produce problems as a result of its other constituents and should also be drunk in moderation.

The biological half-life of caffeine is increased in pregnancy. It crosses the placenta and low concentrations are found in breast milk. Although no conclusive evidence suggests that caffeine has an adverse effect on the foetus, it may be prudent for pregnant women to reduce their intake. Oral contraceptives also increase the half-life of caffeine.

Theobromine   Theobromine is a muscle stimulant and about 200 mg is present in a cup of drinking cocoa; it is also present in tea and coffee. Chocolate bars also contain theobromine but the concentrations are unlikely to cause problems in the average amounts ingested.

Herbal teas   Herbal teas are frequently considered to be 'healthy' because they are claimed not to contain caffeine or tannins; they are therefore considered by

---

* Boiled coffee contains considerably more caffeine than filtered or percolated coffee.

some as substitutes for tea or coffee. However, they too may present problems if ingested in large quantities, and the constituents should be examined critically. For example, maté contains caffeine, and blackberry contains tannins. Some herbs (e.g. juniper, pennyroyal, and raspberry) stimulate the uterus and, if ingested in large quantities during pregnancy, may induce abortion. Volatile oils that may cause kidney damage are present in juniper and pennyroyal. Lovage and yarrow contain coumarins, which may potentiate the action of anticoagulants. Chamomile, golden rod, marigold, and yarrow have been associated with hypersensitivity reactions in susceptible people. Comfrey, larkspur, hawthorn, and uva-ursi all contain potentially toxic compounds.

2.3 DIETARY NEEDS OF SPECIFIC GROUPS

Infants, children, and adolescents

Infants obtain most of the nutrients they require from milk alone during the first few months of life. Those nutrients present in only small quantities in milk (e.g. iron and copper) are stored in sufficient quantities in the liver to last until a more complete diet is introduced. Milk may be either breast milk or an infant formula milk (modified cows' milk or one derived from soya protein). It is generally considered that breast milk is the preferred alternative provided that the mother herself is well nourished. Unmodified cows' milk has very little copper in it and, occasionally, copper deficiency may occur in infants fed on this alone once their initial reserves have been depleted. Boiling cows' milk to render it sterile for infant consumption was formerly responsible for infantile scurvy, but this is rarely now reported in the UK because all infant formula milks are supplemented with ascorbic acid. The energy requirements of infants increase with age (Table 2.2) and, in proportion to body size, the need is greater than that of adults.

The kidneys of very young infants are unable to cope with excessive amounts of sodium, and salt should not, therefore, be added to their feeds. Sugar in any form should also be used conservatively because it has no nutritional value other than as a source of energy. Excessive sugar consumption either causes malnourishment because the child is satiated and does not feel the need for more nutritious foods, or paves the way for obesity in later life by laying down early fat deposits. Dietary sugars are also the cause of dental caries (*see* Section 3.3). Salt and sugars are not necessary in a balanced diet, and the general recommendations for the

TABLE 2.2
EARS for energy and RNIs for protein for infants

Age range in months	EAR for energy MJ/day (kcal/day)	RNI[a] for protein g/day
Boys		
0 to 3	2.28 (545)	12.5
4 to 6	2.89 (690)	12.7
7 to 9	3.44 (825)	13.7
10 to 12	3.85 (920)	14.9
Girls		
0 to 3	2.16 (515)	12.5
4 to 6	2.69 (645)	12.7
7 to 9	3.20 (765)	13.7
10 to 12	3.61 (865)	14.9

(a) These figures, based on egg and milk protein, assume complete digestibility.

The figures for this table are derived from DoH, Dietary reference values for food enegy and nutrients for the United Kingdom, *Report on Health and Social Subjects No. 41*, London: HMSO, 1991.

population are to reduce consumption. As food taste is based largely on habit, parents may help their offspring considerably by restricting the availability of these items in the diet.

The digestive system of infants takes several months to develop, and solid weaning foods should not be introduced until the child is at least four months of age. Weaning is a gradual process and infants should continue to receive milk. Infant formula milks, follow-up milks, or whole cows' milk may be used. Alternatively, breast-feeding may continue, although vitamin supplements will be required by breast-fed infants over six months of age. After 12 months of age, follow-up milks or whole cows' milk should be used. Whole cows' milk is a valuable energy source for young children and should not be replaced with skimmed milk in the diets of children under five years of age (*see* Section 2.2.2). However, it has been suggested by the DHSS (1988) that the gradual introduction of semi-skimmed milk from two years of age onwards is acceptable provided that sufficient energy and fat-soluble vitamins are derived from other dietary sources. From two years of age, the infant should be able to digest and metabolise a diet similar to the rest of the family. A special diet is not necessary for young children provided that they receive sufficient nutrients and dietary energy for growth. Inadequate nutrition during infancy and childhood results in stunted physical growth and possibly mental retardation, although this is more of a problem in

developing countries than western nations. The demand for most nutrients increases with age up to adult levels, and should be adequately provided by a varied diet. Some nutrients are required in greater amounts during childhood and adolescence.

The RNI for calcium for infants up to 12 months of age is 525 mg/day, and thereafter 350 mg/day (1 to 3 years), 450 mg/day (4 to 6 years), and 550 mg/day (7 to 10 years). Adolescents have the greatest requirement of all at 1000 mg/day (males) and 800 mg/day (females). Calcium deficiency is the cause of rickets in developing countries, but in western nations, particularly those in the northern hemisphere, the cause is usually vitamin-D deficiency because of inadequate exposure to sunlight during the winter months. This was a severe problem in industrial towns in the UK around 1900, and 70% of children living in such areas developed rickets because the dense smog that filled the air further reduced the available sunlight. This led to the current practice of fortifying margarine and some milk products with vitamin D. Cows' milk has less vitamin D than breast milk and, consequently, all infant formula milks are also fortified. However, cows' milk is a valuable source of calcium and should be encouraged in the diets of children over 12 months of age, and adolescents.

The RNI of vitamin D is 8.5 μg/day for infants under 6 months of age, and 7 μg/day for children up to three years of age. Supplements of vitamin D are recommended for weaned infants and children (especially vegans, *see below*), particularly during winter months. Vitamin D is toxic in excess (*see* Section 2.2.4) and the recommended dose should not be exceeded. In general, supplements are unnecessary for breast-fed babies unless there is a risk of low levels in the mother's milk, or for infants receiving fortified formula milks. Formula milks also contain vitamin A, although deficiency of this vitamin is rare in the UK and further supplements are unnecessary. Premature infants may also need supplements of some vitamins because they have insufficient body stores to last until weaned. The DHSS (1988) recommends the administration of children's vitamin drops containing vitamins A, D, and C from six months to two years of age (preferably up to five years of age, particularly in winter and early spring). It is considered that older children and adolescents do not need vitamin D supplements provided that they have adequate exposure to sunlight. For more detailed information on infant feeding, breast and formula milks, and feeding problems, the reader is referred to Child health and immunisation in Harman RJ, ed., *Handbook of pharmacy health-care: Diseases and patient advice*, 1990. For the effect of fluoride on prevention of dental caries, and the recommendation of fluoride supplements for infants and children, *see* Section 3.4.

The RNI of iron for adolescent males is 11.3 mg/day, which is greater than that for adult men; female adolescents require 14.8 mg/day and even more if they suffer regular heavy menstrual losses. A good mixed diet should provide enough, although deficiencies may arise in vegetarian diets (*see below*). The requirements for some of the vitamin-B group also increase above the adult level during adolescence. Again, these extra nutritional demands should be met by the diet, and deficiencies are unlikely. Problems may, however, arise out of bad eating habits, such as regularly missing meals and indulging in inappropriate snacks ('junk' food) rich in refined carbohydrates, fats, and sugars, and deficient in proteins, vitamins, and minerals.

Psychological problems may occur in some adolescents as a result of undesirable weight. Fat deposits are laid down at puberty, particularly in females, and may initially be the cause of severe distress. Reassurance and counselling on appropriate diets may be of benefit at this stage. The increased energy demands of adolescence and a consequent increase in appetite may cause excessive fat deposits if inappropriate foods are eaten. Dietary management is essential at this stage to avoid obesity in adulthood. Anorexia nervosa is a condition that may occur in adolescents, particularly in females, and reflects a distorted perception of body size. Undereating causes dramatic weight loss, and is a serious clinical problem requiring medical intervention and, in some cases, psychiatric counselling.

Pregnant and breast-feeding women

The total nutritional and energy requirements of a growing foetus must be supplied by the mother. If these extra demands are not met, her own body stores will be depleted.

It has been calculated that up to 293 MJ (70 000 kcal) of additional energy is required during the nine months of pregnancy. However, considerable reductions occur in physical activity during pregnancy, which may compensate for the increased needs. The DoH (1991) recommends an increase in EAR for energy of 0.8 MJ/day (200 kcal/day) for the final trimester. Women, who were underweight at the start of pregnancy may need to eat more. Up to 4 kg of fat may remain at the end of the pregnancy to supplement the extra demands of lactation. A gain in weight above the extra weight contributed by the foetus is necessary during pregnancy for the well-being of both mother and child; for a non-obese woman, the increase in weight should be of the order of 12.5 kg.

For most women, the fat gained during pregnancy will be lost afterwards, particularly if they breast-feed. This may not be the case in obese women, and they do not need to provide as much extra energy in their diets as non-obese women. They do, nevertheless, have the same requirements for an adequate supply of essential nutrients. Slimming during pregnancy without medical supervision is to be discouraged because it may result in a low birth-weight infant. Dieting too soon after parturition may prove stressful for the mother, and should preferably be delayed until she has stopped breast-feeding. The mother's diet during pregnancy and lactation should consist of foods rich in starch, and vitamins and minerals. Foods containing sugars, fats, and refined carbohydrates should be avoided. A marginal increase in protein intake is recommended during pregnancy and an extra 6 g a day of mixed proteins should be added to the RNI for non-pregnant women (45 g/day), making a total of 51 g/day.

Women who have several pregnancies and breast-feed each infant may suffer large losses of calcium and develop osteomalacia. In developed countries, however, this is more likely to be a consequence of vitamin-D deficiency. Lack of calcium or vitamin D in the mother may also lead to rickets in the infant (*see above*). The RNI for vitamin D during pregnancy is 10 μg/day, and since dietary sources may not supply this amount, supplements are recommended. Calcium absorption increases during pregnancy, and no additional calcium is generally needed. Calcium is widely distributed in food, and a good balanced diet should therefore supply a sufficient quantity. For examples of good dietary sources of calcium, *see* Section 2.2.5. The needs of the pregnant adolescent are, however, particularly high.

The RNI for vitamin A increases to 700 μg/day during pregnancy. The amount present in a good balanced diet is considered sufficient to meet the demands of the mother, and to lay down stores in the liver of the foetus. There is evidence to suggest that ingestion of excessive amounts of vitamin A during pregnancy may have an adverse effect on the foetus. Although there are, as yet, no reported cases of adverse effects in the UK, the DoH has advised that all women who are, or who may become, pregnant should not take vitamin A supplements except under medical supervision. The advice also extends to excluding liver or liver products (e.g. liver pâté and liver sausage) from the diet because animal liver contains extremely high levels of vitamin A. Good dietary sources of vitamin A include dairy products, eggs, margarine, carrots, green vegetables, and tomatoes and other fruits. Vitamin A is generally combined with vitamin D in supplements, and often occurs naturally with vitamin D (e.g. fish-liver oils); this must be taken into consideration if vitamin-D supplementation is required (*see above*). There are marginal increases in the RNIs of some of the B-group vitamins but these are likely to be met from the diet. However, folic acid deficiency may arise in pregnancy as a result of the increased demands made by erythropoiesis. Supplements are generally recommended to prevent megaloblastic anaemia. The RNI for folate during pregnancy is 300 μg/day. The increased needs for iron caused by pregnancy should be met without a further increase in iron intake because of cessation of menstrual losses and by mobilisation of maternal stores and increased intestinal absorption. Supplements may be required by women with low iron stores. Women who stop eating liver during pregnancy should be advised to substitute other types of lean red meat and meat products as good dietary sources of iron; other sources of iron include bread, vegetables, and fortified breakfast cereals. It has been suggested by some workers that pregnant women may need supplements of pyridoxine, although there is no official recommendation. Megadoses may even be harmful to the foetus (*see* Section 2.2.6). The amount of ascorbic acid ingested should be increased during pregnancy, and the RNI is 50 mg/day. This can readily be met from the diet by increasing the amount of fresh fruits and vegetables consumed, or by supplementation.

The surplus fat remaining at the end of pregnancy is used during the first weeks of lactation to meet some of the increased energy requirements but additional energy intake, over and above pre-pregnancy intakes, is needed during lactation. As soon as weaning begins, the mother's energy needs begin to return to their pre-pregnancy levels and two different groups are defined for the purpose of assessing EARs for energy: Group 1 mothers are those whose breast milk supplies all or most of the infant's food for the first 3 months, and Group 2 mothers, whose breast milk supplies all or nearly all the infant's food for 6 months. EARs during lactation are:

	MJ/day (kcal/day)	
up to 1 month	1.9 (450)	
1 to 2 months	2.2 (530)	
2 to 3 months	2.4 (570)	
	Group 1	Group 2
4 to 6 months	2.0 (480)	2.4 (570)
over 6 months	1.0 (240)	2.3 (550)

The actual amount will vary between women depending on the weight gained during pregnancy and those nursing more than one infant have greater requirements. To meet the increased demands, the quantity of food consumed should be increased, taking into account the same recommendations for dietary adjustments during pregnancy (*see above*). Protein consumption should increase and the RNIs during lactation are 56 g/day for the first four months of breast-feeding, and 53 g/day for the next four months.

The RNI of vitamin D is the same during lactation as for pregnancy (*see above*) but the requirement for calcium increases and the RNI during lactation is 1250 mg/day; the RNI for vitamin A increases to 950 μg/day. A further increase in some of the B-vitamins is necessary, and may be provided in the diet. The RNI of folate is 260 μg/day, which is less than during pregnancy, but still above the RNI for non-pregnant women. The RNI of ascorbic acid increases to 70 mg/day.

The elderly

The overall nutritional requirements of the elderly are the same as those of younger adults. However, the basal metabolic rate decreases with age as a result of the decrease in the fat-free mass (*see* Section 2.1), which together with a reduction in physical activity, generally results in a decrease in total energy requirements. In order to avoid an increase in weight, elderly people must decrease their total intake of energy but without upsetting the recommended contributions made by the various components (i.e. carbohydrates, fats, and proteins, *see* Section 2.2). The RNI for protein for the elderly is the same as for younger adults (*see* Section 2.2.3) but because of the small amount of lean body mass per kg body weight in the elderly, the resultant figure per unit lean body mass is higher than in younger adults. Inexpensive protein sources include milk, eggs, and pulses. The requirements for vitamins and minerals do not decrease with age and an adequate intake must be maintained.

Scurvy in the elderly is not common but many do have low reserves of ascorbic acid and, as a consequence, may have symptoms of depression, fatigue, myalgia, and weakness. Wound healing may be impaired and skin may bruise easily. The deficiency may arise as a result of poor understanding of dietary requirements, restricted income, or an inability to chew fruits and vegetables. These problems could be overcome by explaining the necessity of ascorbic acid in the diet, and suggesting food sources that are inexpensive or require minimal or no chewing (e.g. soft seedless fruits, and fruit juices). Vitamin-D deficiency may arise in the elderly, especially the housebound. The DoH (1991) has set the RNI for vitamin D at 10 μg/day for all people over 65 years of age. As there are few dietary sources, supplements may be necessary to achieve this level.

Elderly people, particularly those with physical disabilities (e.g. poor vision, loss of teeth, or arthritis) may have difficulty in preparing and eating food. Those living alone may have little incentive to prepare food for themselves, and financial problems may make good food prohibitively expensive for some. Malnourishment may occur as a consequence of a monotonous and nutritionally incomplete diet. Those with difficulties should be encouraged to consume nutritious foods that require minimal preparation (e.g. bread, breakfast cereals, cheese, eggs, fruit, milk, and salads). Consumption of NSP-rich foods should also be encouraged to help prevent constipation. If possible, there should be one cooked meal a day, and relatives may be able to help with the provision of this. Alternatively, a daily visit from a meals-on-wheels service could be organised. Local luncheon clubs fulfil a dual role of providing a cooked meal and an opportunity for the lonely to meet other people.

Friends, relatives, neighbours, or home-helps, may be called upon to do the shopping of elderly housebound or disabled people, and this provides a good opportunity to directly influence their diets. Helping elderly people to make shopping lists, explaining why some foods should be added and others rejected, could increase their nutritional knowledge and interest in food, with a consequent improvement in nutritional status.

Vegetarians

A vegetarian diet in its most basic form is one that excludes meat; most vegetarians will also not eat fish. Lacto-vegetarians allow milk and milk-products in their diet, ovo-vegetarians allow eggs, and ovo-lacto-vegetarians allow both. A vegan diet totally excludes all animal products, but the most restrictive diet of all is that of fruitarians, which allows only raw fruit and nuts.

Vegetarian diets may be adopted for reasons of health, religion, or an aversion to using animals to satisfy human needs. Some studies undertaken to compare the health of vegetarians with non-vegetarians have shown a decreased incidence of cardiovascular disease, gallstones, and gastro-intestinal disorders in the former group. However, these results may be attributed to an overall difference in life-style and a greater awareness of health issues among vegetarians, as much as to dietary differences. A parameter, however, that can be scientifically measured is the plasma-cholesterol concentration, and this is generally lower in vegans than non-vegetarians; vegetarians either show no difference or an intermediate level. This may be attributable to the fact that, in a vegan diet, saturated fats contribute less than 10% to the total dietary energy, which is considerably less than that of the general population. Lacto-vegetarians consume more saturated fatty acids in dairy products, although the exact amount depends on whether whole or low-fat milk is used. High plasma-cholesterol concentrations are associated with an increased risk of ischaemic heart disease.

Meat contains much fat, which is a concentrated source of energy. Avoiding all meat, therefore, reduces total dietary energy, which must be compensated for by increasing the amounts of other foods eaten. Fruits and vegetables contain mostly water and supply little energy unless eaten in great quantity, whereas cereals and dairy products are high in energy. A reduction in dietary energy may be beneficial to some adults, particularly if overweight, but it is not desirable in growing children. Consequently, a great deal of thought and planning must go into devising vegetarian diets (especially vegan diets) for the young (see below). Vegetarians and vegans generally consume less refined sugars than non-vegetarians, although their total sugar consumption may be similar as a consequence of the natural sugar content of fruits. Starch and NSP intake is also higher and reflects the reduction in fat consumption. Plant proteins have a lower biological value than animal proteins (see Section 2.2.3), and are thus unable to supply all the essential amino acids unless a mixed variety, preferably from different food groups, is consumed. For example, baked beans on toast is a combination of a pulse and a cereal, and the combination of the constituent proteins has a high biological value.

Vegans may be at risk of low calcium intake because of the lack of milk in their diets. Many non-animal foods do contain calcium (e.g. leafy vegetables and nuts), and judicious selection should ensure adequate dietary intake. Problems may, however, arise because oxalic acid present in some plants, and phytic acid in nuts and cereals (particularly whole grain cereals) bind with calcium and reduce absorption. Phytic acid also binds with other minerals, including iron and zinc. These minerals may already be deficient in vegan diets because the principal dietary sources are meat, eggs, and dairy products. Ascorbic acid enhances iron absorption, and consequently consumption of foods rich in ascorbic acid at the same time as plant sources of iron increases the amount absorbed. In many cases, ascorbic acid and iron occur together in plant foods.

Vegans who have inadequate exposure to sunlight run the risk of vitamin-D deficiency. The few available dietary sources are all animal products and are consequently denied to them. Supplements may be necessary, especially during the winter months. Similarly, as the only natural sources of vitamin B_{12} are meat, fish, and dairy products, vegans are advised to take supplements (which are of bacterial origin). Yeast extracts, meat substitutes (e.g. derived from soya), and a number of commercially produced vegan foods are fortified with vitamin B_{12}.

Well planned vegetarian and vegan diets should not pose any threat to health, and are thought to reduce the risks of some diet-related diseases common in the western world. Pregnant and breast-feeding women, and children on such diets should not suffer any adverse effects provided that the extra requirements for energy and nutrients are met (*see above*). Some authorities consider that infants should not be fed vegan diets, although others disagree. A full understanding of how the particular nutritional needs of infants and young children may be met by a vegan diet is necessary. Weaning should start at the same age in vegan infants as non-vegetarians (*see above*), but the diet should be supplemented with breast or soya infant formula milks up to two years of age to avoid calcium deficiency. The high energy requirements of young children will not be satisfied by vegetable foods unless large amounts are eaten, and this may require an increase in the number of meals per day. Alternatively, fats may be added to the diet. Riboflavine and vitamins B_{12} and D are likely to be deficient and may need supplementation, and ascorbic acid with each meal should increase the absorption of iron from food. This vitamin is widely present in fruits and vegetables, but additional supplementation may be beneficial.

The elderly may safely continue with their chosen form of diet, although adjustments may have to be made in the actual foods eaten to take into account some of the feeding problems associated with old age (*see above*). This may be more of a problem for vegans because milk and eggs, which are inexpensive, nutritious, and easy to eat, are not available in their diet.

The change from a meat diet to a vegetarian diet should be gradual. Red meat should be cut out first, then white meat followed by fish, and finally eggs and dairy products, if required, adding in sufficient vegetarian foods to compensate at each stage. A sound knowledge of the nutritional requirements of the body is essential, particularly if planning diets for vulnerable groups. A wide variety of foods must be consumed to ensure that the diet provides all the necessary amino acids, vitamins and minerals, and use of food tables (*see* Section 2.1) may be of help.

Immigrants

Immigrants to a foreign country may face dietary problems. They may have special needs dictated by habit, culture, or religion, or the non-availability or expense of their traditional foods, or both.

Some non-white races do not consume milk after weaning, which results in the disappearance of lactase (the enzyme required to digest lactose) from the gastro-intestinal tract. Subsequent challenge with milk causes lactose intolerance, which is characterised by watery diarrhoea and abdominal discomfort. The only remedy is to avoid milk and milk products.

Asian women and children are particularly at risk of developing osteomalacia and rickets. Vegetarian diets, sometimes coupled with inadequate exposure to sunlight, may lead to vitamin-D deficiency. As dietary sources of this vitamin are largely unavailable in vegetarian diets, supplements are necessary and absolutely essential for pregnant and breast-feeding women. Some traditional non-meat diets may be low in iron, and children are particularly at risk if they develop iron-deficiency anaemia (*see also* Vegetarians above).

The sick and convalescent

Disease or trauma (e.g. burn injuries or surgery) may result in reduced nutritional status and, if long-term, malnutrition. Metabolic losses of nitrogen may occur, particularly during infections, and disorders involving the gastro-intestinal tract may cause malabsorption of some nutrients (e.g. vitamins and minerals). Repair of tissues increases the requirements for nutrients, especially proteins. However, appetite is often poor in illness, and this further reduces the levels of essential nutrients. Consequently, body stores are depleted and tissues may become wasted.

The requirements for all nutrients increase during convalescence and are similar to those needed for growth. However, a poor appetite may not allow these demands to be met in full. Foods must be selected with care in order to satisfy the criteria of low bulk, high levels of proteins, vitamins, and minerals, and sufficient energy to meet the metabolic demands of repair and replenishment. Variety is also important to stimulate an interest in food. Convalescents may appreciate small but frequent meals, rather than being overwhelmed by large amounts of food all at once. Difficult cases who do not appear to be regaining their normal appetite, and especially those continuing to lose weight, may need referral. Dietary supplements may be indicated, and are available for oral, nasogastric, and intravenous routes (BNF 9.3, 9.4, and BNF Appendix 7).

Slimmers

Ideally, the energy provided in the diet should match exactly the amount of energy expended, and this is controlled fairly accurately by appetite. Problems arise when individuals fail to adjust their diets to take into account reduced requirements occasioned by reduced activity, or increasing age, or both. Previous habits are maintained, resulting in a steady, and sometimes insidious, increase in weight. An intake in excess of requirements of only 0.042 MJ (10 kcal) per day for one year would cause a weight increase of 0.5 kg. Fat is laid down under the skin and around internal organs. The physiological function of fat deposits is to provide a reserve energy supply for times of increased need. In affluent nations, such episodes rarely occur, and therefore as long as energy intake exceeds energy expended, fat will continue to accumulate.

The degree of body fatness can be measured by calculating the Body Mass Index (BMI), which is expressed as:

$$\frac{\text{weight (kg)}}{\text{height (m)}^2}$$

A BMI between about 20 and 25 represents the normal range, between 25 and 30 may be described as overweight, and over 30 is recognised as obesity. Various authorities publish charts relating ideal weight to height, which are often used by life insurance companies to assess risk of early death because studies have shown a correlation between excessive weight and ischaemic heart disease, diabetes mellitus, and hypertension. Correlations have also been made with conditions that may not prove fatal, but nevertheless decrease the quality of life (e.g. gallstones, gout, joint disorders, and varicose veins). Being overweight may also increase the risk of complications in pregnancy or surgery. All these risks increase with excessive amounts of body fat. A heavy body-weight caused by build up of muscles (e.g. in athletes) does not appear to be associated with increased risks from these diseases, provided that body fat is not also increased.

Actual gain in weight will eventually cease if the individual's energy intake becomes equal to output, but no weight will be lost until the equation is reversed. There may be a variety of reasons to account for the initial weight gain, not the least of which may be bad eating habits started during childhood. Many women blame pregnancy, but the fat laid down should be utilised during the third trimester and lactation (see Section 2.3); once breast-feeding has ceased, there should be no significant gain in weight above the pre-

pregnancy level provided that consumption of the extra food required for pregnancy and lactation stops. In some people, compulsive overeating may have a psychological cause (e.g. anxiety, depressive disorders, or emotional disturbances), and medical help may be necessary to treat such conditions before initiating a weight-reducing diet. If boredom is the reason, a change in life-style as well as diet is likely to be successful. Overweight people are generally physically inactive, and a gradual and programmed increase in exercise is often of benefit (see Chapter 8).

Weight will be lost by providing less energy in the diet than is expended. It has been estimated that each kilogram of excess weight represents 29.3 MJ (7000 kcal) of stored energy. Reducing the daily dietary energy intake by 4.2 MJ (1000 kcal) will result in a loss in weight of up to one kg/week. However, simply reducing the total amount of food eaten without any thought given to nutrient content is not recommended, and may be dangerous if drastic reductions are continued long-term. Only the energy provided by food must be reduced; the requirement for all other nutrients remains the same. An increase in physical activity (see Chapter 8) is also beneficial for weight control, although exercise without dietary modification will not produce significant weight loss.

Any food is fattening if enough is eaten. The difference lies in the energy density: fat-rich foods have a high energy density whereas fruits and vegetables have a low energy density. The most effective way of retaining a nutritious balance in a weight-reducing diet is to cut out as many energy-rich foods as possible. Alcohol and non-milk extrinsic sugars should not be consumed at all because they may contribute a significant amount to total dietary energy. The amount of visible fats in the diet (e.g. butter, margarine, cooking oils, and fat on meat) should be reduced as much as possible, and foods with a high content of invisible fats (e.g. red meat and whole milk) should be avoided. As overweight people are at increased risk of developing ischaemic heart disease and hypertension, they are also advised to follow the general recommendations made by the DoH (1991) for reduction of saturated fatty acids and salt in the diet (see Section 2.2).

Some food energy is required, and this may be provided by complex carbohydrates (e.g. bread, pasta, potatoes, and rice). NSP-rich carbohydrates (e.g. whole grain cereals and wholemeal bread) are particularly beneficial because some people on weight-reducing diets complain of constipation. It has been postulated that NSP is also of direct benefit because it has a high satiety value and reduces the craving for other 'filling' foods, although the evidence for this is inconclusive. Fruits and vegetables are a good source of vitamins and minerals, and some NSP, and contribute little energy. The protein requirement remains the same, but low-fat sources should be chosen (e.g. lean meat and fish, low-fat cheeses, and skimmed milk).

When there is a negative energy balance, fat stores are depleted, but there is also some loss of non-fat tissues. These tissues, referred to as the fat-free mass (FFM) (*see* Section 2.1), comprise the body organs, bones, and muscles. The amount lost from the FFM increases disproportionately to the degree of the energy deficit, and can be considerable in very low calorie diets (*see below*). The basal metabolic rate is determined by the metabolic requirements of the FFM and consequently decreases as the FFM is reduced. In addition, the energy expended as heat in response to food intake decreases as intake decreases. The net result is a decrease in energy demands, which may be perceived by the individual as failure of the diet (i.e. despite strictly adhering to it, the rate of weight-reduction slows down or ceases). A further reduction in dietary energy intake is necessary to effect further weight losses. This may be offset to some extent by increasing the levels of physical activity.

Very low calorie diets (VLCDs) are used to reduce weight rapidly by severely restricting the daily energy intake to below 2.5 MJ (600 kcal), and are intended to be used as a complete replacement for all food intake. Early VLCDs were associated with sudden death, particularly as a result of ventricular arrhythmias. It has been suggested that the cause might have been a rapid loss of protein from vital tissues as a result of too drastic a reduction in the FFM (*see above*). Such diets require careful formulation to ensure adequate amounts of good quality proteins, and vitamins and minerals. The DHSS (1987) has laid down guidelines on VLCDs in obesity. VLCDs should provide a minimum of 1.68 MJ (400 kcal) and 40 g of protein per day for women, and 2.1 MJ (500 kcal) and 50 g of protein per day for men; the vitamin and mineral content should also be adequate. The use of VLCDs should be restricted to the severely obese. It is absolutely essential that the instructions for use of these products are strictly followed.

VLCDs should not be used as the sole nutritional source for longer than 3 to 4 weeks, and medical advice and supervision is necessary before prolonging this period or repeating the diet. People wishing to lose weight are recommended to try traditional methods first, and should consult their doctor before embarking on a VLCD. Medical supervision, perhaps under hospital conditions, is recommended for anyone suffering with cancer, cardiovascular disease (including hypertension), diabetes mellitus, kidney disease, or any other major clinical condition. Extreme caution should be exercised

for those with abnormal psychological states. VLCDs are not recommended for infants, children, adolescents, pregnant or breast-feeding women, or the elderly, and all members of these groups should only undertake weight-reduction under medical supervision.

It should be emphasised that the use of VLCDs does not contribute to the changes in eating behaviour necessary to maintain the reduced weight once the programme has been completed. People become over-weight by consuming excessive quantities of food at meal-times, or eating a lot of snacks between meals, or both. Such habits must be completely broken, which may initially be difficult. Dividing the total daily food allowance into several small meals rather than eating 1 or 2 large ones may be of benefit. However, it must be emphasised that strict control of quantities consumed must be exercised. It may be helpful, particularly when first embarking on a weight-reducing diet, to calculate the food allowance for the day and then divide it into portions to be consumed throughout the day. This helps establish a new routine and educates the individual with regard to the quantities that may be consumed. Once the desired weight has been reached it must be maintained, and former eating habits must not be resumed. Permanent weight-reduction, therefore, involves a total change in eating habits.

Non-compliance with a weight-reducing diet or inappropriate diets are generally the reasons for failure to lose weight. It should be stressed, particularly to people taking part in group weight-reducing schemes, that comparisons between individuals of weight lost against daily calories should not be made. Individuals vary greatly in their requirements, and a good weight-reducing diet should be designed on a personal basis. The best guide to a successful diet is loss of weight; if this ceases, dietary energy must be further reduced, while still maintaining adequate levels of nutrients for health. Patience is also essential as learning new eating habits and reduction in weight takes time.

2.4 FOOD SAFETY

Microbial contamination

Food may be responsible for illness by being the vehicle for transmission of pathogenic micro-organisms, and contamination may occur at any stage of its production. The most common infecting micro-organisms are *Salmonella* spp., *Staphylococcus aureus*, *Campylobacter* spp., and *Clostridium perfringens*.

Salmonella and *Campylobacter* spp. are present in the faecal flora of many animals, and intensive farming methods increase the likelihood of contamination of meat and other animal products. In the UK, there has been a dramatic increase in contamination of hen's eggs with *Salmonella enteritidis* DT4, which infects the genital tracts of hens. Although the actual proportion of contaminated eggs is still likely to be small, the risk of salmonellosis may be high because, nationally, a large number of eggs are consumed each day. This is a particular problem in vulnerable groups (e.g. the very young and old, pregnant women, and the chronically sick). The chicken carcass itself may also be contaminated. Duck's eggs are also contaminated with *Salmonella* spp. *Listeria monocytogenes* is ubiquitous, and infections in humans have increased. People at risk include the elderly and immunocompromised. This micro-organism is particularly hazardous for pregnant women because of adverse effects on the foetus. Pigs may be an important source of *Yersinia enterocolitica*, although this micro-organism could potentially contaminate many other foods as it is widely distributed in environmental water. A toxin produced by *Clostridium botulinum* causes botulism; although rare, the condition may be fatal, and is associated with improperly canned or bottled food. Other micro-organisms implicated in food-borne infections include *Bacillus cereus* and *Vibrio parahaemolyticus; Escherichia coli* is often responsible for traveller's diarrhoea (*see* Section 9.3).

Animals may contract infections initially from feedstuffs, grazing on contaminated land, or from water, and may show clinical symptoms or be asymptomatic carriers. Transmission from other infected animals, birds, or humans may occur at any stage of production (e.g. on the farm, in transit to market, or in the slaughterhouse). Subsequent bad practices in handling carcasses may cause cross-contamination or additional contamination with other micro-organisms right up to the moment the meat is purchased by the consumer. Thereafter, the consumer may introduce further micro-organisms or unwittingly cross-contaminate other foods if poor practices of storage and preparation of food are adopted (*see below*).

Pathogenic micro-organisms in the human gastro-intestinal tract may be transmitted by the faecal-oral route during illness or convalescence, to both animals or food. Some individuals may remain asymptomatic carriers for years. *Staphylococcus aureus* is present as part of the normal flora in the nares, skin, and perianal area of many people. This micro-organism is also found in skin lesions (e.g. boils, carbuncles, and ulcers). Animals may be responsible for direct transmission of micro-organisms to food if they are allowed in food preparation areas, or via humans who prepare food with unwashed hands after handling them. Insects (e.g. flies and cockroaches) may be responsible for transporting bacteria to food, and people may pick up bacteria from fomites (e.g. towels, door handles, taps, or lavatory flush chains and handles). Poor sewage and rubbish disposal allows insects and scavenger animals to come into contact with many micro-organisms.

Food-borne gastro-intestinal infections are often referred to as food poisoning, although this term also refers to poisoning with non-bacterial toxins such as solanine in badly stored potatoes, organophosphate contamination of food, and inherently toxic foods such as fungi (e.g. *Amanita* spp.). Conversely, some food-borne gastro-intestinal infections are not traditionally classified as food poisoning (e.g. dysentery and typhoid fever). Infective cases of food poisoning that are thought to have been caused by food bought or eaten from a public place must, by UK law, be notified to the Environmental Health Officer of the local council. Dysentery and typhoid fever must also be notified, although they are covered under a different Act of Parliament.

In many cases, the inoculum required to cause clinical symptoms is large. Therefore, contamination with a few micro-organisms is unlikely to have any adverse effect. However, if food is left to stand unrefrigerated for several hours, bacteria will rapidly divide and sufficient numbers will quickly build up; under optimum conditions over two million bacteria could result after seven hours from one bacterium. Some sporing bacteria (e.g. *Clostridium perfringens* and *Bacillus cereus*) are even able to form spores at high temperatures. Cooking, therefore, will kill vegetative cells but not destroy spores, and subsequent storage at optimum growth temperatures allows the spores to germinate and multiply. *Bacillus cereus* favours warm, moist conditions, and has been found to be a particular problem in cooked rice left for long periods at room temperature.

Food hygiene

It is the responsibility of everyone concerned with the manufacture and preparation of food to ensure that the risk of its contamination at every stage of production is kept to an absolute minimum. Government legislation controls the food industry (including agriculture) and retail trade, but the consumer also has a responsibility, and there are government guidelines to reduce the level of food contamination in the home. This is especially important for those groups most at risk (*see above*). The appearance, taste, or smell of food is not usually changed by pathogenic micro-organisms (as opposed to spoilage micro-organisms). This makes the task of those responsible for preventing infections doubly difficult, and reinforces the need for scrupulous practices of hygiene.

Stringent controls are necessary to reduce the level of contamination of raw foods, and to prevent cross-contamination between foods and recontamination of cooked food. Commercial food handlers must be well trained, and should not be allowed to prepare food if suffering from a gastro-intestinal infection. Retailers must also lay down strict guidelines covering hygiene for their premises and staff. Consumers should avoid making purchases in those food stores that do not appear to be cleaned regularly and where the staff have dirty overalls, hands, and fingernails. Careful selection of food is essential, and damaged packages, dirty or cracked eggs, and food from overfilled freezers should be avoided. Dents in cans may damage the inner lacquer and allow leaching of tin particles into the food. Rusty or faulty seams may disrupt the integrity of the can, and swollen ends indicate the presence of gas inside, which could indicate contamination with *Clostridium botulinum*. The batch code stamped on the can indicates the canning date. It consists of a four-figure number, of which the first three digits indicate the day of the year (i.e. out of 365), and the fourth digit is taken from the last figure of the year (i.e. 0591 is the code for 28 February 1991). Raw food should appear fresh and use-by dates for all foods observed.

The optimum temperature for growth of pathogenic bacteria is 37°C, although the range for most is 15 to 45°C. Some may grow at even higher temperatures, albeit at a reduced rate. Most bacteria are killed above 60°C, but this does not destroy spores or toxins. Bacteria are not killed by low temperatures or freezing but most do cease multiplication below 5°C, and refrigerators should be kept below this temperature. A notable exception is *Listeria monocytogenes*, which can multiply slowly at 4°C. Freezers should be maintained at −18°C and defrosted regularly because this helps them to run more efficiently and economically.

Food must be transported home from the shops as quickly as possible. This is particularly important for frozen food, which must not be allowed to defrost. Fresh food is also at risk, especially on warm days or if kept in hot cars or offices for any length of time before going home; bacteria may multiply to a significant level after only one hour. Cooked food and food intended to be consumed raw should be kept well away from raw meat and fish at all times. This point is particularly important when storing food in a refrigerator. Raw meat and fish should be stored on plates or drip trays at the bottom of the refrigerator so that the juices cannot drip onto other food.

If cooked food is not intended to be eaten straight away it must be cooled quickly and refrigerated or frozen to reduce the chances of recontamination or germination of spores. Not all bacteria are killed by cooking, and survivors start to multiply as soon as the optimum temperature is reached. Cooling to a temperature suitable for refrigeration must not take more than one hour. Warm food placed in a refrigerator will raise the internal temperature. Similarly, warm food should never be put straight into a freezer. Cooked food should not be kept for longer than 1 to 2 days, and it must be reheated thoroughly and once only. This is particularly important with purchased cook-chill food, which has been associated with *Listeria monocytogenes* contamination. All preserved foods, once opened, should be treated in exactly the same way as fresh food.

Some foods are intended to be cooked from frozen, but dense bulky foods (e.g. meat) must thaw completely before cooking to allow even temperature distribution to ensure that the centre is fully cooked. It is better to thaw food in a refrigerator than at room temperature to limit bacterial multiplication. Once thawed, food must not be refrozen without first cooking it. Bacteria start to multiply during thawing, and the population reached will become dormant if refrozen. Multiplication continues during the second thaw, so that the final population could well approach the numbers required to cause illness.

It is essential to wash all vegetables and salads thoroughly, paying particular attention to those intended to be eaten raw. *Listeria monocytogenes* has been associated with ready-to-eat salads, and it is recommended that vulnerable groups avoid these. Consumption of raw meat and fish is not advised and, because of the increase in incidence of contamination of eggs with salmonella, it is also recommended that raw eggs or products made with them should not be consumed by anybody. Additionally, vulnerable groups should not consume any dish prepared with fresh eggs unless both the white and yolk are hard, which signifies that they are thoroughly cooked. This does not apply to pasteurised eggs. Some soft cheeses (e.g. Brie and Camembert) and blue-vein cheeses have been associated with contamination by *Listeria monocytogenes* and should be avoided by pregnant women and immuno-compromised people. It is also recommended by the DHSS (1988) that unpasteurised milk should not be given to infants and young children.

A strict stock rotation system should be followed, and all food storage cupboards and shelves kept scrupulously clean. Bacteria can multiply in food spills and may be transferred to other food in the kitchen by flies or human hands. Pets may contaminate food by transferring bacteria from their coats, paws, or saliva onto work surfaces, and should be kept out of food preparation areas. Work surfaces should be cleaned regularly, and especially between preparing meat and other food. If possible, a separate chopping board and knife should be reserved for raw meat. All cleaning cloths and tea-towels should be regularly cleaned and kept solely for use in the kitchen. Separate cleaning cloths should be used for the floor, dustbin, and work surfaces, and disposable cloths and scourers changed frequently. Scrubbing brushes used to clean crockery and cutlery should not be used to scrub vegetables. Hands should always be washed before preparing food, and after touching the dustbin, pets, soiled nappies, or visiting the lavatory. All cuts, grazes, and open wounds should be covered with dressings.

Home-canning or bottling of meat and vegetables is discouraged because of the difficulties involved in generating the high temperatures required to destroy the spores of *Clostridium botulinum*. However, home-bottling of most fruits may be quite safe because spores do not survive in acidic environments less than pH 4.5.

For information on prevention of food-borne and water-borne infections during travel, *see* Section 9.3.

Food additives and contaminants

The safety of food may be compromised by the presence of additives used during commercial processing or residues of chemicals used during agricultural production, and legislation exists to control these factors.

Food additives

Food additives are used in commercial food processing for a variety of reasons. Some are necessary for the safety and stability of the product (e.g. preservatives and antoxidants) whereas others are required to facilitate processing methods. Some are not absolutely necessary and merely serve to influence the appearance or enhance the flavour of the product. Many processed products available today would simply not exist without additives and, for many others, the appearance would be considered unappetising.

In the UK, only approved additives may be used in commercially processed foods, and it is illegal to add anything that is considered unsafe. Serial numbers have been given to many of the approved additives (Table 2.3); numbers prefixed with an E have also been approved by the European Community. Food additives must be listed on food labels by category together with the serial number or chemical name, or both. UK approved additives that have not been allocated a number must be listed on food labels by their chemical name. Unpackaged food, beer, spirits, and wine are not covered by this legislation. Not all food additives are synthetic chemicals, and many natural substances have been given E-numbers. Thus, a statement on a food label implying that the product is free from artificial additives may still have E-numbers listed (e.g. E440(a) is pectin used in jam-making). Some additives may even have a nutrient value (e.g. E300 is L-ascorbic acid).

Studies have demonstrated a relationship between additives in food and some allergic conditions (e.g. asthma and urticaria). The claimed association with behaviour disorders in children, notably hyperactivity, has been well publicised. Wide coverage of these issues in the media has led to the erroneous belief that additives with E-numbers are unsafe. The reverse, in fact, is true, and additives with E-numbers are those that have been approved for use. However, it is accepted that some individuals may react to certain approved additives, and should avoid them. Some preservatives (e.g. sulphites, E220-E227) can precipitate attacks in asthmatics, and may also cause skin rashes. Colours and antoxidants may also induce skin rashes, and tartrazine has been linked with asthma. Large doses of colours have been associated with hyperactivity in children, although the evidence is conflicting because the aetiology of behaviour disorders is probably multifactorial. It is often assumed that natural products are safer than synthetic chemicals, but this is not always the case. One study has shown that annatto (E160b), a natural food colour, precipitates more adverse reactions than the artificially produced tartrazine (E102). People who must avoid a specific additive should be familiar with both its name and number because either may be used on a food label.

Food contaminants

Modern methods of agriculture and animal husbandry are designed to increase the yield of food in the most economic way. For crops, this may involve the use of fungicides, herbicides, or insecticides. Residues may remain on the crop after harvesting, and possibly also in the soil to contaminate future crops. Continued productivity relies on the use of artificial fertilisers, which have a tendency to seep away from fields and pollute water with phosphates and nitrates. This same water may eventually find its way back to other crops if used for irrigation, or may end up as drinking water. Fruits and vegetables may be treated with chemicals after harvesting to improve the appearance and increase the shelf-life. Animals are exposed to similar chemical contaminants in their feeds or pasture, and this may represent an indirect route to humans who subsequently eat the animal products. Growth promoters (e.g. antibiotics) are used extensively in animal feeds because

TABLE 2.3
Serial numbers of food additives approved for use in the UK

Colours

E100	curcumin		155	brown HT (chocolate brown HT)
E101	riboflavin		E160(a)	alpha-carotene; beta-carotene; gamma-carotene
101(a)	riboflavin-5'-phosphate		E160(b)	annatto; bixin; norbixin
E102	tartrazine		E160(c)	capsanthin; capsorubin
E104	quinoline yellow		E160(d)	lycopene
E110	sunset yellow FCF		E160(e)	beta-apo-8'carotenal
E120	cochineal		E160(f)	ethyl ester of beta-apo-8'-carotenoic acid
E122	carmoisine		E161(a)	flavoxanthin
E123	amaranth		E161(b)	lutein
E124	ponceau 4R		E161(c)	cryptoxanthin
E127	erythrosine		E161(d)	rubixanthin
128	red 2G		E161(e)	violaxanthin
E131	patent blue V		E161(f)	rhodoxanthin
E132	indigo carmine		E161(g)	canthaxanthin
133	brilliant blue FCF		E162	beetroot red (betanin)
E140	chlorophyll		E163	anthocyanins
E141	copper complexes of chlorophyll and chlorophyllins		E171	titanium dioxide
			E172	iron oxides; iron hydroxides
E142	green S		E173	aluminium
E150	caramel		E174	silver
E151	black PN		E175	gold
E153	carbon black (vegetable carbon)		E180	pigment rubine (lithol rubine BK)
154	brown FK			

Preservatives

E200	sorbic acid		E221	sodium sulphite
E201	sodium sorbate		E222	sodium hydrogen sulphite (sodium bisulphite)
E202	potassium sorbate		E223	sodium metabisulphite
E203	calcium sorbate		E224	potassium metabisulphite
E210	benzoic acid		E226	calcium sulphite
E211	sodium benzoate		E227	calcium hydrogen sulphite (calcium bisulphite)
E212	potassium benzoate		E230	biphenyl (diphenyl)
E213	calcium benzoate		E231	2-hydroxybiphenyl (orthophenylphenol)
E214	ethyl 4-hydroxybenzoate (ethyl para-hydroxybenzoate)		E232	sodium biphenyl-2-yl oxide (sodium orthophenylphenate)
E215	ethyl 4-hydroxybenzoate, sodium salt (sodium ethyl para-hydroxybenzoate)		E233	2-(thiazol-4-yl) benzimidazole (thiabendazole)
			234	nisin
E216	propyl 4-hydroxybenzoate (propyl para-hydroxybenzoate)		E239	hexamine (hexamethylenetetramine)
			E249	potassium nitrite
E217	propyl 4-hydroxybenzoate, sodium salt (sodium propyl para-hydroxybenzoate)		E250	sodium nitrite
			E251	sodium nitrate
E218	methyl 4-hydroxybenzoate (methyl para-hydroxybenzoate)		E252	potassium nitrate
			E280	propionic acid
E219	methyl 4-hydroxybenzoate, sodium salt (sodium methyl para-hydroxybenzoate)		E281	sodium propionate
			E282	calcium propionate
E220	sulphur dioxide		E283	potassium propionate

Antoxidants

E300	L-ascorbic acid		E309	synthetic delta-tocopherol
E301	sodium L-ascorbate		E310	propyl gallate
E302	calcium L-ascorbate		E311	octyl gallate
E304	6-O-palmitoyl-L-ascorbic acid (ascorbyl palmitate)		E312	dodecyl gallate
E306	extracts of natural origin rich in tocopherols		E320	butylated hydroxyanisole (BHA)
E307	synthetic alpha-tocopherol		E321	butylated hydroxytoluene (BHT)
E308	synthetic gamma-tocopherol		E322	lecithins

Table 2.3 continued

Emulsifiers and stabilisers

E400	alginic acid
E401	sodium alginate
E402	potassium alginate
E403	ammonium alginate
E404	calcium alginate
E405	propane-1,2-diol alginate (propylene glycol alginate)
E406	agar
E407	carrageenan
E410	locust bean gum (carob gum)
E412	guar gum
E413	tragacanth
E414	gum arabic (acacia)
E415	xanthan gum
416	karaya gum
432	polyoxyethylene (20) sorbitan monolaurate (Polysorbate 20)
433	polyoxyethylene (20) sorbitan mono-oleate (Polysorbate 80)
434	polyoxyethylene (20) sorbitan monopalmitate (Polysorbate 40)
435	polyoxyethylene (20) sorbitan monostearate (Polysorbate 60)
436	polyoxyethylene (20) sorbitan tristearate (Polysorbate 65)
E440(a)	pectin
E440(b)	amidated pectin; pectin extract
442	ammonium phosphatides
E460	microcrystalline cellulose; alpha-cellulose (powdered cellulose)
E461	methylcellulose
E463	hydroxypropylcellulose
E464	hydroxypropylmethylcellulose
E465	ethylmethylcellulose
E466	carboxymethylcellulose, sodium salt (CMC)
E470	sodium, potassium and calcium salts of fatty acids
E471	mono- and di-glycerides of fatty acids
E472(a)	acetic acid esters of mono- and di-glycerides of fatty acids
E472(b)	lactic acid esters of mono- and di-glycerides of fatty acids
E472(c)	citric acid esters of mono- and di-glycerides of fatty acids
E472(e)	mono- and diacetyltartaric acid esters of mono- and di-glycerides of fatty acids
E473	sucrose esters of fatty acids
E474	sucroglycerides
E475	polyglycerol esters of fatty acids
476	polyglycerol esters of polycondensed fatty acids of castor oil (polyglycerol polyricinoleate)
E477	propane-1,2-diol esters of fatty acids
E481	sodium stearoyl-2-lactylate
E482	calcium stearoyl-2-lactylate
E483	stearyl tartrate
491	sorbitan monostearate
492	sorbitan tristearate
493	sorbitan monolaurate
494	sorbitan mono-oleate
495	sorbitan monopalmitate

Sweeteners

E420	sorbitol; sorbitol syrup	E421	mannitol

Other permitted sweetening agents (*see* Section 2.2.1) do not have serial numbers and must be listed on a food label by their category and chemical name. For example, saccharin would be listed on a food label as: Artifical Sweetener (Saccharin). Non-artificial sweeteners (e.g. hydrogenated glucose syrup) do not have a category name and are listed by chemical name only.

Others

Acids, Anti-caking agents, Anti-foaming agents, Bases, Buffers, Bulking agents, Firming agents, Flavour modifiers, Flour bleaching agents, Flour improvers, Glazing agents, Humectants, Liquid freezants, Packaging gases, Propellants, Release agents, Sequestrants and Solvents

E170	calcium carbonate
E260	acetic acid
E261	potassium acetate
E262	sodium hydrogen diacetate
262	sodium acetate
E263	calcium acetate
E270	lactic acid
E290	carbon dioxide
296	DL-malic acid; L-malic acid
297	fumaric acid
E325	sodium lactate
E326	potassium lactate
E327	calcium lactate
E330	citric acid
E331	sodium dihydrogen citrate (monosodium citrate); disodium citrate; trisodium citrate
E332	potassium dihydrogen citrate (monopotassium citrate); tripotassium citrate
E333	monocalcium citrate; dicalcium citrate; tricalcium citrate
E334	L-(+)-tartaric acid
E335	monosodium L-(+)-tartrate; disodium L-(+)-tartrate
E336	monopotassium L-(+)-tartrate (cream of tartar); dipotassium L-(+)-tartrate
E337	potassium sodium L-(+)-tartrate
E338	orthophosphoric acid (phosphoric acid)
E339	sodium dihydrogen orthophosphate; disodium hydrogen orthophosphate; trisodium orthophosphate

Table 2.3 continued

E340	potassium dihydrogen orthophosphate; dipotassium hydrogen orthophosphate; tripotassium orthophosphate	529	calcium oxide
E341	calcium tetrahydrogen diorthophosphate; calcium hydrogen orthophosphate; tricalcium diorthophosphate	530	magnesium oxide
350	sodium malate; sodium hydrogen malate	535	sodium ferrocyanide
351	potassium malate	536	potassium ferrocyanide
352	calcium malate; calcium hydrogen malate	540	dicalcium diphosphate
353	metatartaric acid	541	sodium aluminium phosphate
355	adipic acid	542	edible bone phosphate
363	succinic acid	544	calcium polyphosphates
370	1,4-heptonolactone	545	ammonium polyphosphates
375	nicotinic acid	551	silicon dioxide (silica)
380	triammonium citrate	552	calcium silicate
381	ammonium ferric citrate	553(a)	magnesium silicate synthetic; magnesium trisilicate
385	calcium disodium ethylenediamine-*NNN'N'*-tetra-acetate (calcium disodium EDTA)	553(b)	talc
E422	glycerol	554	aluminium sodium silicate
E450(a)	disodium dihydrogen diphosphate; trisodium diphosphate; tetrasodium diphosphate; tetrapotassium diphosphate	556	aluminium calcium silicate
		558	bentonite
		559	kaolin
		570	stearic acid
E450(b)	pentasodium triphosphate; pentapotassium triphosphate	572	magnesium stearate
		575	D-glucono-1,5-lactone (glucono delta-lactone)
E450(c)	sodium polyphosphates, potassium polyphosphates	576	sodium gluconate
500	sodium carbonate; sodium hydrogen carbonate (bicarbonate of soda); sodium sesquicarbonate	577	potassium gluconate
		578	calcium gluconate
		620	L-glutamic acid
501	potassium carbonate; potassium hydrogen carbonate	621	sodium hydrogen L-glutamate (monosodium glutamate; MSG)
503	ammonium carbonate; ammonium hydrogen carbonate	622	potassium hydrogen L-glutamate (monopotassium glutamate)
504	magnesium carbonate	623	calcium dihydrogen di-L-glutamate (calcium glutamate)
507	hydrochloric acid	627	guanosine 5'-disodium phosphate (sodium guanylate)
508	potassium chloride	631	inosine 5'-disodium phosphate (sodium inosinate)
509	calcium chloride	635	sodium 5'-ribonucleotide
510	ammonium chloride	636	maltol
513	sulphuric acid	637	ethyl maltol
514	sodium sulphate	900	dimethylpolysiloxane
515	potassium sulphate	901	beeswax
516	calcium sulphate	903	carnauba wax
518	magnesium sulphate	904	shellac
524	sodium hydroxide	905	mineral hydrocarbons
525	potassium hydroxide	907	refined microcrystalline wax
526	calcium hydroxide	920	L-cysteine hydrochloride
527	ammonium hydroxide	925	chlorine
528	magnesium hydroxide	926	chlorine dioxide
		927	azodicarbonamide

Food additives must be listed on food labels by category together with the serial number or chemical name, or both. There are other food additives approved for use in the UK which have not been assigned a serial number; these must be listed on food labels by chemical name.

Numbers prefixed with an E have also been approved by the European Community.

they can increase the body-weight by up to 5% and improve feed conversion efficiency. This is an important economic advantage although much concern has been expressed over their use. Drugs used to treat farm animals may also be a source of contamination in the products intended for consumption.

Legislation exists to control the use of chemicals and veterinary drugs in farming practices, and to minimise the levels of residues in food. A withdrawal period is sometimes specified for licensed veterinary preparations, to indicate the time after cessation of treatment before the animal or any of its products can be used as human food. However, there is still widespread concern about the long-term effects of chemical or drug residues in food, and there is a growing trend towards food produced by so-called 'organic' methods. These methods preclude the use of any synthetic chemicals or growth promoters. It takes time for an organic farm to become viable if starting on land that was previously farmed by conventional methods and, at present, the demand for 'organic' food exceeds the supply. It is difficult to avoid consuming food that is not contaminated in some way with residues of chemicals or drugs. Even home-grown 'organic' food may become contaminated by drift of chemical spray from neighbouring allotments or gardens. Control of any atmospheric pollutants that may contaminate food is out of the hands of the individual and can only be undertaken by government legislation on a national scale. International policies may be the only means of controlling the levels of some substances.

2.5   THE ROLE OF THE PHARMACIST

Diet has become a confusing issue to the public, and is a problem likely to be presented on many occasions and in different ways to pharmacists. Prevention of diet-related diseases and overall health improvements may be facilitated by following government recommendations to reduce the intake of fats (particularly saturated fats), salt, non-milk extrinsic sugars, and refined carbohydrates in favour of unrefined NSP-rich carbohydrates, and fruits and vegetables. DRVs have been quoted as a guide, but as it is not practical in a domestic setting to weigh all food to be eaten, or to attempt calculation of the dietary constituents, translation of the guidelines into a working diet may, at first, seem impossible.

The pharmacist may be called upon to explain why the changes are necessary and how, in practical terms, they may be effected. It should be borne in mind when recommending life-style adjustments of any sort that people are, by nature, resistant to change. Habits may be firmly entrenched, and it may seem that change requires a lot of hard work and effort. The idea that 'anything that is good for you is bound to be unpleasant' may remove the incentive to even attempt a change. All of these obstacles may be removed by careful and thoughtful counselling. The changes do not have to be made overnight, and for many, a gradual transition may be preferable, dealing with one component at a time.

The pharmacist should also be aware that there is a limit to how much information a person can assimilate at once. For many people, the ideas discussed by the media and the recommendations made are too numerous and, in some instances, extremely vague. It is all very well to state that consumption of an item should be increased or reduced, but by how much? Acceptance of change is more likely if the number of recommendations are kept to a minimum, and if specific messages are conveyed. It is also important not to suggest too many negative changes without qualifying them in some way. If a particular component of the diet is to be avoided, the pharmacist should suggest alternatives, and thereby encourage a positive attitude with a greater chance of compliance.

Diet is largely based on habit, both in terms of the food eaten, and when it is eaten. One of the causes of a bad diet is missed or irregular meals. The quickest way to satisfy hunger in busy life-styles is to resort to ready prepared snack foods, but unfortunately most of those that are widely available contain a high proportion of fats, or sugars, or both, and few nutrients. Additionally, such foods may be low in bulk and though they may meet the energy requirements, they do not necessarily satiate. When making dietary changes, it is essential to avoid long periods without food because growing hunger may reduce will-power and cause a regression into bad habits. The value of regular meals cannot be overemphasised, and perhaps the first stage in effecting dietary changes is to establish a good routine that fits in with an individual's life-style. There is a growing trend towards snack meals and away from the traditional idea of sitting down 2 or 3 times a day to a full meal. There is evidence that several small meals a day may be more beneficial than a smaller number of large meals, provided that the foods consumed are selected with care and that the total daily dietary energy requirements are not exceeded.

It may be necessary, initially, to allow more time to plan and shop for food, so that alternatives to items in the former diet may be sought. However, it should be stressed that it is not necessary to shop exclusively at 'health food' or 'whole food' shops. In fact, some of the snack foods available in such stores may be just as high in sugars and fats as any other type of snack food. Supermarkets have been changing their policies to make available more healthy foods, with a wide variety of breads, fruits, and vegetables. Careful selection of food is necessary, relying heavily on fresh unprocessed foods and taking note of the product labels on processed foods. The pharmacist can be of great help in this field by explaining how to interpret the data and clarifying the various claims on labels. New recipes may be required to meet the adjustments or alternatively old ones could be adapted. Eventually, new ways will themselves become habits, and the time spent in planning and preparing meals should revert back to what it was previously.

Foods should not be considered in isolation as being healthy or unhealthy. A diet consisting solely of oranges would be just as harmful as one made up entirely of chocolate. The most important factors in a healthy diet are variety and balance. In many instances, food is used as a reward or a comfort, and the types of food chosen for this function are generally high in fats and sugars. To abolish these items totally from the diet would be quite unacceptable to many, and unnecessary in most cases. As long as such foods do not form the major part of a diet, and are really only used as infrequent treats, they are not harmful.

The most important change to be made is reduction of total fat intake and alteration of the balance between polyunsaturated fatty acids and saturated fatty acids (*see* Section 2.2.2). The amount of non-milk extrinsic sugars ingested in the diet should also be reduced (*see* Section 2.2.1). Reducing the consumption of fats and sugars should automatically lead to the desired changes in other aspects of diet. The reduced energy intake will cause hunger, and the deficit should be made up with complex carbohydrates. Once fruits and vegetables are added to increase variety and interest, then most of the major adjustments will have been made; there is also an added advantage in that the intake of vitamins and minerals should increase.

It is recommended that the amount of NSP in the diet should be increased (*see* Section 2.2.1). However, NSP should not be thought of as a separate component in itself, but rather as a constituent of those foods of plant origin. The amount present in different sources varies widely and more is found in cereals than fruits and vegetables. As the intake of complex carbohydrates increases with decreasing fat consumption, NSP intake will automatically increase if the carbohydrate sources are chosen carefully. The emphasis should be towards those foods that utilise whole grains and have undergone minimal processing. A variety of NSP-rich carbo-hydrates should be chosen; there is no nutritional advantage to be gained by merely sprinkling all food with wheat bran. An increase in NSP intake may result initially in reduced absorption of some minerals (*see* Section 2.2.1), but this is not considered a problem for those consuming a mixed diet. Fruits and vegetables also provide NSP, especially those in which the skins are eaten. Nuts are also a good source but meat provides absolutely none.

The pharmacist should be aware of the nutritional needs of specific groups, and these are discussed in detail in Section 2.3. In general, however, if the recommen-dations for the population as a whole are followed, then these groups will receive an adequately balanced diet.

The main differences are focused on energy require-ments (*see* Section 2.1), which must either be increased during periods of active growth, or reduced in the overweight and obese. The pharmacist should take an active role in helping those having difficulty with any dietary adjustments, and encourage them to discuss their problems. Those on restricted diets (e.g. vegetarians, *see* Section 2.3) may need to pay particular attention to the food sources of some of the nutrients that may be lacking in their diets, particularly if they are raising young children, and advice from the pharmacist may be welcome.

The pharmacist is often asked to counsel and advise the overweight, and this group, in particular, are faced with an overwhelming amount of material from the media. Being overweight can be extremely distressing both psychologically and physically, and attempting weight-reduction requires a lot of support from family, friends, and health-care professionals. The pharmacist is in an ideal position to play an active role and should encourage such people in every possible way. The pharmacist should explain the principles of energy balance and draw attention to the dangers of obesity (*see* Sections 2.1 *and* 2.3). Each person's life-style is individual and it is necessary to consider how changes may best be effected with minimal disruption. Greater compliance may be achieved if the individual is actively involved in decision-making and develops an interest in nutrition. Effective dieting is a long-term commitment, and once the novelty has worn off, it is essential that bad practices are not resumed. The pharmacist should make it clear that they are always on hand for advice if necessary; compliance could be encouraged by arranging weekly 'weigh-ins' if there are suitable weighing scales on the premises. This would provide an opportunity to offer praise if weight has been lost and thus give an incentive to carry on, or to re-evaluate a diet if there has been no loss or even a gain in weight.

The pharmacist may be consulted about the problems relating to contamination of food with residues of chemicals and drugs used in agriculture, or micro-organisms. Food additives used in commercial processing are also of great concern to many. These issues are discussed in Section 2.4.

2.6 USEFUL ADDRESSES

BRITISH DIABETIC ASSOCIATION (BDA)
10 Queen Anne Street
London W1M 0BD
Tel: 071-323 1531

THE BRITISH DIETETIC ASSOCIATION
7th Floor
Elizabeth House
22 Suffolk Street Queensway
Birmingham B1 1LS
Tel: 021-643 5483

THE BRITISH NUTRITION FOUNDATION
15 Belgrave Square
London SW1X 8PS
Tel: 071-235 4904

FOOD AND CHEMICAL ALLERGY ASSOCIATION
27 Ferringham Lane
Ferring
West Sussex BN12 5NB
Tel: (0903) 41178

THE FOOD COMMISSION
88 Old Street
London EC1V 9AR
Tel: 071-253 9513; 071-250 1021

HENRY DOUBLEDAY RESEARCH ASSOCIATION
Ryton Gardens
Ryton-on-Dunsmore
Coventry CV8 3LG
Tel: (0203) 303517
This organisation is involved in the research and promotion of organic growing methods, principally for gardeners.

HYPERACTIVE CHILDREN'S SUPPORT GROUP
71 Whyke Lane
Chichester
West Sussex
PO19 2LD
Tel: (0903) 725182

THE INSTITUTE OF FOOD SCIENCE & TECHNOLOGY (UK)
5 Cambridge Court
210 Shepherd's Bush Road
London W6 7NL
Tel: 071-603 6316

THE MINISTRY OF AGRICULTURE, FISHERIES, AND FOOD (MAFF)
Whitehall Place
London SW1 2HH
Tel: 071-270 8080

SOIL ASSOCIATION
86 Colston Street
Bristol BS1 5BB
Tel: (0272) 290661

THE VEGAN SOCIETY LTD
7 Battle Road
St Leonards-on-Sea
East Sussex
TN37 7AA
Tel: (0424) 427393

THE VEGETARIAN SOCIETY (UK) LTD
Parkdale
Dunham Road
Altrincham
Cheshire WA14 4QG
Tel: 061-928 0793

WEIGHT WATCHERS (UK) LTD
Kidwells Park House
Kidwells Park Drive
Maidenhead
Berks SL6 8YT
Tel: (0628) 777077

WOMEN'S NUTRITIONAL ADVISORY SERVICE
incorporating
THE PRE-MENSTRUAL TENSION ADVISORY SERVICE
PO Box 268
Hove
East Sussex BN3 1RW
Tel: (0273) 771366

2.7 FURTHER READING

Bender AE, Bender DA. *Food tables*. Oxford: Oxford University Press, 1986.

Clements FW, Rogers JF. *Nutrition handbook for pharmacists*. The Pharmaceutical Society of Australia, 1983.

DHSS. Present day practice in infant feeding: Third report. *Report on Health and Social Subjects No. 32*. London: HMSO, 1988.

DHSS. The use of very low calorie diets in obesity. *Report on Health and Social Subjects No. 31*. London: HMSO, 1987.

DoH. *Clean food. Food handlers guide*. London: HMSO, 1990.

DoH. *Dietary reference values. A guide*. London: HMSO, 1991.

DoH. Dietary reference values for food energy and nutrients for the United Kingdom. *Report on Health and Social Subjects No. 41*. London: HMSO, 1991.

DoH. Dietary sugars and human disease. *Report on Health and Social Subjects No. 37*. London: HMSO, 1989.

FAO/WHO. Evaluation of certain food additives and contaminants: thirty-third report of the joint FAO/WHO expert committee on food additives. *WHO Tech Rep Ser 776* 1989.

FAO/WHO. Evaluation of certain veterinary drug residues in food: thirty-fourth report of the joint FAO/WHO expert committee on food additives. *WHO Tech Rep Ser 788* 1989.

Harman RJ. Dietary products. In: *Patient care in community practice. A handbook of non-medicinal health-care*. London: The Pharmaceutical Press, 1989: 107-38.

Harman RJ, ed. Child health and immunisation. In: *Handbook of Pharmacy Health-care. Diseases and patient advice*. London: The Pharmaceutical Press, 1990: 389-403.

Hobbs BC, Roberts D. *Food poisoning and food hygiene*. 5th ed. London: Edward Arnold, 1987.

The Institute of Food Science & Technology (UK). Nutritional enhancement of food. (Benefits, hazards and technical problems). *IFST Technical Monograph No. 5* 1989.

MAFF. *Manual of nutrition*. 9th ed. London: HMSO, 1985.

Paul AA, Southgate DAT. *McCance and Widdowson's The composition of foods.* 4th ed. London: HMSO, 1978.

Paul AA, *et al. Amino acids, mg per 100 g food. Fatty acids, g per 100 g food. 1st supplement to McCance and Widdowson's The composition of foods.* London: HMSO, 1980.

Tan SP, *et al. Immigrant foods. 2nd supplement to McCance and Widdowson's The composition of foods.* London: HMSO, 1985.

Holland B, *et al. Cereals and cereal products. 3rd supplement to McCance and Widdowson's The composition of foods.* Nottingham and London: The Royal Society of Chemistry and MAFF, 1988.

Holland B, *et al. Milk products and eggs. 4th supplement to McCance and Widdowson's The composition of foods.* Cambridge and London: The Royal Society of Chemistry and MAFF, 1989.

Holland B, *et al. Vegetables, herbs and spices. 5th supplement to McCance and Widdowson's The Composition of foods.* Cambridge: The Royal Society of Chemistry and MAFF, 1991.

US National Research Council Food and Nutrition Board. *Recommended dietary allowances.* 10th ed. Washington DC: National Academy Press, 1989.

WHO. *Food irradiation. A technique for preserving and improving the safety of food.* Geneva: WHO, 1988.

WHO. Diet, nutrition, and the prevention of chronic diseases: report of a WHO study group. *WHO Tech Rep Ser 797* 1990.

Chapter 3

DENTAL HEALTH-CARE

3.1 INTRODUCTION

It is now a reasonable expectation that a person's complete set of permanent teeth should last their entire life, which is in stark contrast to the situation only a generation ago when it was accepted that most, if not all, teeth would have to be removed and replaced by dentures well before old age. Loss of teeth, other than by accident, is caused by two different pathological processes, dental caries and periodontal disease. Dental disease is not generally life-threatening, although this has not always been the case and, in the 19th century, acute dental infection did sometimes prove fatal. The treatment of dental disease may produce adverse effects, or even death, in susceptible individuals. Certain pre-existing medical conditions dramatically increase the risks of treatment. Haemophiliacs are at risk of severe haemorrhage after dental procedures, and subacute bacterial endocarditis may occur in susceptible individuals (e.g. those with a history of rheumatic fever)

as a result of a bacteraemia derived from extractions, calculus removal (scaling), or other invasive dental procedures. Dental health-care in such individuals is, therefore, extremely important. However, for most people, dental disease is more of a social embarrassment and inconvenience rather than a serious health risk; at its worst, it may reduce the quality of life if many teeth are lost.

In terms of the effects of dental disease on the community, its treatment is costly, and extensive treatment results in loss of time from school or work. Approximately £800 million is spent on dental health-care annually but, unfortunately, the majority of this is on treatment of established dental disease rather than disease prevention. In the UK, a staggering 8 million teeth are extracted every year. A few extractions are unavoidable (e.g. to reduce overcrowding) but the majority are a direct result of dental disease. An even greater number of teeth undergo some form of restorative treatment. A dedicated commitment to prevention of dental disease by the individual is of far greater benefit than treatment.

The link between dental caries and diet has long been recognised. The incidence of dental caries increased significantly after the 17th century, and there was a further dramatic increase in the late 19th century. This has been attributed to an increase in consumption of refined carbohydrates, particularly sugars. The prevalence in developing countries has, up until recently, been low compared to western nations, but is now increasing as western-style diets are adopted. Conversely, the prevalence in western nations was high, reaching a peak in the 1960s, but is now on the decline as a result of improved dental health education and the use of fluoride, especially fluoride-containing toothpastes (*see* Section 3.4).

Surveys were conducted in England and Wales in 1973 and 1983 to assess the dental health of children. The results showed that the number of children of 5 years of age with dental caries had fallen from 72% in 1973 to 49% in 1983, and the incidence of caries in the permanent dentition of the population had fallen by 30%. A subsequent survey carried out in England and Wales in 1985 to 1986 did not show any further significant decrease in overall prevalence of dental caries in children. These figures illustrate that, although the trend with respect to dental caries in the UK is declining, the prevalence is still too high. There is still room for much improvement, and there is no reason why the scales cannot be tipped so that the presence of restored teeth in a child's mouth becomes the exception rather than the rule.

Periodontal disease, although generally considered a disease of adults, also occurs in children, and the results from the 1983 survey showed that 19% of children of 5 years of age and 50% of children over 9 years of age had some degree of gingival inflammation. Surveys conducted to assess the dental health of adults in the UK have shown that the majority of adults over 35 years of age with some natural teeth exhibited evidence of periodontal disease, and that the proportion of edentulous adults (i.e. those with no teeth at all) over 16 years of age was 30%. As the incidence of dental caries decreases, and the number of teeth that are retained well into adulthood consequently increases, periodontal disease will assume more importance as a cause of tooth loss. Periodontal disease has, in the past, been thought to be a normal process of ageing, and the gingival recession that is often a feature of the disease is responsible for the expression 'getting long in the tooth', meaning getting old.

Dental health-care is not a new fad, and people have attempted to clean their teeth with a wide variety of abrasive substances throughout history. There is evidence that the ancient Egyptians used mixtures of burnt egg shells, myrrh, ox hoof ashes, and pumice; the ancient Greeks used granulated alabaster stone, coral powder, emery, pumice, rust, and talcum; and the ancient Romans used bones, hooves, horns, shells (e.g. crabs, oysters, or eggs), and myrrh. Some civilisations have even used honey. Mouthwashes also have been used throughout history to ensure dental health- care, and ancient Chinese writings advocate the use of urine to treat periodontal disease. Toothbrushes or toothpicks in a variety of forms have been used for thousands of years. Modern dental health-care products have evolved as knowledge of the mechanism of dental disease, and the necessary preventive measures, has increased. By tradition, these products have always been sold through community pharmacies, and the pharmacist, therefore, has the potential to make a significant contribution towards dental health education. However, a sound knowledge of the properties, actions, and uses of the products available, together with a basic understanding of dental anatomy and the aetiology of dental disease and its prevention are essential. These subjects and the role that pharmacists may play are discussed in the ensuing sections.

This Chapter is concerned only with diseases that affect the teeth and gums, and for diseases of the other tissues in the oral cavity, the reader is referred to Disorders of the ear, nose, and oropharynx in Harman RJ, ed., *Handbook of pharmacy health-care, Diseases and patient advice*, 1990.

3.2 DENTAL ANATOMY AND PHYSIOLOGY

The oral cavity is the area between the cheeks, the lips, the hard and soft palates, and the pharynx; the floor of the oral cavity is formed from the tongue and its associated muscles, and salivary glands. The structures of the oral cavity have several important functions, which involve:

- mastication of food
- initiation of digestion of food by salivary enzymes
- swallowing of food, fluid, and saliva
- respiration
- speech.

Gingivae

The gingivae (gums) cover the alveolar ridges, which are bony horseshoe-shaped projections of the maxillae

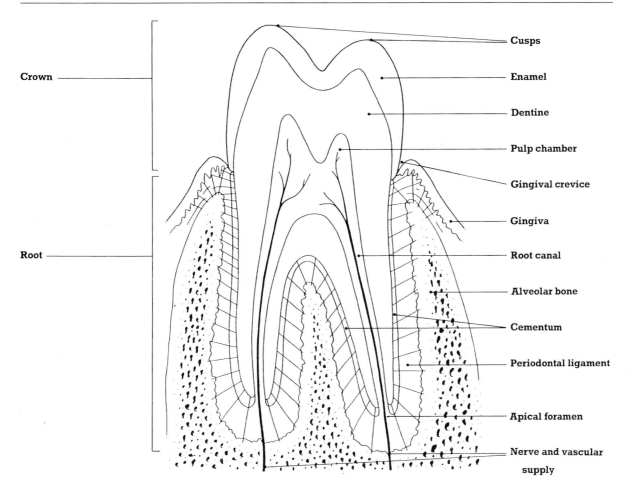

Crown

Root

Cusps

Enamel

Dentine

Pulp chamber

Gingival crevice

Gingiva

Root canal

Alveolar bone

Cementum

Periodontal ligament

Apical foramen

Nerve and vascular supply

Fig. 3.1
Section through a molar to show the anatomy of a typical tooth.

(upper jaw bone) and mandible (lower jaw bone). The gingival epithelium is continuous with the mucous membrane of the inner surface of the lips and cheeks and with the epithelium of the hard palate and the floor of the oral cavity. In health, the gingivae are pink and the oral mucous membrane is red. Folds of soft tissue (called fraena) run between the alveolar ridges and the lips and cheeks; the largest is found in the midline. Gingival connective tissue forms a collar around each tooth, and is attached to the tooth surface by junctional epithelium. There is a shallow trough (the gingival crevice, *see* Fig. 3.1) between the crest of gingival tissue and the tooth, which in health is between 0.5 and 1 mm in depth.

Teeth

The teeth are supported on the upper and lower alveolar ridges, and are important structures required for

mastication; they also profoundly affect speech, and facial appearance and expression.

Anatomy and morphology

Each tooth consists of the crown, which projects through the gingivae into the oral cavity, and a root or roots, which anchor the tooth in the socket of the alveolar ridge (Fig. 3.1). There are different types of teeth (Fig. 3.2), reflecting their varied functions: incisors are chisel-shaped teeth used for cutting into food; canines (cuspids) have a pointed surface (the cusp) used for tearing and shredding food; premolars (bicuspids) have two cusps used to chew food; and molars have four cusps for crushing and grinding.

The cusps of premolars and molars are separated by fissures, and the whole biting surface of these teeth is called the occlusal surface; the other important surfaces are the lingual surface nearest to the tongue, the labial

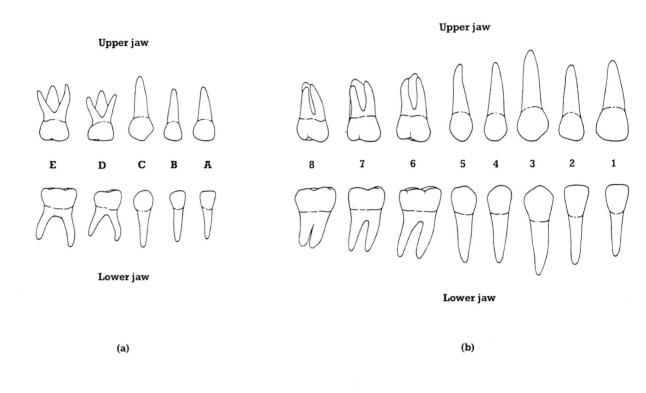

Fig. 3.2
Morphology of teeth: (a) Primary dentition. (b) Permanent dentition. (*See* Fig. 3.4 for key to identification of teeth.)

surface nearest to the lips, and the buccal surface nearest to the cheeks. The surfaces in apposition with adjacent teeth are also important as they are associated with dental caries and early periodontal disease (*see* Section 3.3). To be effective, each tooth must meet with its opposing tooth in the opposite jaw, and if one of the pair is missing, the remaining tooth is less effective as a chewing surface because it has nothing to work against. The incisors, canines, and premolars have only one root, with the exception of the upper first premolar, which usually has two roots, although occasionally these may be fused to form only one root. The lower molars have two roots and the upper molars have three roots except the third molars, which may have one, two, or three.

The principal component of a tooth is dentine, which in the crown is covered with enamel and in the root with cementum. Dentine surrounds a cavity containing pulp; in the crown, the cavity is termed the pulp chamber, and in the root, it becomes the root canal.

Dentine   Dentine is a hard yellowish substance consisting of a complex calcium salt called hydroxyapatite, water, and an organic matrix, which is composed of collagen and mucopolysaccharides. Dentine is extremely sensitive, although the exact reason why pain is felt when this tissue is touched is not known. Dentine is deposited continuously throughout life and gradually reduces the size of the pulp cavity. This is a normal physiological process and proceeds at a relatively slow rate compared to the secondary deposition of dentine following loss of tooth substance (e.g. as a result of dental caries, *see* Section 3.3, excessive wear, or cavity preparation).

Enamel   Enamel is the hardest substance in the human body (and indeed in the animal kingdom), and consists mainly of hydroxyapatite; the remainder is composed of water and an organic matrix similar in structure to keratin. The function of enamel is to protect the teeth from the rigours of mastication, which would otherwise eventually wear them away. Enamel also insulates teeth from sensations of heat, cold, or other pain-producing stimuli. Enamel is, however, brittle and requires the support of dentine; if this support is lost (e.g. as a result of dental caries) it will readily fracture. The enamel is thinnest at the point where it approaches the root of the tooth, but at the cusps (or edges of incisors) it may be up to 2.5 mm thick. The colour of enamel is governed by its thickness, and appears lightest and almost translucent at the tip of a tooth. If the layer is thin, the colour appears yellow because the dentine beneath shows through. Colour, however, is not an indicator of the strength of teeth, and those that are yellowish are not necessarily weaker than very white teeth or vice versa; teeth also tend to darken with age.

Cementum   Cementum is softer than dentine. It is a bone-like substance consisting of hydroxyapatite and an organic matrix composed of collagen and mucopolysaccharides. Cementum is laid down continuously, and the thickness may treble throughout life; some cementum is also resorbed, although these areas are repaired by further deposition. Cementum attaches the tooth to the alveolar bone of the socket by means of the periodontal ligament (*see below*).

Pulp   Pulp is composed of loose areolar connective tissue, and is richly supplied with blood vessels, lymphatics, and nerves, which reach the tissue through the apical foramen. The nerve supply consists of sympathetic nerves and sensory nerves, but as the only sensory receptors in pulp are pain receptors, all stimuli are perceived as pain. The pulp becomes more fibrous and less vascular with age, and is reduced in overall size as dentine is laid down throughout life (*see above*). These changes combine to reduce the sensitivity of teeth with age.

Periodontal ligament   A tooth is suspended firmly in the socket by the periodontal ligament, which connects the cementum to the underlying bone. The function of the periodontal ligament is to support the tooth, and protect both tooth and bone from excessive pressures generated during chewing and biting. The periodontal ligament is composed of collagenous fibrous connective tissue, and has a rich vascular supply, which provides essential nutrients to the cementum. The nerve supply to periodontal fibres includes both touch and pain receptors, which are important in controlling mastication. The periodontal ligament also contains cementoblasts and osteoblasts, responsible for laying down new cementum and bone, respectively, throughout life.

Dentition

Dentition refers to the natural teeth and their position in the alveolar ridges. In humans, there are two dentitions: the primary dentition (deciduous teeth, baby teeth, or milk teeth) and the permanent dentition. There are 20 primary, and 32 permanent, teeth. To aid identification of the different teeth in their positions in the alveolar ridges, the two dental arches are divided into four quadrants, the upper left and right, and the lower left and right (Fig. 3.3). The dentitions are represented diagrammatically by using key-coded numbers or letters arranged in four quadrants (Fig. 3.4).

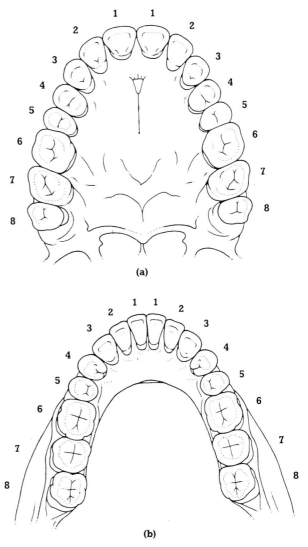

(a)

(b)

Fig. 3.3
Permanent dentition: (a) Upper jaw. (b) Lower jaw. (*See* Fig 3.4 for key to identification of teeth.)

EDCBA	ABCDE	87654321	12345678
EDCBA	ABCDE	87654321	12345678

A central incisor
B lateral incisor
C canine
D first molar
E second molar

1 central incisor
2 lateral incisor
3 canine
4 first premolar
5 second premolar
6 first molar
7 second molar
8 third molar (wisdom tooth)

(a) Primary dentition. (b) Permanent dentition.

Fig. 3.4
Diagrammatic representation of the dentitions: (a) Primary dentition. (b) Permanent dentition.

Teeth start to erupt at about 6 months of age with the emergence of the central incisors, which are followed at about 8 months of age by the lateral incisors. The first molars appear at about 12 months of age, the canines at about 18 months of age, and the second molars at about 24 months of age, although there is wide individual variation. Contrary to popular belief, there is little evidence to suggest that eruption of teeth in children causes systemic illness. As teeth move through the jaw of a child and begin to erupt, the shape of the jaw bone changes. Suckling, before eruption, also influences the shape of the jaw bone, and many authorities advocate breast-feeding as a possible means of ensuring optimal dental development. Premature loss of any of the primary teeth may adversely affect the subsequent spacing of the permanent teeth and the shape of the jaws.

Teeth are mineralised before eruption so that they are hard enough to withstand the rigours of mastication immediately. Secondary maturation takes place after eruption and is an important process in increasing the strength of teeth and their resistance to dental caries (see Section 3.3); fluoride is particularly important in this process (see Section 3.4).

Teeth may become intrinsically stained during development as a result of the systemic administration of some drugs (e.g. tetracyclines), ingestion of high levels of fluoride (see Section 3.4), or systemic illness (e.g. chickenpox or measles). These are intrinsic stains and cannot be removed from the tooth substance. Pathological lesions (e.g. dental caries or pulp necrosis, see Section 3.3) may cause intrinsic stains in developed teeth.

The entire set of primary teeth is lost between 6 and 12 years of age, and replaced by the permanent dentition; this permanent set is not, however, completed until adulthood. The first of the permanent teeth to erupt are the first molars at about 6 years of age, followed by the central incisors at about 7 years of age. The lateral incisors appear at about 8 years of age, and the canines, first premolars, and second premolars between 9 and 11 years of age. The second molars erupt at about 12 years of age, and the third molars (wisdom teeth) between about 17 and 21 years of age. Human evolution has resulted in a jaw that may be too small to accommodate the full dentition and, in many cases, the third molars do not erupt at all but remain impacted; if they cause pain and infection, they must be removed surgically. In some cases, the third molars fail to develop at all.

Saliva

Approximately 0.5 to 1.5 litres of saliva is secreted each day from three pairs of salivary glands: the sublingual and submandibular glands located in the floor of the oral cavity, and the parotid glands (the largest) located below each external auditory meatus. Salivary flow is affected by several factors including age, sex, nutritional and emotional states, time of day, and season of the year. Over 50% of unstimulated saliva (resting saliva) is secreted from the submandibular glands, whereas more than half of the stimulated saliva is derived from the parotid glands. Saliva is formed from serum and is composed of water (99.5%) containing dissolved proteins and inorganic ions. The proteins in saliva include glycoproteins (mucin), albumins, globulins, and enzymes. One of the major protein components of saliva is the enzyme, amylase, which initiates digestion of starch in the oral cavity; antibacterial enzymes are also present. The watery and mucinous character of saliva is important for lubrication of the mucous membranes of the oral cavity, and to facilitate chewing and swallowing; saliva also assists speech. The inorganic component of saliva includes bicarbonate, calcium, chloride, magnesium, phosphate, potassium, sodium, and sulphate. The proportions of the salivary components vary with the source of the saliva, and also with the flow rate. This has the effect of changing the pH of submandibular saliva from 6.47 (flow rate of 0.26 mL/minute) to 7.62 (flow rate of 3.0 mL/minute), and of parotid saliva from 5.8 (flow rate of 0.1 mL/minute) to 7.8 (flow rate of 3.0 mL/minute).

Saliva plays a role in maintaining oral hygiene and preventing dental disease in several ways:

• the bicarbonate and phosphate content acts as a buffer in acidic environments

- antibacterial enzymes (e.g. lysozyme and lactoperoxidase) control the oral bacterial population
- the inorganic component assists in the remineralisation of tooth enamel and thus helps prevent dental caries
- water and mucin in saliva assist the tongue in clearing food debris and bacteria from the gingivae and teeth.

Saliva is continuously secreted in response to parasympathetic stimulation to keep the mucous membranes moist, although the flow increases dramatically in response to stimulation by food (by taste, sight, or smell). The heavy secretion of saliva continues after food has been swallowed to clean the mouth and buffer any acidic components. Sympathetic stimulation in response to fear or anxiety causes the glands to stop secreting saliva, and the characteristic feelings of a dry mouth are experienced. Secretion of saliva may be reduced as a result of some medical conditions (e.g. anaemia or diabetes mellitus) or as a side-effect of some drugs (e.g. adrenergic neurone blocking drugs, antidepressant drugs, antihistamines, antimuscarinics, anxiolytics, diuretics, hypnotics, or lithium), causing xerostomia. Radiotherapy to the head and neck may also reduce salivary flow, although it usually returns to normal after a period of some months. The dry mouth may be relieved by the administration of Artificial Saliva DPF, which is an inert, slightly viscous, aqueous liquid containing sodium chloride, hypromellose '4500', benzalkonium chloride, saccharin sodium, thymol, peppermint oil, spearmint oil, and amaranth solution; alternative formulations may be used and several commercial preparations are available. Frequent sips of cool drinks or sucking pieces of ice or sugar-free pastilles may also be of value.

3.3 DENTAL DISEASE

There are two distinct dental diseases that may ultimately result in loss of teeth, and these are dental caries and periodontal disease. Both diseases can occur at any age but, in general, dental caries is more prevalent in children whereas periodontal disease is more likely to be the cause of tooth loss in adults. The aetiology of each disease is different, although the common factor present to both is the presence of bacteria in plaque.

Plaque

Plaque is a film of soft material that forms on the teeth, the gingivae, restorations, and orthodontic appliances; it is composed predominantly of micro-organisms. Other constituents include:

- dietary carbohydrates
- organic acids formed as a result of bacterial metabolism of carbohydrates
- glucans (dextrans) formed from the metabolism of dietary carbohydrates by streptococci
- proteins (including enzymes) from saliva
- leucocytes
- toxins from Gram-negative bacteria.

The first stage of plaque formation is the development of the salivary pellicle, which is a thin layer of mucoproteins derived from the glycoproteins of saliva. Mucoproteins are unstable in solution and adsorb to hydroxyapatite in tooth enamel. Formation of the pellicle commences immediately after cleaning the teeth, and the whole of the crown, with the exception of areas exposed to friction, becomes covered. The pellicle readily takes up extrinsic stains (*see below*), which, although not necessarily harmful to the teeth, are unattractive and generally considered socially unacceptable. The pellicle is very quickly colonised by commensal bacteria and plaque is formed.

Streptococcus spp. are usually the first bacteria to form colonies on the salivary pellicle after about 3 to 8 hours, and *S. mutans* is of particular importance; *Actinomyces* spp. may also be found at this stage. After 24 hours, other species, including Gram-negative anaerobes, are attracted to the plaque and start to multiply. The bacterial composition continues to become more complex, and the earlier species of colonising micro-organisms assume less importance. Plaque reaches its final mature state after about seven days. Micro-organisms make up about 70% of plaque, although the exact composition varies from one area of the oral cavity to another, even around a single tooth, and is dependent on the micro-environment and the accessibility of the various regions for cleaning. Mature plaque has a different composition from new plaque and a different role in the aetiology of dental disease.

Food is not essential for plaque formation, although the presence of dietary sugars, especially sucrose, increases its rate of formation and thickness. Bacteria utilise sugars as an energy substrate and produce extracellular mucilaginous polysaccharides (glucans) in the process. The glucans provide the plaque matrix and facilitate the firm adhesion of plaque to the tooth surface.

Plaque is highly tenacious and cannot be removed from the teeth by water or saliva alone, but only by mechanical means (*see* Section 3.4). Plaque forms rapidly over all surfaces after cleaning, and is always present in areas that are difficult to clean. Plaque may only be detected during the early stages of formation if disclosing agents (*see* Section 3.4) are used, but eventually, if the deposits are allowed to build up, it becomes clearly visible. Plaque that is in the early stages of development is thought to be cariogenic whereas mature plaque is more likely to influence the development of periodontal disease. Bacterial toxins and enzymes in plaque cause gingivitis (inflammation of the gingivae), which results in enlargement of the gingivae and produces a greater surface for the deposition of more plaque.

Staining of the salivary pellicle or plaque may occur, although such extrinsic stains can be removed and should not be confused with permanent intrinsic stains that are part of the tooth substance (*see* Section 3.2). The most common extrinsic stain is tar from tobacco, which is usually found on the lingual surfaces of the teeth and ranges in colour from light brown to black. The degree of staining generally reflects the standard of oral hygiene rather than the amount of tobacco smoked. Brown-black stains may also occur on teeth following use of chlorhexidine mouthwashes, or plaque may become stained a dull yellow by food dyes. Children sometimes have black or green stains, which may be associated with the remnants of the primary enamel cuticle and are thought to be derived from chromogenic bacteria.

Calculus

Dental calculus (tartar or scale) is mineralised plaque, and may occur in any area of the mouth where plaque develops. Its prevalence is high in most populations and increases over 30 years of age. Calculus is composed of inorganic salts (70%) plus organic material and micro-organisms (30%). The composition of calculus varies with location in the oral cavity and the age of the calculus. The organic constituents of calculus are similar to those in plaque, and the micro-organisms comparable to those found in mature plaque.

Plaque acts as an organic matrix essential for calculus formation, although the exact mechanism of mineralisation is unknown; it is possible that a component of the plaque acts as a seeding agent. Calculus is not harmful to teeth, but it does provide a hard rough surface for the formation of plaque. Plaque is difficult to remove from calculus because the bacteria present in plaque reside within the porous structure of calculus. Plaque on calculus may itself become calcified and, in this way, incremental layers of calculus are built up. Calculus formation may commence any time between 2 and 14 days after the start of plaque development, or even as early as 4 to 8 hours in some individuals, and does not appear to be dependent on diet.

Calculus above the gingival margin is called supragingival calculus, and is formed from minerals derived from saliva. It is especially prevalent on the teeth opposite the ducts of the principal salivary glands (i.e. on the lingual surface of the lower front teeth and on the buccal surface of the upper back teeth). Supragingival calculus is moderately hard and usually white or pale yellow in colour, although it may become stained by tars from tobacco or pigments from food. Subgingival calculus occurs below the gingival crest. It contains fewer micro-organisms than supragingival calculus and is very hard and difficult to remove. Subgingival calculus is stained a dark colour by the breakdown products of blood derived from the ulcerated periodontal pocket. It used to be thought that calculus was the cause of periodontal disease, but it is now considered that subgingival calculus is merely an indicator of its presence. However, calculus indirectly influences the development of periodontal disease by virtue of the plaque deposits present on its surface.

Dental caries

Definition and aetiology

Dental caries is a disease that destroys the mineralised portion of the tooth, and is one of the most common diseases in western society; the prevalence in the UK is particularly high. Once established, caries is irreversible and, unless treated, proceeds inexorably to ultimate destruction of the tooth. Dental caries is a disease of the modern world, and numerous studies have shown conclusively that a high sugar diet is implicated in its aetiology, although the exact mechanism remains unclear. However, it is known that sugars alone do not cause dental caries but rather the combination of sugars in the oral cavity with plaque on the teeth. Dietary sugars dissolved in saliva readily diffuse into the film of plaque, and bacteria present in plaque (particularly streptococci in early plaque) ferment the sugars to produce organic acids (e.g. lactic acid). The acids demineralise tooth enamel and dentine, enabling bacteria to invade and cause infection and inflammation. The infection progressively destroys the dentine until the pulp is reached. This is the most damaging stage and, if unchecked, eventually results in pulp death. The infection then spreads through the apical foramen to involve the apical part of the periodontal ligament and an abscess may result.

The frequency of sugar consumption is more important than the quantity consumed, although the quantity consumed is important in increasing plaque thickness and rate of formation (*see* Plaque above). The incidence of new dental caries is higher in children and adolescents than adults because secondary maturation of dental enamel over several years increases the resistance of teeth to acid attack. Fluoride also appears to increase the resistance of enamel.

There are several host factors that may influence the development of caries or the rate of decay. The structure of teeth varies between individuals, and the presence of deep fissures and pits predisposes to caries formation. The chemical structure of the enamel also varies, and some people have teeth that are more resistant to acid attack than others. Crowded or malaligned teeth render good plaque control difficult and, consequently, these areas may be more susceptible to dental caries.

Dental caries may attack any surface of the tooth, although more than 50% of all lesions affect the occlusal surfaces of the back teeth, with marginally more occurring in the upper dental arch than the lower. The first molars appear to be more susceptible to caries than other teeth, in contrast to a low prevalence in the lower incisors and canines. There are three types of caries:

- Pit and fissure caries

  Carious lesions that occur in the pits or fissures are the most common type. The initial break in the enamel is seen as a small black pit, which may extend as far as the dentine. Dentine is destroyed at a faster rate than enamel and eventually a bluish-white area surrounding the initial pit shows through the enamel. The enamel collapses as more of the underlying dentine is destroyed, and the later stages are marked by an open cavity.

- Smooth surface caries

  Smooth surface caries is the least common type and occurs on any smooth surface, particularly on the adjacent surfaces between teeth. Lingual surfaces are affected less frequently than buccal or labial surfaces. The initial appearance of the lesion is chalky-white, becoming gradually roughened as the enamel starts to break down. The subsequent stages of formation are as described above, under Pit and fissure caries.

- Cervical caries

  Cervical caries attacks exposed parts of the dentine of the tooth and is more common in older people. There is no enamel at this point of the tooth and an open cavity is formed during the initial stages. The subsequent stages of formation are as described above, under Pit and fissure caries.

On average, it takes about 2 years for a cavity to be clinically visible in the permanent teeth, although there is wide individual variation and the timespan may be as short as three months in primary teeth.

Rampant caries ('dummy' caries or 'bottle' caries) occurs in infants allowed to suck comforters (dummies) coated with sugary substances (e.g. honey, jam, or undiluted fruit syrups); drinking concentrated sweetened liquids from feeding bottles produces the same effect. Such practices allow prolonged contact between the teeth and sugar, resulting in severe and extensive caries affecting several teeth, particularly the upper incisors. The newly erupted teeth of infants are particularly prone to decay because they have not yet undergone secondary maturation processes.

The properties of saliva (e.g. mineral composition, viscosity, and rate of production) vary between individuals, which affects susceptibility to dental caries. Saliva is the body's natural means of cleaning and buffering the oral cavity, and is also involved in the remineralisation of enamel, which can reverse early dental caries (see below). Xerostomia, caused by a reduction in salivary secretion (see Section 3.2), is associated with an increased incidence of dental caries.

Dental erosion   Erosion of dental enamel may occasionally occur as a result of frequent ingestion of dietary acids (e.g. from citrus fruits or fruit juices) or from chronic contact with gastric acid as a result of vomiting or regurgitation (e.g. in bulimia nervosa associated with anorexia nervosa, or prolonged morning sickness in pregnancy). However, enamel attack by dietary or gastric acids will not result in dental caries if the oral bacterial population is kept to a minimum by good plaque control.

Symptoms

The early stages of dental caries are asymptomatic. Pain is first felt when the dentine is exposed during the open-cavity stage, although there is wide variation in the degree experienced; the dentine may be protected from pain sensation by a layer of diseased tissue or food debris. Short-term pain on exposure to heat, cold, or sweet substances during the initial stages of tooth decay indicates that prompt treatment of the tooth may save the pulp from irreversible damage.

Pulpitis produces swelling of the pulp in an enclosed area, which sometimes results in a throbbing pain that is exacerbated by heat and relieved by cold. If the pain lasts for some time (e.g. up to 20 minutes), it is likely that the pulp damage is irreversible. Severe pain that is unconnected with any stimuli or disturbs sleep signifies extensive decay. If untreated, the pain eventually ceases when pulp necrosis occurs because of the degeneration of the nerve supply. However, this does not indicate the end of the problem as the infection may spread through the apex and cause inflammation of the apical tissues.

An apical abscess may occur, and is painful during the acute phase as a result of pressure build-up in the enclosed space around the apical foramen. The pain is exacerbated by pressure on the tooth and subsides once the pus has discharged.

Treatment

Early dental caries may be reversible because minerals present in saliva allow remineralisation of the enamel to take place. The organic matrix is still intact during the initial stages of demineralisation, which allows deposition of further crystals. Once the matrix collapses, remineralisation is impossible. Remineralisation is more likely to be successful if further acid attack is kept to a minimum, which entails strict plaque and dietary sugar control. Fluoride is highly beneficial in remineralisation (see Section 3.4).

Treatment of irreversible caries comprises restorations (fillings), and may involve root canal treatment (endodontics), the fitting of crowns or bridges, or in severe cases extraction of the tooth itself. Analgesics may be given for pain relief until dental treatment is available, but it should be stressed that controlling the pain is not, in any way, controlling the disease, and dental referral should not be delayed longer than necessary. For measures to prevent dental caries, see Section 3.4.

Periodontal disease

Definition and aetiology

Periodontal disease (gum disease or pyorrhoea) comprises several inflammatory disorders that affect the periodontal tissues and may eventually destroy the underlying bone, resulting in tooth loss. It is one of the most common diseases in the world, and virtually everyone suffers from it at some stage in their life. Chronic periodontal disease is a slow, insidious, and usually painless process, which may take as long as 30 years to complete. It is more serious in terms of tooth loss than dental caries because the supporting structures cannot be repaired as effectively as teeth can be restored.

Like dental caries, periodontal disease is caused by the bacteria in plaque. However, diet is not thought to be an important factor in the development of periodontal disease, and dental caries itself is also not a cause; it is possible to lose completely undecayed teeth. Plaque deposits on the teeth around the gingival margin and within the crevice are most important in the aetiology of periodontal disease.

If the inflammation is confined to the gingivae only, the condition is called gingivitis whereas inflammation of the periodontal ligament and alveolar bone is termed periodontitis. Chronic gingivitis and chronic periodontitis were formerly thought to be different stages of the same disease, and that one inevitably led to the other. It is now considered that they are separate disease entities, although they are still grouped together under the collective heading of periodontal disease. Chronic gingivitis precedes chronic periodontitis, but does not always lead to it, although the reason why some cases do progress and why others do not, is not known. Prevention of chronic gingivitis will therefore prevent chronic periodontitis. Gingivitis may also be an acute condition but, unlike chronic gingivitis, it is always painful.

Chronic gingivitis

Definition and aetiology

Chronic gingivitis arises as a result of inflammatory changes produced in the gingivae by endotoxins and enzymes from the bacteria present in plaque. Undisturbed plaque deposits may cause the initial inflammatory reaction within 2 to 4 days.

There are some medical conditions (e.g. diabetes mellitus, leukaemias, and scurvy) that may increase the risk of chronic gingivitis. The precise mechanism is unknown, but increased susceptibility may arise as a result of altered host response to bacterial products (e.g. toxins and enzymes) present in plaque. Administration of some drugs (e.g. cyclosporin, nifedipine, oral contraceptives, or phenytoin) may also predispose to gingivitis and, in some cases, may result in severe gingival hyperplasia in which the gingivae may cover most of the crown of the tooth. Any disorder or drug that reduces salivary secretion and therefore causes a dry mouth, increases the susceptibility to chronic gingivitis (see also Dental caries above). People who have a habit of keeping their lips apart, particularly when asleep at night, show a greater susceptibility to inflammation of the front gingivae, which is most likely to be a result of excessive drying of the tissues. Smokers are also more susceptible to chronic gingivitis, but it is not certain whether this is caused by a component present in tobacco smoke or poor oral hygiene, which has been shown to be greater in smokers than non-smokers.

Pregnant women are more susceptible to gingivitis ('pregnancy gingivitis') as a result of hormonal changes that affect connective tissues, including those of the gingivae. Some pregnant women may even complain of loose teeth, which is a result of softening of the connective tissues in the tooth socket. Scrupulous oral hygiene will prevent pregnancy gingivitis, and the tissues revert to normal after parturition. Puberty is also commonly associated with an increased incidence of gingivitis, but again it is not clear whether this is associated with hormonal changes or poor standards of oral hygiene.

Symptoms

Inflammation of the tissues results in oedema and causes the gingival crevice to deepen, and pockets develop between the gingivae and the teeth. At this stage, these are called 'false pockets', and should not be confused with the true periodontal pockets of chronic periodontitis (*see below*). The epithelium of the crevice becomes ulcerated. Subgingival plaque accumulates in the deepened crevices and bacterial products produce further inflammation. A vicious cycle is set up, which causes the crevices to enlarge further. In the presence of gingivitis, gingival crevicular fluid exudes through the junctional epithelium into the gingival crevice. This cannot be detected by the patient but the amount of exudate can be measured using crevicular strips (small filter paper strips), and is an indicator of the extent of inflammation. Crevicular fluid contains immunoglobulins (IgA, IgG, and IgM) and neutrophils (polymorphonuclear leucocytes), which may exert a protective effect against dental disease.

The outward symptoms of chronic gingivitis are mild so that many sufferers do not realise that they have the condition. Established chronic gingivitis is marked by changes in appearance of the gingivae, which become reddened, glossy, soft, and swollen; halitosis may also be present. Pain is usually absent although abrasive food or vigorous toothbrushing may produce discomfort. The cardinal symptom is bleeding gums, which is, all too often, attributed to toothbrushing trauma and therefore ignored.

Treatment

Mild chronic gingivitis can be treated by good plaque control (*see* Section 3.4). Dental treatment may not be necessary other than instruction in oral hygiene, although it would be wise to refer patients for a check-up if it is some time since their last one. In many cases, scaling, which involves the removal of plaque and calculus from the crown and exposed root surfaces using small curettes, may be necessary. The surfaces are then finally polished to remove any rough areas that may attract plaque accumulations. For measures to prevent chronic gingivitis, *see* Section 3.4.

Chronic periodontitis

Definition and aetiology

Chronic periodontitis is always preceded by chronic gingivitis and results in irreversible damage to the periodontal ligament and alveolar bone. It is rare in children under 13 years of age but becomes more common from late teens onwards; it is the most common reason for loss of teeth over 30 years of age.

Symptoms

Inflammation spreading through the gingival crevice eventually destroys the periodontal ligament, and the junctional epithelium moves downwards onto the root. A pocket is formed, called the periodontal pocket, and gingival recession may occur, exposing the upper portion of the roots. As the periodontal pockets deepen, plaque and debris can collect within them, exacerbating the inflammatory process already at work. The depth of the periodontal pocket may be measured using a dental probe and is an indication of the progression of the disease. Further spread of inflammation to the supporting bone causes resorption, which eventually loosens the teeth.

Many of the symptoms of chronic gingivitis are present, although as the periodontal pockets deepen, the swelling and reddening of the gingivae may subside leading to the mistaken belief by the patient that the gingivitis has resolved; the inflammation is still present but much deeper in the tissues. Chronic periodontitis does eventually cause extensive irreversible damage, and patients should seek treatment at the earliest opportunity.

Treatment

Treatment of chronic periodontitis is similar to the treatment of chronic gingivitis (*see above*) and involves thorough scaling and polishing, usually over several appointments. Root planing to clean the roots and remove infected cementum is usually necessary. In severe cases, where the periodontal pockets are very deep, surgery may be required. Surgery to reshape the gums may be necessary in advanced disease to facilitate routine plaque removal by the patient, although this procedure is not carried out as often as it used to be. Chlorhexidine mouthwash or gel may be useful to control plaque deposition, but it should be not be used as a substitute for toothbrushing. It is not recommended for long-term use, and it should, therefore, be restricted to the treatment phase only. It may stain the teeth. Oral administration of tetracycline may be required in refractory cases.

Treatment of chronic periodontitis may be a long

process, and relies heavily on improvements in home dental health-care by the patient. Oral hygiene measures alone will not arrest advanced chronic periodontitis, but they will serve as a valuable adjunct to periodontal treatment and, if continued afterwards, prevent further disease. Corrective measures (e.g. restorations or orthodontic procedures) in areas prone to plaque accumulation may be beneficial in preventing further periodontal disease. For measures to prevent chronic periodontitis, *see* Section 3.4.

Periodontal abscess

Definition and aetiology
A periodontal abscess may develop from a periodontal pocket if it becomes blocked with exudate or a foreign body (a lateral periodontal abscess). Alternatively, it may develop if infection of the pulp spreads through the apical foramen (periapical periodontal abscesses).

Symptoms
Both types of periodontal abscess present with a throbbing pain that is exacerbated by pressure on the tooth and pus is discharged. The gingivae in the area of the abscess become reddened and swollen, which may spread to surrounding tissues (e.g. the cheeks or lips). Once the pus has discharged, the acute phase subsides and, if untreated, results in a painless chronic abscess, which may continue to exude pus. Abscesses cause further resorption of the surrounding bone.

Treatment
Treatment of periodontal abscesses comprises drainage, mouthwashes and, in severe cases, administration of antibacterial drugs. Subsequent treatment may include extraction of the tooth or periodontal surgery.

Juvenile periodontitis

Definition and aetiology
Juvenile periodontitis (periodontosis or periodontitis complex) is a chronic periodontal disease occurring in adolescents and young adults, and its development appears to be independent of the level of oral hygiene. It is not known what causes severe chronic periodontal disease to develop so early in life, although it has been suggested that the bacterial flora present in the mouths of sufferers may be excessively virulent.

Symptoms
The features of juvenile periodontitis are superficially similar to chronic periodontitis but its early onset and the associated bone loss make it a more serious condition. Pain is usually absent unless a lateral periodontal abscess develops. The most common presenting features are

drifting of teeth and localised periodontal pockets around specific teeth. These are usually only apparent during dental examination; radiographs may also show severe bone loss. The course of the disease is often relentless despite dental intervention, and the prognosis for the teeth is not good.

Treatment
Treatment is similar to chronic periodontitis but more follow-up examinations are required to monitor the progress of the disease. Periodontal surgery is not always successful, and treatment may have to rely on strict plaque control measures together with frequent scaling, root planing, and polishing. Chlorhexidine solution is only of value if it penetrates the periodontal pockets, which in juvenile periodontitis are very deep. Rinsing is, therefore, unlikely to be effective, and use of a syringe with a suitable nozzle may be necessary.

Primary herpetic gingivostomatitis

Definition and aetiology
Primary herpetic gingivostomatitis is a form of acute gingivitis that occurs mainly in children around three years of age. It is caused by a primary infection with herpes simplex virus type 1 (HSV 1). On recovery, the virus lies dormant in the ganglia of the trigeminal nerve and produces latent herpes labialis (cold sore or fever blister) in response to various stimuli (e.g. emotional disturbances, fever, menstruation, sunlight, or local trauma).

Symptoms
The infection is usually asymptomatic, but if symptoms do occur, they include fever, malaise, gingivitis, pharyngitis, and generalised adenopathy. Vesicles appear all over the oral cavity and on the lips, rupturing to form excessively painful ulcers. Accompanying symptoms may include increased salivation and halitosis. The child appears unwell, irritable, unable to eat, and has a high temperature.

Treatment
The condition is self-limiting and untreated ulcers heal without scarring within 14 to 21 days. Treatment is not generally given for primary HSV 1 infection but measures that may be taken to relieve the discomfort include paracetamol for pain, bland mouthwashes, and soft food. Chlorhexidine mouthwash or gel may be of value as an alternative to toothbrushing until the pain subsides.

Vincent's infection

Definition and aetiology
Vincent's infection (acute ulcerative gingivitis, acute necrotising ulcerative gingivitis, trench mouth, or Vincent's disease) is an acute, destructive, ulcerative condition affecting the gingivae. It occurs most commonly between 14 and 30 years of age. The micro-organisms most often present are fusiform bacilli and spirochaetes, although it is not conclusive that these are the only causative agents.

Symptoms
Vincent's infection is of sudden onset, and usually begins in the gingival papillae between the teeth and may extend throughout the gums. It is characterised by general malaise, marked gingival bleeding, inflammation, and swelling. Fever is generally absent, but the pain may be so severe as to render eating and talking impossible. Halitosis and excessive salivation are also common. Characteristic 'punched-out' gingival ulcers that bleed readily often develop. These ulcers develop a pseudomembrane, composed of a necrotic grey slough.

Treatment
Treatment of Vincent's infection comprises the administration of metronidazole or nimorazole in conjunction with local debridement of necrotic and infected tissue. Hydrogen peroxide mouthwashes may be used between dental appointments, and the patient should be fully instructed in good oral hygiene procedures. All patients should be followed-up regularly because the extent of permanent destruction may make subsequent plaque removal in some areas difficult.

Gingival recession

Definition and aetiology
Gingival recession may occur in the absence of periodontal disease in healthy mouths, even in the young. Recession takes place around teeth with thin bone covering them or where there are bony defects. Trauma produced by over-zealous toothbrushing may exacerbate this process.

Symptoms
The gingivae are pushed back and the cementum is worn away to expose the dentine. This may cause increased sensitivity and pain, particularly on exposure to heat, cold, or sweet substances. Gingival recession may increase the risk of developing root caries.

Treatment
Desensitising toothpastes (*see* Section 3.4) may be used to reduce the sensitivity of the dentine. Topical application of a small amount of such a toothpaste directly to the sensitive area after toothbrushing may also be beneficial. Fluoride varnishes may be applied topically by the dental surgeon to promote remineralisation of the exposed dentine. The patient should be encouraged to adopt a less vigorous toothbrushing technique to prevent further recession.

Halitosis

Definition and aetiology
Halitosis (bad breath) is characterised by an offensive unpleasant breath odour. It is highly prevalent and is a source of social embarrassment to many.

Halitosis is commonly a symptom of periodontal disease but abnormal breath odours are produced by elimination of certain substances via the lungs, and may be a symptom of disease (e.g. ketones are detected in the breath in uncontrolled diabetes mellitus, or ammoniacal compounds in uraemia; liver cirrhosis is also associated with bad breath). Malodorous breath may also arise as a result of smoking, alcohol consumption, or ingestion of certain foods (e.g. garlic). However, in the majority of cases, halitosis is not caused by systemic disease, and the offensive odour does not arise from the lungs or gastro-intestinal tract.

Halitosis is usually caused by anaerobic bacterial putrefaction in the oral cavity. The offending bacteria may be present anywhere in the mouth but particularly on the tongue and in the gingival crevices and interdental spaces. The main substrate for putrefaction is blood arising from periodontal pockets, although retained food debris, especially meat, fish, and dairy products, may also provide suitable substrates. Halitosis is common on waking. During sleep, salivary flow ceases and mouth and tongue movements are minimal, which increases the activity of the local oral flora; volatile foul-smelling sulphur compounds (e.g. dimethyl sulphide, hydrogen sulphide, and methyl mercaptan) are produced by bacterial action.

Treatment
Halitosis may be controlled by keeping the oral bacterial population to a minimum, and all the measures advocated to reduce the level of gum disease and hence bleeding (*see* Section 3.4) will concomitantly improve breath odour. Brushing the tongue without toothpaste may also be beneficial, and will improve its appearance in those prone to tongue 'furring'. Removal of food debris will also reduce the level of halitosis.

Mouthwashes (*see* Section 3.4) are often used to freshen the breath, although their value in treating halitosis is questionable.

3.4 PREVENTION OF DENTAL DISEASE

Dental disease may not be life-threatening but it can severely affect the quality of life. Loss of many or all of the permanent teeth necessitates the use of dentures, which may seem, at first sight, an end to all dental health-care problems. However, wearing dentures can create a different set of problems, and they still have to be kept as scrupulously clean as natural teeth. For the young, the social stigma of wearing dentures is now much greater than it was in the past when wholesale loss of teeth was much more common.

Loss of teeth that are not replaced by dentures creates problems for the remaining teeth, and may even alter the shape of the jaw. Adjacent teeth often drift into the remaining gaps, which may alter the biting pattern. Loss of one tooth from a complementary pair may limit chewing movements because the remaining tooth has nothing to work against in the opposite jaw. There is, in addition, the psychological aspect of altered appearance to be considered since gaps in the permanent dentition are not generally considered attractive. Premature loss of primary teeth may affect the spacing of the subsequent permanent teeth and can influence jaw development.

Decayed teeth may be restored if treated in time but scrupulous dental health-care is still essential to save them from further damage. It is rare that even the best filling in a tooth is perfect, and secondary caries may form around the margins or underneath the filling if bacteria and sugar can gain access. If this does happen, the tooth must be refilled. Subsequent fillings are always larger, and eventually the walls of the teeth may become so thin that they collapse and the tooth must be crowned or even extracted.

It is absolutely essential that the gingivae are in peak condition before crowns or bridges are fitted or any form of cosmetic dentistry is carried out because the position of the gingival margins is used as a reference point. Inflamed gingivae may be swollen and thus lie higher on the crowns of the teeth than normal. If the inflammation subsequently subsides as a result of improvements in dental health-care, the margins may recede to a more normal position and thus spoil the alignment of the dental work.

Almost all dental disease is completely preventable, although effective preventive measures do require a high degree of motivation on the part of the individual; the only passive measure available is water fluoridation, which reduces the incidence of dental caries but not periodontal disease. Both dental caries and chronic periodontal disease are painless conditions until the later stages when irreversible damage has already occurred. Many people are unable to perceive that a problem may exist if there are no outward signs and symptoms and, consequently, cannot easily be convinced of the need to take preventive measures. This represents one of the greatest barriers to be overcome in dental health education.

Primary prevention involves measures taken to ensure that disease does not occur at all; it must be started at an early age and continued throughout life to be totally effective. Secondary prevention involves the detection and arrest of disease in the early stages. Tertiary prevention is the treatment of advanced disease together with measures to prevent further destruction.

Plaque control

Plaque control is the basis of prevention of dental disease, although its role in the development of dental caries and periodontal disease is different. Plaque bacteria, particularly those of mature plaque, are responsible for the vast majority of periodontal disease, and prevention is aimed at keeping its level on all hard surfaces within the oral cavity to an absolute minimum. The area between the teeth, which is extremely susceptible to periodontal disease, is also unfortunately one of the most difficult areas of the mouth to clean. Similarly, crowded or malaligned teeth, or orthodontic and prosthetic appliances present cleaning problems and increase the risk of both periodontal disease and dental caries.

The role of plaque in dental caries is more complex because it is the combination of sugar with plaque that results in tooth decay (*see* Section 3.3). In theory, if plaque is removed from the teeth immediately before consuming sugar, dental caries would not develop. However, for the majority of people, this is impractical and impossible. It is also unlikely that the teeth could ever be considered to be completely plaque-free because plaque forms extremely rapidly after cleaning, and there are some areas that are inaccessible (e.g. the fissures on the occlusal surfaces). Prevention of dental caries must, therefore, be a combination of good plaque control and sugar control.

The most effective means of removing plaque from the hard surfaces within the oral cavity is by using a toothbrush; invariably, a toothpaste is used as well. Regular toothbrushing is a habit adopted by many people when young and continued throughout life. However, in many cases, the adopted toothbrushing regimen is inadequate for complete plaque control. There are some areas of the dentition that a toothbrush cannot reach and additional methods (e.g. dental floss or interproximal brushes) must be employed; use of these does not parallel the widespread use of toothbrushes.

Disclosing agents

Plaque cannot readily be seen on teeth, and it might be difficult to convince an unwilling or sceptical person of its presence. A disclosing agent that stains plaque should be recommended. Reapplication after brushing serves to illustrate the effectiveness of brushing technique and highlights areas where changes may be required. Any food dye applied on a cotton bud may be used; erythrosine is particularly popular and is incorporated into some proprietary disclosing tablets or fluids. Agents that can distinguish between new and mature plaque, staining each a different colour, are also available. Patients should be advised to smear white soft paraffin on their lips to prevent discoloration by the dye.

Toothbrushing

Toothbrush design   Selecting a toothbrush can be a daunting prospect when faced with the vast array of designs available, which may be backed up by impressive claims from the manufacturers. In reality, there is no general consensus of opinion or experimental evidence to suggest which might be the best design for a toothbrush, and the ultimate selection is based on personal preference. However, consideration of certain factors may help when making a choice.

Nylon bristles are preferable to natural bristles because they do not absorb fluids or harbour micro-organisms as readily, and the control of bristle quality during manufacture is easier. Natural bristle toothbrushes also have the disadvantage that they become soft (and therefore less effective in plaque control) when wet. Multi-tufted, small bristles are better than fewer, larger bristles. Rounded-ends to the filaments offer no major advantage over cut ends, because cut ends will 'round-off' after a short time in use and have not been proved detrimental to teeth anyway; rounded-end filaments may, however, be of value in preventing soft tissue injury in over-enthusiastic toothbrushers.

Soft brushes are less efficient in removing plaque than medium brushes, although they may be of value for those with sensitive teeth, painful gum disorders, or gingival recession. Hard brushes should be avoided because they may cause gingival recession. Large-headed brushes are unable to reach awkward areas, and small-headed brushes require longer brushing time to ensure effective plaque removal. A medium-sized brush-head with multi-tufted nylon bristles of medium texture is probably the best choice for most adults.

Interproximal brushes or brushes shaped like miniature bottle brushes may be required for extremely awkward areas (e.g. malaligned teeth or bridges) or large interdental spaces. Mechanical brushes may be of value for people with mental or physical handicaps, but there is no evidence that, when used by the able-bodied, they are superior to manual toothbrushes; rechargeable mechanical toothbrushes are considered preferable to battery-operated brushes, which lose torque quickly.

Toothbrushes should be renewed much more frequently than they are on average. A worn toothbrush cannot effectively remove plaque, and is absolutely useless once the bristles are bent. There is, however, no simple means of visually detecting when a toothbrush is past its prime; a brush with very obviously bent bristles has long exceeded its useful life. It has been estimated that the lifespan of a toothbrush being used properly and regularly is probably less than a month.

Toothbrushing technique   The aim of toothbrushing is to remove plaque and not, as once firmly believed, solely to remove food debris; it is also a means of delivering topical fluoride in toothpastes to the teeth. Toothbrushing technique, like toothbrush design, has been the subject of much argument and many suggestions have been put forward. However, different dentitions may require different techniques, and as long as the technique adopted results in good plaque control without causing any damage to the teeth or soft tissues, there can be no right or wrong method.

The most important factor in toothbrushing is that every surface should be thoroughly cleaned during each session. Most people concentrate on the buccal and labial surfaces, which are easy to reach, but often forget the lingual surface. It is also most important that the occlusal surfaces are well brushed. It is helpful to divide mentally the dentition into sections and concentrate on one area at a time, making sure that each surface has been brushed thoroughly before moving onto the next section. Initially, this routine will require a little extra time and thought to ensure that it has been completed satisfactorily, but eventually it will become a habit. Patients who are concerned that their toothbrushing technique may not be adequate should be referred to their dental surgeon for evaluation; they may then, if necessary, be trained by a dental hygienist.

Toothbrushing frequency   There are no hard and fast rules about toothbrushing frequency, although the most widely accepted routine is once in the morning and once at bedtime; some also advocate brushing the teeth in the middle of the day after lunch, although this is probably not practical for many people. The thoroughness of plaque removal is more important than the frequency, and there is nothing to be gained by several cursory attempts at toothbrushing throughout the day.

Toothbrushing before going to bed is important in the prevention of dental disease because of the effects of reduced salivary flow during sleep, which allows the build up of thick plaque deposits. Thus, removing as much plaque and debris as possible before sleeping will considerably reduce the overnight plaque levels. In theory, the best time to brush teeth during the day would be before eating because sugar is only cariogenic in the presence of plaque. However, in practice, unless plaque control is of the highest standard, it is unlikely to be removed completely, and so it is probably wise to continue to recommend toothbrushing after meals, which will remove plaque and sugars together.

Toothbrushing immediately after consuming acidic foods or drinks, or after vomiting should be avoided because the enamel is in a particularly delicate state during the first stages of acid attack; after a while, the enamel is stabilised as a result of remineralisation.

Toothpaste

A toothpaste (dentifrice) is applied with a toothbrush to clean the teeth, although the action of the toothbrush itself is more important than the toothpaste. It has even been suggested that a toothpaste is not necessary at all for plaque removal. However, toothbrushing with water alone is of little benefit in stain removal. Toothpastes also serve to polish the surface of the tooth, and it has been demonstrated that plaque forms less readily on smooth surfaces than rough surfaces. Many people like to use a toothpaste purely and simply for the freshening effect it has in the mouth, particularly first thing in the morning. Toothpastes are composed of the following ingredients:

- Humectants

   Humectants (e.g. glycerol or sorbitol) prevent the formulation from drying out and provide a vehicle to which the other constituents can be added; humectants also have the ability to control microbial growth by making water unavailable to micro-organisms, and therefore preclude the need for preservatives to be added to toothpaste formulations.

- Abrasives

   Abrasives (e.g. calcium carbonate, calcium pyrophosphate, or hydrated aluminium oxide) polish the surface of the tooth and remove debris, plaque,

and stains; highly abrasive agents (e.g. in smokers' toothpastes) may damage teeth and surrounding structures, and regular use of these should be avoided.

- Surface-active agents

   Surface-active agents (e.g. sodium lauryl sulphate) loosen debris and facilitate its removal; these agents produce the foaming action of toothpastes and some may have antimicrobial action.

- Binders and thickeners

   Binders and thickeners (e.g. cellulose derivatives or gums) prevent separation of the aqueous and non-aqueous constituents and thicken the formulation; these agents influence the appearance and texture of the toothpaste.

- Flavourings

   Flavourings improve consumer acceptability and therefore increase the likelihood of maintaining a good plaque control regimen; mint flavours with a sweetener (e.g. saccharin) are commonly used.

- Colourings

   Colourings improve appearance and consumer acceptability.

Toothpastes may act as vehicles for active ingredients, and about 95% of all toothpastes sold in the UK contain fluoride (*see below*), either in the form of sodium fluoride or sodium monofluorophosphate (MFP), or both together. The fluoride content of toothpaste is usually about 0.1%. Fluoride-containing toothpastes deliver fluoride to the enamel surface, which is extremely important in preventing dental decay in children, and is also of value in reducing root decay and secondary decay around fillings in adults. Desensitising toothpastes contain formaldehyde or strontium chloride, which block the perception by dentine of painful stimuli. Chlorhexidine (*see below*) inhibits plaque formation on the teeth and is included in toothpastes indicated for the control of gingivitis.

Most people cover the entire brush head with toothpaste, which is far in excess of the quantity needed; all that is really required is an amount the size of a pea. Too much toothpaste generates a lot of foam, which induces a premature desire to spit and rinse; for many people, this signals the end of toothbrushing. Use of too much fluoride toothpaste by children, who tend to swallow a lot more than adults, may result in fluorosis, particularly if fluoride supplements are also being administered.

Dental floss and interdental woodsticks

Dental floss and interdental woodsticks are used to remove plaque from the areas between the teeth (embrasures) where a toothbrush cannot reach. It is necessary to clean these areas regularly but not every time the teeth are brushed; once a day should be sufficient.

Dental floss   Dental floss is available in waxed or unwaxed forms, and the choice is one of personal preference. Unwaxed floss splays out when in contact with the tooth surface and may be more efficient at removing plaque; it may also be easier to pass through tight interdental spaces. However, the loose threads may tear against the margins of fillings, in which case, waxed floss may be preferred. Dental tape, which is wider than dental floss, is also available, and there are special types of floss manufactured for cleaning bridges. Correct use of floss may also remove some subgingival plaque.

A long piece of floss (approximately 30 cm) should be wound around the first two fingers of each hand leaving a length of approximately 10 cm in between. The floss is held taut and inserted carefully into the space between two teeth, and moved up and down to remove the plaque. This procedure is repeated until all the teeth have been cleaned. A floss threader may be required to pass the end of the floss through the gaps where the biting surfaces of the teeth are effectively joined together as a result of dental work. An alternative method of using dental floss involves tying a length of floss (approximately 15 cm) into a loop. The lower teeth are cleaned by holding the floss between both index fingers whereas the left thumb and right index finger are used to clean the upper left quadrant, and the right thumb and left index finger to clean the upper right quadrant.

Interdental woodsticks   Interdental woodsticks should not be used without proper instruction from a dentist because they can cause tissue damage. They are not as effective as floss and do not remove subgingival plaque; they should not be used in tight spaces. However, they are useful for those unable to master the use of floss or who refuse to devote the time that floss requires. The elderly or handicapped might also find woodsticks easier to use than dental floss. Hard woodsticks are less likely to break off and become stuck between the teeth than soft woodsticks. Interdental woodsticks should not be confused with toothpicks, which are used to remove food debris from between the teeth and are not shaped for effective plaque removal. Similarly, woodsticks are not intended to be used as toothpicks.

Water irrigation

Water irrigation units direct jets of water at and between the teeth, and are promoted for plaque removal. However, plaque is an extremely sticky, tenacious substance and unlikely to be removed by water alone, even if expelled under force. Water irrigation units are ineffective in removing stains from tooth surfaces. They do, however, remove debris from orthodontic appliances and fixed prosthetic devices. They may potentially be of value as a means of delivering chemical antiplaque agents (e.g. chlorhexidine) to specific areas, although the effectiveness of this technique has not been fully evaluated. It is possible that the power of the water jet may be sufficient to force bacteria into the crevicular epithelium and into the underlying connective tissue. Resultant bacteraemia poses a serious risk for patients predisposed to bacterial endocarditis (e.g. those with rheumatic fever).

Mouthwashes

Mouthwashes are liquid preparations that contain many of the same constituents as toothpastes (*see above*). Essential differences are the exclusion of abrasives and thickening agents. They may, in addition, contain antibacterial agents, astringents, demulcents, or ethanol.

Some studies have demonstrated that antibacterial mouthwashes do have an effect in reducing supragingival plaque but not subgingival plaque, and therefore may be of benefit in controlling gingivitis but not periodontitis. However, the evidence is not conclusive, apart from in the case of chlorhexidine. Mouthwashes do assist in the removal of debris, tenacious mucus, and purulent secretions, and the cleansing of traumatised areas (e.g. aphthous ulcers). Although the solution is present in the mouth for only a few minutes, the effects may last considerably longer, particularly if eating, drinking, and smoking is avoided after rinsing. Patients using mouthwashes to treat oral lesions should be referred to their doctor or dental surgeon if the condition has not resolved after seven days; severe cases should be referred immediately. Antiplaque mouthwashes intended to loosen plaque before toothbrushing have been developed, although the evidence for their effectiveness when compared to toothbrushing alone is inconclusive. Benzalkonium chloride, benzethonium chloride, cetylpyridinium chloride, sodium lauryl sulphate, volatile oils (e.g. in thymol glycerin), and zinc salts have all been used as antimicrobial agents in mouthwashes.

Chlorhexidine   Chlorhexidine is a cationic antibacterial agent available in a mouthwash or dental gel. Chlorhexidine gluconate has proven activity against the bacteria in dental plaque and is used to prevent build up of plaque deposits, although it is not effective as a substitute for toothbrushing except for short-term use in painful oral conditions (*see* Section 3.3). In some cases, chlorhexidine stains the teeth a yellow-black colour, which may require removal by a dental surgeon, and has not been evaluated for long-term use.

Hydrogen peroxide   Hydrogen peroxide is rapidly decomposed by enzymes present in oral tissues and saliva to release oxygen. The formation of gas bubbles exerts a debriding effect and cleanses tissues. The antimicrobial action of hydrogen peroxide is negligible.

Carbamide peroxide   Carbamide peroxide (urea peroxide or urea hydrogen peroxide) is degraded to hydrogen peroxide (*see above*).

Sodium chloride   A sodium chloride solution may be used as a mouthwash, and can be prepared by dissolving half a teaspoon of salt in a tumblerful of warm water, or by diluting Compound Sodium Chloride Mouthwash (BP) in an equal volume of warm water.

Sodium perborate   Sodium perborate is degraded to sodium metaborate and hydrogen peroxide. It is useful in removing tenacious mucus, an action facilitated by the alkaline medium of the solution. Concern has been expressed by some authorities about the safety of this compound because it is a derivative of boron, which is toxic. However, it was concluded that a dose of 1.2 g dissolved in 30 mL of water and used as a mouthwash did not pose any threat provided that it was not used for more than seven days; it should not be swallowed or administered to children under six years of age.

Sodium bicarbonate   Sodium bicarbonate may be used as a 2% solution to rinse the mouth. Its alkalinity renders it an effective mucolytic agent but it does not have any antibacterial action.

Prevention of dental caries

Dietary management

Dental caries is unlikely to be prevented by plaque control alone, and a reduction in sugar consumption is important. Soft, sticky foods are able to release sugars into the oral cavity over a long period of time because they cling to the tooth surfaces. Also, different sugars affect the drop in pH to varying degrees; lactose and galactose have been shown to cause a smaller fall in pH than glucose, maltose, sucrose, or fructose. There is no difference in cariogenic potential between refined and unrefined sugars, or some 'natural' (e.g. honey) and processed products, and all should be avoided. Apples (and other fibrous fruits and vegetables), contrary to popular belief, are not effective in cleaning the teeth. However, fruits and vegetables are a preferred alternative to cakes, biscuits, puddings, confectionery, and any other similar type of food with a high sugar content.

Results from animal studies suggest that complex carbohydrates may be cariogenic, although to what extent is not known. However, to suggest that these too should be avoided would be to contradict the advice given to prevent other disorders, which is that complex carbohydrates should be consumed in preference to refined carbohydrates and fat (*see* Section 2.2). A compromise must be made so that the health of the body as a whole is considered, and not just one part of it. It is therefore recommended that the frequency of carbohydrate consumption rather than the amount should be reduced. If snacks between meals are eaten, they should consist of non-sticky savoury rather than sticky sweet foods, although it must be borne in mind that sugar is also present in many processed savoury foods (*see* Section 2.2.1).

Non-cariogenic sugar substitutes (*see* Section 2.2.1) may be used in place of sugar, although it is probably wiser to attempt to alter dietary habits and do without sweet foods and drinks altogether. Sugar alcohols (e.g. sorbitol, mannitol, and xylitol) may be used as sugar substitutes, and are not as cariogenic as sugars because the bacteria in plaque are less able to utilise them as substrates to produce energy. However, large quantities of sugar alcohols do cause osmotic diarrhoea, and the daily intake should not exceed 50 to 80 g. Hydrogenated glucose syrups are licensed for use in foods in the UK, and the available evidence suggests that they are less cariogenic than sucrose. Starch hydrolysates (e.g. glucose syrup, corn syrup, or corn sweetener) are commercially produced from the starch contained in cereals and potatoes. They are used in place of sucrose in some processed foods, which, as a consequence, may be labelled sucrose-free.

Fluoride

It was noted in certain areas of America in the early 1900s that the inhabitants had mottled teeth, which was eventually found to be caused by increased levels of fluoride in the local drinking water; the condition was therefore called fluorosis. It was also observed that these people had a lower prevalence of dental caries than the population as a whole. Similar observations were made in the UK and other parts of the world, where children living in areas supplied with water containing a high level of natural fluoride had healthier teeth than those living in areas supplied with water with a low fluoride content. The role of fluoride in the prevention of dental caries was investigated and, in the UK in the 1950s, selected test areas were studied to assess the effects of fluoridation of the water supply. It was seen after five years that the children living in the areas with a fluoridated water supply showed a 50% reduction in incidence of dental caries compared to nearby control areas. World-wide epidemiological studies have confirmed that the prevalence of dental caries is reduced in areas where the water supply contains at least 1 mg/litre (1 ppm) of fluoride. However, concentrations of fluoride above 1 mg/litre may cause fluorosis. Fluoride is also present in many foodstuffs but significant amounts are present only in tea and the bones of sea-fish.

There is a strong anti-fluoridation lobby in the UK, which objects to fluoridation of water supplies on the grounds that it is dangerous, unnecessary, uneconomic, and of negligible benefit. Careful and controlled studies have refuted all these claims and fluoridated water has been shown to be safe and effective in preventing dental caries. However, in the UK, most of the population does not benefit from fluoridated water supplies. This is in stark contrast to other nations (e.g. Russia and the USA) where fluoridation is widespread; it is mandatory in the Republic of Ireland.

Fluoride is effective both topically and systemically, and it is now considered that perhaps the topical effect is more important than the systemic effect because the greatest concentrations of fluoride are found at the surface of the tooth. There are several theories explaining the mode of action of fluoride. The most popular theory is that hydroxyapatite in dental enamel is replaced by calcium fluorapatite, which has a lower critical pH and therefore increases the resistance of the enamel to acid attack. Fluoride is also important in remineralisation and reversal of early caries. Fluoride can block the enzymes of bacteria in plaque and may have an inhibitory action in the metabolic conversion of sugars to acids. Fluoride is more effective in reducing the incidence of smooth surface caries than pit and fissure caries. Application of topical fluoride can remineralise enamel and is able to reverse completely the development of early carious lesions; it may also arrest, or slow down, the progress of later lesions.

Oral fluoride supplements containing sodium fluoride may be given to children living in areas where the level of fluoride in the water is less than 1 ppm. Pharmacists should check the level of fluoride in the local water supply with the water authority, and issue the following guidelines when selling fluoride supplements. Doses are expressed as the amount of fluoride ion to be taken daily. These guidelines are for temperate climates, and the dose may be less in tropical climates where more water is likely to be consumed.

- Fluoride level less than 300 μg/litre (0.3 ppm)

  6 months to 2 years of age – 250 μg
  2 to 4 years of age   – 500 μg
  more than 4 years of age   – 1000 μg

- Fluoride level of 300 to 700 μg/litre (0.3 to 0.7 ppm)

  less than 2 years of age   – no supplementation
                                              required
  2 to 4 years of age   – 250 μg
  more than 4 years of age   – 500 μg

- Fluoride level above 700 μg/litre (0.7 ppm)

  no supplementation required

These doses take into account the small amount of fluoride that may be ingested by children during toothbrushing. The daily dose should preferably be administered as two divided doses to avoid the plasma concentration peaking to a value that might cause fluorosis. However, it is recognised that this requires a high degree of motivation for full compliance, and the once daily administration (preferably in the evening) is an effective compromise; forgotten doses should not be doubled the following day. Fluoride tablets should be sucked or dissolved in the mouth rather than swallowed whole, which allows a topical as well as a systemic effect. Although some authorities advocate fluoride supplements for pregnant women, there is no conclusive evidence that this influences the developing teeth of the neonate. In the UK, fluoride supplementation is now considered unnecessary for infants under 6 months of age irrespective of local water concentrations.

Additional protection may be provided for those at increased risk of developing dental caries by the use of fluoride rinses or by the application of fluoride gels. Rinses may be used daily or weekly, although daily use of a less concentrated rinse is more effective than weekly use of a more concentrated one. A concentration of 0.05% sodium fluoride may be used for daily rinsing, and 0.2% for weekly or fortnightly rinsing. The mouth should be rinsed for one minute; the rinse should not be swallowed, and eating and drinking should be avoided for 15 minutes after use. Gels must be applied by a dental surgeon on a regular basis, usually twice a year; extreme caution is necessary to prevent the child from swallowing any excess. Less concentrated gels have recently become available for home use. Fluoride varnishes are also available for application by the dental surgeon; they are particularly valuable for young or handicapped children since the varnish adheres to the teeth and sets in the presence of moisture.

It should be borne in mind that fluoride does not confer complete protection against dental caries on its own, and minimal sugar consumption together with good plaque control are still essential measures to prevent dental decay.

Dental intervention

The most important preventive measures are those routinely undertaken by the individual at home. However, regular visits to the dental surgeon are necessary to identify early caries, some of which may be reversed; for lesions that cannot be reversed, restorative treatment limits the amount of the tooth that is lost. X-ray examination is essential to detect some cavities, especially those between teeth, and will also show periapical disease and early periodontal bone destruction.

Some individuals are more susceptible to dental caries than others, and some of the factors responsible may be outside their personal control (e.g. those that are genetically inherited or occur during tooth development, see Section 3.3). The risks may be minimised by strict attention to oral hygiene and use of fluoride products. In some cases, however, dental intervention may be necessary to ensure effective plaque control (e.g. orthodontic procedures, which involve moving teeth into more favourable positions under mild pressure, or extraction of healthy teeth to reduce overcrowding). Orthodontic appliances provide a surface for plaque build up and are a source of irritation to the gingivae; they may, themselves, increase the susceptibility to dental disease, and must be kept scrupulously clean.

The fissures on the occlusal surfaces of the molars and premolars are most prone to dental caries, and fluoride is not as effective in preventing dental caries as in other areas of the tooth (see above). Sealants may be applied to teeth with very deep fissures. This involves filling the fissures and pits with a plastic substance (e.g. bis-glycidyl-methacrylate resins). If applied properly, there should not be any decay in the sealed tooth as long as the sealant remains in place. The technique has only been in use since the early 1970s, and data are not yet available to ascertain the long-term effectiveness. Sealants should be applied as soon as possible after eruption of teeth. The method is painless but time-consuming, and may therefore be difficult if the child is uncooperative.

Regular dental check-ups are also important for adults to detect and reverse periodontal disease at as early a stage as possible. The dental surgeon is able to offer advice and training in good plaque control techniques.

It is generally recommended that the dental surgeon should be visited every six months for a routine check-up, although some young children may benefit from visits every four months; adults with good plaque control may only need a check-up once a year because their teeth are more resistant to dental caries and periodontal disease is a much slower process. It must be stressed that regular dental check-ups are not a substitute for good oral hygiene.

Prevention of dental disease in children

Dental caries is more of a problem in children than periodontal disease, and dental health-care measures should be directed towards reducing tooth decay. However, the practices and habits adopted during childhood will also aid the fight against periodontal disease if continued into adulthood.

Instilling good dietary habits (see above) is essential in the early years, together with fluoride supplementation (see above), if necessary, during the tooth development phase. Parents should not add sugar to feeding bottles or coat dummies with sweet substances. Children should be discouraged from adding sugar to foods or drinks (e.g. cereals, fruit, tea, or coffee). A taste for savoury foods rather than sweet foods should be encouraged because, once attained, a 'sweet tooth' is very difficult to lose.

Toothbrushing should be started as soon as the first tooth erupts, and the child encouraged to take an active part in the routine as soon as capable. The reasons for thorough cleaning of the teeth should be explained, and the presence of plaque demonstrated using a disclosing agent. Children's toothbrushes with small heads and short handles should be used. Use of dental floss is not usually necessary in children, and would be difficult because of lack of full manual dexterity. However, flossing should be started as soon as possible in adolescence. Thumbsucking may alter the alignment and spacing of the front teeth, and should be discouraged.

Children should be introduced to the dental surgeon at an early age, preferably as soon as all the primary teeth have erupted, and should never be made to fear either the dental surgeon or the surgery. Good oral hygiene practices will reduce the necessity for traumatic treatment and therefore ensure that a child builds up a good relationship with the dental surgeon right from the start.

Care of dentures

Anyone who has to wear a complete set of dentures has obviously lost all their teeth, and may therefore assume that it is too late to worry about dental health-care. However, plaque accumulates on dentures in exactly the same way as on natural teeth, and must be removed regularly to avoid mucosal inflammation. Removal of plaque and food debris also reduces the likelihood of bacterial putrefaction and resultant offensive mouth odours. Plaque on dentures is subject to the same risks of staining (e.g. coffee, tea, tobacco, or red wine) as natural teeth, and regular cleaning will maintain an attractive appearance. It is imperative that partial dentures are kept scrupulously clean in order to preserve the remaining natural teeth. Dentures should always be cleaned out of the mouth, once or twice a day. They are not usually worn at night, when they should be placed in a bowl of water to prevent them drying out and risk of distortion of shape.

Dentures are generally made of acrylic materials that are softer than enamel, and equipment and products designed for use with natural teeth should not be used. Some partial dentures are metal, cobalt-chrome alloy being the one most commonly used. Denture brushes differ from ordinary toothbrushes, and resemble nail brushes on long handles. There is very often a thick tuft of bristles on the opposite side of the head, and this is used to clean any awkward areas that cannot be reached by the larger brush. Toothpastes specifically designed for use with dentures should be used, and highly abrasive cleansers avoided because of the risks of scratching; household bleach, disinfectants, or antiseptics should never be used. Alternatively, brushing with soap and water can be just as effective. Disclosing solutions may be used to detect plaque on dentures and assess the thoroughness of cleansing routines in exactly the same way as on natural teeth. Tablets or powders that release oxygen when dissolved in water may be used to soak the dentures to remove plaque; a stronger acidic cleanser may be required for stubborn stains. Soaking, however, is not an effective substitute for brushing. Any metal parts on dentures may corrode in certain solutions, and the manufacturer's instructions should always be consulted before soaking. Some dentures have soft linings, and the dental surgeon should be consulted about the safest way to clean these.

Dentures are extremely fragile and should be handled with great care; it is usually recommended that they are cleaned over a bowl of water or soft surface in case they are dropped. Denture repair kits are available to carry out emergency repairs, and household adhesives should not be used; the dentures should be taken to a dental surgeon or dental technician for complete repair as soon as possible.

Once a tooth is lost, the surrounding alveolar bone is gradually resorbed, the rate of resorption varying dramatically between different individuals. Dentures must sit on the alveolar ridge and a large loss of bone with advancing age therefore results in a poor fit. Loose dentures affect eating and speaking, and the effects may be severe enough to make the wearer withdraw socially. Eating may also be painful because the soft gingivae are crushed between the dentures and the shrivelled bone. The hard palate in the roof of the oral cavity provides a wide surface over which the weight of the upper denture is distributed whereas the lower dentures can only be fitted onto the jaw bone itself because the floor of the oral cavity is taken up by the tongue and its associated muscles. Consequently, lower dentures are more difficult to wear than upper dentures. Denture fixatives, usually containing either karaya gum or tragacanth, are used by many people to ensure that their dentures fit securely. However, anyone having problems should be referred to their dental surgeon, although there are those who, even with a good set of dentures, may feel more confident if they apply a little fixative.

The risk of developing oral lesions is increased in the presence of some disorders, and the pharmacist should always enquire for any underlying condition when a patient presents with denture problems (e.g. there is an increased incidence of oral candidiasis in diabetics). A dry mouth may also make the wearing of dentures difficult and uncomfortable, and pharmacists should be aware of the conditions and drugs that reduce salivary secretion (see Section 3.3); the patient may need to be referred to their doctor as well as their dental surgeon.

Dentures will not last a lifetime and must be renewed periodically. Denture wearers should visit their dental surgeon every 1 to 3 years (or every six months if they have partial dentures) to have their dentures checked and the fit re-evaluated. New dentures may take a little getting used to, especially if it is the first time that dentures have been worn. They may produce gum discomfort and even sores or ulcers. An oral preparation containing a local anaesthetic may be applied to the gums in the short-term to cover the settling-in period, but severe or prolonged cases should be referred to the dental surgeon.

3.5 THE ROLE OF THE PHARMACIST

The pharmacist, by tradition, has always been involved in the sale of dental products to the public, and is therefore in an ideal position to reinforce the health education messages put forward by the dental profession and other dental health-care authorities. In addition, the pharmacist can recognise disorders affecting the oral cavity and refer patients to general practitioners or dental surgeons as appropriate. Dental health-care is essential for a healthy life-style, and should be placed equally among other forms of life-style modification. It is not the intention that the pharmacist should take over the role of dental health education from the dental surgeon, but rather to augment it, and much could be achieved if dental surgeons and pharmacists liaised together. This would also ensure that the pharmacist was issuing the same dental health-care advice as endorsed by the dental profession.

In most cases, the sale of dental health-care products is a passive process. It would not be practical to become actively involved in every sale, but there are occasions when a pharmacist may perceive that a problem exists (e.g. by noticing repeat purchases of mouthwashes by a customer or a customer's difficulty in making a decision when selecting a toothbrush or toothpaste). Dental health-care products should be positioned in the pharmacy in such a manner that the pharmacist can observe customers, and therefore be in a position to offer help when necessary. In large pharmacies with more than one cashpoint, locating the dental health-care section close to the dispensary will serve to raise the status of dental products in the eyes of the public from mere toiletries to essential health-care items.

The pharmacist should be aware of the importance of sugar control in the prevention of dental caries, and make a habit of only counter-prescribing non-cariogenic liquid medicines, particularly for children. Mouth and throat lozenges may also contain cariogenic sugars, a fact which should be pointed out to patients. The pharmacist has little control over medicines supplied on prescription unless generic items are requested. However, a discussion with the local doctors to make them aware of any sugar-free alternatives available may be of value. The pharmacist should also check the manufacturer's information to see if alternative diluents to syrup may be used when dispensing reduced-strength preparations.

Whenever the opportunity arises, the pharmacist should stress the insidious and painless nature of dental disease, and that prevention is not only better than cure, but that complete prevention is totally feasible; regular dental check-ups are essential at any age. It should also be emphasised that periodontal disease is not a normal ageing process but a pathological disease that can be prevented by good oral hygiene. Children should be encouraged to adopt good habits from as early an age as possible, and should not be made to fear the dental surgeon.

Some diseases and drugs may increase the susceptibility to dental caries or periodontal disease. The pharmacist should be familiar with these (*see* Section 3.3) and offer counselling on preventive measures where appropriate. It is imperative, however, that pharmacists do not compromise a patient's confidence in their prescribed medicine, or increase their anxiety over a disease state. The discussion needs to be handled with tact and sensitivity, maintaining a positive attitude throughout and emphasising that there is nothing difficult about good routine dental heath-care. In some cases, there is no alternative to the prescribed medicine, and it may seem that a patient's medical health is more important than their dental health. While this may be true, it is not necessary that either should be compromised at the expense of the other and, in most cases, dental health can be maintained with good plaque and sugar control. If a patient is over-anxious, the pharmacist should discuss the matter with the patient's doctor and dental surgeon in an attempt to resolve the difficulty. Pregnant women are prone to gingivitis and should be counselled that good plaque control will reduce problems to a minimum. It is also essential that pregnant women and children do not take tetracyclines because these cause intrinsic discoloration of children's permanent teeth during the developmental stages.

There may be occasions when a patient consults a pharmacist about emergency dental treatment because the local dental surgeries are closed (e.g. at the weekends and over bank holidays). If a patient is unable to obtain emergency treatment from his own dental surgeon, the pharmacist should supply the address and telephone number of the nearest emergency dental service, even if it is located some distance away; a patient in severe pain may be willing to travel a long way for treatment. Analgesics may be administered in the interim, but it is important to stress that the problem does not disappear with the pain, and dental treatment must be sought at the earliest available opportunity. Oil of cloves is a traditional remedy that has been used to relieve toothache; 'toothache tinctures' containing varying proportions of clove oil, camphor, chloroform, menthol, and phenol are also available, but these can have an irritant effect on adjacent mucosal surfaces, causing ulceration, and their value in pain relief is doubtful. They should be applied carefully and never used long-term. There is a belief that placing an aspirin tablet against the offending tooth will relieve toothache, but this practice is to be deprecated because of the risk of extensive mucosal ulceration; aspirin is of greater benefit in pain relief if taken systemically. Gutta percha may be used as a temporary filling material to plug cavities when a filling has fallen out; proprietary temporary fillings are also available.

Teeth that have been knocked out in an accident may be successfully reimplanted if treated as soon as possible; the reimplanted tooth may not, however, survive a lifetime, or it may discolour and require crowning at a later date. The tooth should be washed in cold water (never hot), and wrapped in a damp cloth to carry to the dental surgeon; it is absolutely imperative that the root does not dry out and any shreds of tissue clinging to the tooth should not be removed. If the root attachments are not completely severed, the tooth should be gently pushed back into the socket. It is vital that there is the minimum delay possible in seeking dental treatment. If the tooth has fallen onto a dirty surface outdoors, the patient may also need to consult a doctor for immunisation against tetanus if this has not been kept up to date.

People who visit a dental surgeon have been sufficiently motivated to make an appointment. However, there are a large number of people who never see a dental surgeon but, nevertheless, buy dental health-care products, and there are others who may not indulge in any sort of oral hygiene regimen, but still visit a pharmacy for other reasons. The pharmacist, therefore, has the opportunity to interact with a significantly greater number of people than the dental surgeon, and should take advantage of this situation whenever possible; the pharmacist is also in a position to try and persuade reluctant people to see a dental surgeon. The impact of any educational material (e.g. books, leaflets, or posters) in a pharmacy is potentially greater than in a dental surgery, and pharmacists would do well to include dental health information among their health education displays.

3.6 USEFUL ADDRESSES

BRITISH DENTAL ASSOCIATION (BDA)
64 Wimpole Street
London W1M 8AL
Tel: 071-935 0875

BRITISH FLUORIDATION SOCIETY
63 Wimpole Street
London W1M 8AL
Tel: 071-486 7007

BRITISH SOCIETY OF DENTISTRY FOR THE HANDICAPPED
Department of Child Dental Health
Dental School
Framlington Place
Newcastle-upon-Tyne
Tel: 091-222 6000 Ext. 8244

GENERAL DENTAL COUNCIL
37 Wimpole Street
London W1M 8DQ
Tel: 071-486 2171

THE ORAL AND DENTAL RESEARCH TRUST
Keats' House
St. Thomas Street
London SE1 9RN
Tel: 071-955 4699

3.7 FURTHER READING

Besford J. *Good mouthkeeping*. 2nd ed. Oxford: Oxford University Press, 1984.

Collins WJN, *et al. A handbook for dental hygienists*. 2nd ed. Bristol: John Wright & Sons, 1986.

Dental Practitioner's Formulary, 1990–92. London: the British Medical Association and the Royal Pharmaceutical Society of Great Britain, 1990.

Elderton RJ, ed. *Positive dental prevention. The prevention in childhood of dental disease in adult life*. London: William Heinemann Medical Books, 1987.

Forrest JO. *Preventive dentistry*. 2nd ed. Bristol: John Wright & Sons, 1981.

Harman RJ, ed. Disorders of the ear, nose, and oropharynx. In: *Handbook of pharmacy health-care. Diseases and patient advice*. London: The Pharmaceutical Press, 1990: 239–48.

Naylor MN. The role of diet in the prevention of dental caries. In: Turner MR, ed. *Preventive nutrition and society*. London: Academic Press, 1981: 85–94.

Pader M. *Oral hygiene products and practice*. New York: Marcel Dekker, 1988.

Seymour RA, Walton JG. *Adverse drug reactions in dentistry*. Oxford: Oxford University Press, 1988.

Tay WM, ed. *General dental treatment*. Edinburgh: Churchill Livingstone, 1990.

WHO. Prevention methods and programmes for oral diseases: report of a WHO expert committee. *WHO Tech Rep Ser 713* 1985.

Chapter 4

CONTRACEPTION

4.1 FERTILITY AND CONTRACEPTION

Fertility and fertilisation

Males produce sperm at the prodigious rate of about 1000 per second from each testicle, and in the normal ejaculate volume of 3 to 5 mL, there are up to 300 million sperm. Only one of these is necessary to fertilise an ovum but, in practice, the presence of 3 million highly motile and active sperm is necessary to ensure a possibility of fertilisation. Sperm can normally survive for up to six hours in the vagina, although this durability is subject to wide variation. Survival times in the fluids of the cervix, uterus, and Fallopian tubes have been variously estimated as between 3 and 5 days, but can be as long as nine days.

By contrast, women are less prodigious. On average, only one ovum is produced in each monthly cycle (*see below*) and, under normal circumstances, is only capable of being fertilised for about 12 hours (maximum 24 hours) after it is released into the Fallopian tube. Ovulation occurs 12 to 16 days before the next period. The menstrual cycle is traditionally thought to last about 28 days, although it may vary from as short as 21 days to as long as 40 days or more. In practice, many women do not have regular menstrual cycles. Therefore the time of ovulation may be difficult to predict.

The menstrual and ovarian cycles   The stages of a theoretical 28-day regular menstrual cycle, in the absence of fertilisation, are represented in Fig. 4.1. These changes generally occur on a cyclical basis throughout a woman's life, from puberty until the menopause. An ovum is produced within the ovary from a primary oocyte by meiosis (oogenesis). The ovum is formed within the fluid-filled Graafian follicle and at ovulation is released from the follicle into the pelvic cavity. The ovum is guided into the funnel-shaped infundibulum of the Fallopian tube by finger-like ciliary projections (the fimbriae). The remaining cells of the Graafian follicle in the ovary multiply rapidly and form the yellow, highly vascularised corpus luteum. The corpus luteum secretes oestrogens and progesterone, which act on the endometrium to increase its blood supply and thickness in preparation for the receipt of a fertilised ovum.

In normal menstrual cycles, variations occur in the plasma concentrations of the gonadotrophins, follicle-stimulating hormone (FSH) and luteinising hormone (LH), and of the female sex hormones, the oestrogens and progesterone. FSH and LH are secreted by the anterior lobe of the pituitary gland in response to gonadorelin (gonadotrophin-releasing hormone or GnRH) produced by the hypothalamus.

At the start of a cycle, FSH stimulates the development of 20 to 25 ovarian follicles that will ultimately produce one ovum. FSH also stimulates the secretion of oestrogens from the follicular cells. Rising oestrogen concentrations inhibit gonadorelin (and consequently secretion of FSH), but stimulate the secretion of LH (the LH surge). LH stimulates further development of the follicles and, together with oestrogens, stimulates the release of the ovum from the ovary. LH also stimulates the formation of the corpus luteum.

If fertilisation does not occur, the continued secretion of oestrogens and progesterone inhibits the release of gonadorelin and, therefore, the secretion of LH. The corpus luteum remains for about 14 days before it degenerates and consequently concentrations of oestrogens and progesterone decline, and menstruation occurs. Falling concentrations of oestrogens and progesterone cause gonadorelin to be secreted, which in turn stimulates the release of FSH and the start of a new cycle. The main events during the menstrual and ovarian cycles are summarised in Table 4.1.

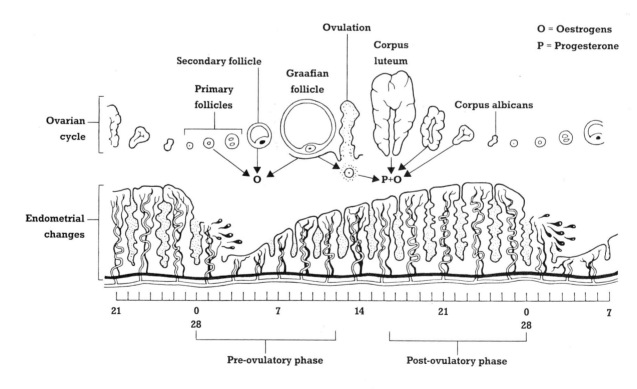

Fig. 4.1
Menstrual cycle in the absence of fertilisation (*see also* Table 4.1).

TABLE 4.1
The stages of the menstrual and ovarian cycles (see also Fig. 4.1)

Days	Events occurring
1–3	FSH stimulates production of approximately 20–25 primary ovarian follicles, which start to secrete oestrogen.
4–5	Approximately 20 of the primary follicles develop into secondary follicles, which continue to secrete oestrogen.
6–13	FSH and LH stimulate further secretion of oestrogen from follicles; oestrogens stimulate repair of the endometrium.
	One of the secondary follicles matures into a Graafian follicle, and oestrogen production continues to increase.
	Small amounts of progesterone start to be secreted at the end of this phase.
	High oestrogen levels inhibit GnRH, which decreases secretion of FSH, but the high oestrogen level increases secretion of LH (the LH surge).
14	LH surge causes release of an ovum into the pelvic cavity, from where it is guided into the Fallopian tube.
15–28	LH secretion stimulates the development of the corpus luteum from the remaining follicular cells of the Graafian follicle; the corpus luteum secretes oestrogen and progesterone; and progesterone prepares the endometrium to receive a fertilised ovum.
	In the absence of fertilisation, LH secretion decreases as a result of the negative feedback effect of rising oestrogen and progesterone levels (from the corpus luteum) on GnRH. As the secretion of LH falls, the corpus luteum degenerates, therefore the secretion of oestrogen and progesterone decreases, and the endometrium is shed (menstruation).
	Falling levels of oestrogen and progesterone cause the release of GnRH, which in turn stimulates the release of FSH, which stimulates the development of ovarian follicles, and a new cycle commences.

Fertile and infertile phases   Combining a knowledge of the survival time of the ovum after ovulation with the survival time of sperm in the female genital tract (*see above*) permits the different stages of the monthly cycle to be considered as infertile or fertile. The first infertile phase of each menstrual cycle begins on the day that menstruation starts. This phase is terminated on the day when sperm can enter the reproductive tract and possibly lead to a pregnancy. The length of this period is determined by the speed at which the ovum is produced by maturation of the primary follicle. The fertile phase includes the one day that the ovum can be fertilised plus the preceding seven days that sperm may survive in the reproductive tract.

A safety margin of an extra day should be allowed. Fertilisation of an ovum can occur if sexual intercourse takes place at any time between days 9 and 17 of a 28-day cycle, but the variability of the time of ovulation produces a much wider range for the possible days on which fertilisation can occur. The presence of sperm already in the Fallopian tubes as an ovum is released from the Graafian follicle produces the greatest likelihood of fertilisation.

The second infertile phase lasts from the day after ovulation until the start of the next menses.

The likelihood of pregnancy resulting from intercourse has been estimated by Drife (1983). If 100 couples have frequent intercourse timed to take place during the most fertile period of the month, 85 of the women will have a fertilised ovum within one month. Of these, 15 will fail to implant; and of the 70 that do become implanted in the uterus, about half will be lost. Chorionic gonadotrophin will be detectable in 36 women, of whom only 24 will fail to menstruate the following month. Of the remaining 24, 3 or 4 will miscarry, leaving an approximate fertility rate of about 20%. The major cause of the high wastage rate is foetal chromosomal abnormalities.

Fertility at puberty   The menarche commonly occurs in healthy young girls between 11 and 12 years of age, although there can be tremendous individual variation. However, the onset of the first period does not necessarily infer that ovulation will regularly occur; indeed, for up to two years after the menarche, ovulation may be infrequent and irregular. More importantly, the occurrence of menarche does not necessarily indicate the onset of fertility, although pregnancies have been reported in girls as young as 11 and 12 years of age.

Amenorrhoea and other menstrual disturbances may develop with the onset of further growth and development during the middle and late teens, particularly if associated with psychological upheavals (e.g. moving away from home). From the point of view of the need for contraception, however, the absence of periods does not preclude ovulation, and pregnancy can still occur.

Contraception

The desire to interrupt the normal physiological events that regulate conception has led to the development of a wide range of contraceptive methods. The usefulness and appropriateness of each of the available methods varies with the circumstances of the woman and her partner, and the age at which contraceptive protection is required; a method that is appropriate at one stage of a woman's life may be unacceptable at another stage.

The methods of contraception chosen at different ages during the fertile lifetime of a woman is also subject to changing trends. A survey of the methods of contraception chosen or recommended at family planning clinics in the UK in 1988 reported that about half of the women attending elected to use oral contraceptives (combined and progestogen-only). This figure had declined from about two-thirds in 1976. The use of the condom had steadily increased from 6 to 15% over the same period.

Condoms are most commonly used as a form of contraception by younger people. This is primarily because condoms are readily available, especially from pharmacies, are easy to use, and are not associated with side-effects. Young people may be unaware of the availability of diaphragms or be reluctant to seek an appointment with a doctor or clinic to have one fitted. The intra-uterine device (IUD) is not recommended for young nulliparous women because of risks of pelvic inflammatory disease and reduced fertility (*see* Section 4.3). There also appears to be a greater awareness of the potential benefits that condoms provide in protecting against the transmission of infections, especially of the human immunodeficiency virus (HIV), and in reducing the risks of cervical cancer. Young people rarely use additional spermicide with condoms.

Young women may approach their doctor to obtain contraceptive preparations, and there are ethical guidelines issued to doctors on their supply to girls under 16 years of age.

4.2 HORMONAL CONTRACEPTION

The introduction of hormonal contraception in the USA in 1960 and in the UK in 1961 revolutionised the techniques of contraception and led to the involvement of medical practitioners in a contraceptive advisory role that they had previously shunned.

The most commonly used form of hormonal contraception is the combined oral contraceptive, which contains an oestrogen and a progestogen in varying strengths. Other forms available are progestogen-only oral contraceptives and progestogen-only injectable contraceptives; progestogen-containing subdermal implants and a vaginal ring are also under development (*see below*). Up to three million women use the combined oral contraceptive in the UK; this represents about 1 in 3 fertile women between 15 and 44 years of age. There are about 65 million users worldwide.

TABLE 4.2

Oestrogens and progestogens contained in oral contraceptive preparations available in the UK

Oestrogens	Progestogens
Ethinyloestradiol	Desogestrel
Mestranol	Ethynodiol diacetate
	Gestodene
	Levonorgestrel
	Norethisterone
	Norethisterone acetate
	Norgestimate
	Norgestrel

The oestrogens and progestogens used in oral contraceptive preparations available in the UK are listed in Table 4.2. The use of combined oral contraceptives in emergency contraception is discussed in Section 4.5.

Combined oral contraceptives

Combined oral contraceptives are indicated in women in whom maximum contraceptive cover is required. They represent the most reliable and appropriate method of contraception for young, healthy, non-smoking women. The failure rate of combined oral contraceptives should be less than one pregnancy per 100 woman years. However, poor compliance may result in failure rates of up to seven pregnancies per 100 woman years. One hundred woman years is equivalent to 100 women using the method for one year.

Types of combined oral contraceptives

A complete list of the combined oral contraceptive preparations available in the UK is given in BNF 7.3.1. A number of factors should be considered when selecting a product, and these include:

- The strength of the oestrogen component

  Combined oral contraceptives are classed as low-dose or high-dose oestrogen. Low-dose oestrogen preparations contain 20 to 35 μg of oestrogen (ethinyloestradiol); high-dose preparations contain 50 μg of oestrogen (either ethinyloestradiol or mestranol). Preparations with as low a dose of oestrogen consistent with effective contraceptive cover are recommended to minimise the incidence of adverse effects (*see below*).

- The strength of the progestogen component

  It is recommended that the lowest effective dose of progestogen with the most appropriate strength of oestrogen should be used.

- Varying the hormone content during the month

  Biphasic and triphasic preparations contain 2 and 3 different hormone combinations respectively in the 21-day dosage schedule.

- Tablets to be taken for 21 or 28 days

  Regular compliance may be enhanced if one tablet is taken each day throughout the month rather than discontinuing administration for seven days to provoke withdrawal bleeding. Some preparations include seven placebo tablets to achieve continuous pill taking while still provoking withdrawal bleeding.

The choice of combined oral contraceptive is based on the lowest oestrogen and progestogen dose compatible with good cycle control. However, different preparations use different progestogens, which have different potencies. Norethisterone acetate and ethynodiol diacetate, however, are metabolised in the body to norethisterone and so may be considered equivalent. It is also difficult to compare the different progestogens because the safety varies with the tissue under study. Some progestogens are more anti-oestrogenic than others and therefore the safety of the combination varies with the strength of each component relative to the other.

The combined oral contraceptive chosen for a first-time user is usually one containing a low dose of progestogen. If, after a few cycles, this is associated with endometrial instability resulting in breakthrough bleeding, a preparation with a higher dose is selected. It is important, however, to reassure patients that breakthrough bleeding is not necessarily associated with failure of contraception, although any patient reporting poor cycle control should be referred to their prescriber.

Mode of action

Combined oral contraceptives act by disturbing the normal release of endogenous hormones and the regulatory feedback mechanisms. The method, therefore, imitates those changes in hormone concentrations that occur at the onset of pregnancy. Combined preparations inhibit ovulation and render the endometrium less favourable to implantation should ovulation occur. These preparations also increase the viscosity of cervical mucus, reducing the ability of sperm to reach the ovum.

Dosage and administration

Combined oral contraceptives are generally taken for 21 days and then stopped for seven days. Withdrawal bleeding occurs during the pill-free week but this is not synonymous with blood loss at menstruation. Withdrawal bleeding is precipitated by removal of exogenous hormones but there is no unfertilised ovum that needs to be discarded and the endometrium does not break down. In theory, there is no need for withdrawal bleeding to take place. Continuous daily administration of combined oral contraceptives can be maintained in the short-term, but the safety profile of long-term, continuous administration is not proven. In practice, however, many women are reassured by the regular monthly loss of blood as it confirms the absence of pregnancy.

During the pill-free week, there may be an increase in endogenous oestrogen concentrations. There is wide individual variation and some women may not exhibit any increase, whereas in others this increase may approach concentrations that could result in an LH surge and, subsequently, ovulation if a follicle is mature at that time (*see* Section 4.1). In these cases, conception is a possibility and could account for rare pill-failures in the presence of perfect compliance. This effect is equally important in the event of any missed doses. If any pill is missed at the beginning or end of the packet, the pill-free week will be increased to beyond seven days. Consequently, there is a risk of endogenous oestrogen concentrations rising to levels that could result in an LH surge.

The procedure for starting the first dose of the first course and the action to be taken in the event of a missed dose, are both outlined in Fig. 4.2a.

Beneficial effects

The primary advantage of combined oral contraceptives, and the main reason why their use has become so widespread, is that they provide an extremely effective form of contraception for women, allied to minimal disruption of life-style. Other subsidiary benefits, which may themselves be primary indications for their administration, are the many improvements in gynaecological conditions produced by combined oral contraceptives.

Effects on menstruation   If a woman's periods are heavy, painful, or irregular, administration of combined oral contraceptives will normally result in lighter, pain-free, and regular withdrawal bleeding. Symptoms of premenstrual syndrome may also be improved.

Combined oral contraceptives

Dosage regimen

The dosage regimen for combined oral contraceptives is usually one tablet daily (at approximately the same time each day) for 21 days followed by a seven-day interval during which withdrawal bleeding occurs. If the first course is started on the fifth day of the cycle, ovulation may not be inhibited during that cycle and additional contraceptive precautions should therefore be taken during the first seven days or when changing from a high to a low oestrogen preparation. Additional contraceptive precautions are unnecessary in the first cycle if the tablets are started on the first day of the cycle, as is now usually recommended.

Phased formulations more closely mimic normal endogenous cyclical hormonal activity. They are generally recommended for a day one start.

Missed-pill guidance

If you forget a pill take it as soon as you remember, and take the next one at your normal time. This may mean taking two pills in one day. Provided that you are no more than 12 hours late in taking the forgotten tablet, contraceptive protection is not reduced.

If you are more than 12 hours late in taking one or more pills you may not be protected. As soon as you remember, take the last missed pill. This may mean taking two pills in one day. Continue to take the pills at your normal time, and either avoid sexual intercourse or use an extra contraceptive method such as a condom for the next seven days. If these seven days run beyond the end of your pack, start the next pack as soon as you have finished the present one. In other words, do not leave a gap between packs. This will mean you may not have a period until the end of two packs but this will not harm you. Nor does it matter if you have some bleeding on days when you take the pill.

If you are in any doubt about these instructions contact your doctor or family planning clinic.

Fig. 4.2a
Dosage regimen and missed-pill guidance for combined oral contraceptives.

Progestogen-only oral contraceptives

Dosage regimen

Oral progestogen-only contraceptives are started on the first day of the cycle and taken every day at the same time (preferably in early evening) without a break. Additional contraceptive precautions are unnecessary when initiating treatment. When changing from a combined oral contraceptive to a progestogen-only preparation, treatment should start on the day following completion of the combined oral contraceptive course so that there is no break in tablet taking.

Missed-pill guidance

If you forget a pill, take it as soon as you remember and take the next one at your normal time. If you are more than three hours overdue in taking a pill, you are not protected. Continue normal pill-taking but you must also use another method of contraception (e.g. the condom) for the next 48 hours. If you have vomiting or very severe diarrhoea the pill may not work. Continue to take it, but you may not be protected from the first day of vomiting or diarrhoea. Use another method of contraception (e.g. the condom) for any intercourse during the stomach upset and for the next 48 hours.

Fig. 4.2b
Dosage regimen and missed-pill guidance for progestogen-only oral contraceptives.

Benign mammary dysplasias   Long-term administration of combined oral contraceptives can also protect against the development of benign, and particularly cystic, breast disease; this is in direct contrast to the postulated link between combined oral contraceptive use and malignant breast disease (*see below*).

Functional ovarian cysts   Administration of combined oral contraceptives has also been reported to reduce the incidence of functional ovarian cysts, primarily as a result of inhibition of ovulation.

Endometriosis   Combined oral contraceptives may

TABLE 4.3
Beneficial effects of administration of combined oral contraceptives

Breast	reduced incidence of benign breast disease
Endocrine system	protection against thyroid disease
Gastro-intestinal tract	protection against peptic ulceration
Genital system	dysmenorrhoea reduced endometriosis controlled functional ovarian cysts controlled menorrhagia controlled menstrual cycle regularity improved pelvic inflammatory disease incidence decreased premenstrual syndrome reduced protection against endometrial and ovarian cancer
Musculoskeletal system	possible protection against rheumatoid arthritis
Skin	acne improved (with oestrogen-dominated pills)

TABLE 4.4
Adverse effects reported with combined oral contraceptive use

Cardiovascular system	Deep vein thrombosis Hypertension Leg pain Myocardial infarction Oedema Pulmonary embolism
Central nervous system	Depression Epilepsy rate increased Headaches and migraine Increase or loss of libido
Endocrine system	Breast cancer Breast discomfort Stunted growth in prepubertal use Worsening of diabetes mellitus
Eyes	Corneal oedema Irritation from contact lenses
Gastro-intestinal tract	Abdominal bloating Appetite increased Crohn's disease Nausea Vomiting (rarely)
Hepatic system	Changes to many liver enzymes Cholestatic jaundice Gall bladder disease Gallstones Hepatic adenomas
Musculoskeletal system	Carpal tunnel syndrome Tenosynovitis
Respiratory system	Allergic rhinitis Asthma Upper respiratory-tract infection
Skin	Acne Chickenpox Chloasma Eczema Erythema nodosum Erythema multiforme Hirsutism Malignant melanoma Neurodermatitis Photosensitivity Rosacea Telangiectasia
Urogenital system	Candidiasis Cervical cancer Urinary-tract infection Vaginal dryness
Miscellaneous	Weight gain

help to suppress endometriosis and prevent the development of endometrial and ovarian cancer; these effects are predominantly seen after administration for more than 2 or 3 years. These beneficial effects can persist for many years after administration of combined oral contraceptives has stopped.

Other beneficial effects can be produced by administration of combined oral contraceptives (Table 4.3).

Adverse effects

The adverse effects reported with combined oral contraceptive use are listed in Table 4.4. The disorders most closely associated with use of combined oral contraceptives are cardiovascular. There is an almost four-fold increase in the risk of deep vein thrombosis and other forms of venous embolism (and in particular pulmonary embolism); the incidence of arterial diseases, including myocardial infarction and thrombotic strokes, is also increased. Most women taking combined oral contraceptives experience a slight rise in blood pressure, and between 2 and 3% become clinically hypertensive. The number of reports of hypertension increases with prolonged administration. The likelihood of the development of cardiovascular complications is closely linked to age, smoking, obesity, and the existence of any conditions predisposing to cardiovascular disease (e.g. diabetes mellitus or hypertension).

The effects of combined oral contraceptives on the incidence of malignant diseases are complex and contradictory. Moreover, an increased incidence of any specific malignancy has not been correlated with combined oral contraceptive use in the general population. Nevertheless, the administration of these hormones may be linked to a higher incidence of cancer in women who are already at increased risk (e.g. as a result of sexual proclivity or a late age of first pregnancy).

Vascular disease   The increased risk of venous thrombosis caused by combined oral contraceptives disappears within a couple of months of stopping administration but the greater susceptibility to strokes has been reported to take up to six years to decline.

The mechanism for predisposition to venous disease is thought to operate through augmented plasma concentrations of clotting factors combined with a reduction in the plasma concentration of a counterbalancing enzyme, antithrombin III; both these effects are caused by oestrogens. Platelet function is also modified. Arterial disease is thought to be a consequence of the metabolic effects of progestogens in promoting atherosclerosis, superimposed upon the oestrogen-induced modifications to blood clotting mechanisms.

Hepatic disease   The passage of steroid hormones through the liver induces changes in physiological function. The range of recorded changes is complex; the activity of some hepatic enzymes is decreased, whereas that of others is increased. These changes may affect the metabolism of some drugs administered at the same time as the combined oral contraceptive (*see below*).

One of the more serious but rare adverse effects associated with combined oral contraceptive use is hepatocellular adenoma, which may have an incidence of 10 to 20 times greater than in non-users. The risk of this benign condition is greatest in older women who have been long-term users of high-dose oestrogens.

Cervical cancer   Cervical cancer has been associated with combined oral contraceptive use, possibly as a result of the exogenous hormones acting as accessories to the pre-malignant and malignant cellular changes. Of equal importance in the development of cervical cancer, however, is the age of first intercourse and the subsequent number of sexual partners. Regular cervical screening is vital to detect any early pre-malignant changes.

Breast cancer   The increased incidence of breast cancer has also been attributed to the use of combined oral contraceptives, and the risk may be increased in those women who started using combined oral contraceptives at an early age. It has been suggested that the risk of breast cancer may be minimised by using the lowest possible dose of oestrogen and progestogen that is consistent with effective contraceptive cover. Women should be advised of the importance of regular breast self-examination to detect any nodules.

Contra-indications

Contra-indications to the use of combined oral contraceptives are listed in Table 4.5.

Drug interactions

A number of potential and proven interactions between combined oral contraceptives and other drugs

TABLE 4.5
Examples of absolute and relative contra-indications to the use of combined oral contraceptives

Absolute contra-indications	Relative contra-indications
Absolute contra-indications are conditions in which combined oral contraceptives should never be used.	Relative contra-indications are conditions in which combined oral contraceptives should not usually be taken, or if they are, careful monitoring is required.
Breast cancer Circulatory diseases (current or former) 　(including deep vein thrombosis, pulmonary embolism, 　transient ischaemic attacks, and any condition 　predisposing to thromboembolism) Endometrial carcinoma History of any serious condition affected by sex 　hormones (including haemolytic uraemic syndrome, 　chorea, and otosclerosis) Hyperlipidaemia Liver conditions 　(including cholestatic jaundice of pregnancy, acute 　infective hepatitis, porphyrias, liver adenoma, 　cirrhosis, and chronic active hepatitis) Migraine (severe or focal) Oestrogen-dependent tumours Pregnancy Thalassaemia major Trophoblastic disease, recent 　(including hydatidiform mole) Vaginal bleeding (undiagnosed)	Asthma Breast-feeding Cardiovascular disorders Depressive disorders Diabetes mellitus Epilepsy Hypertension Immobilisation Major surgery Migraine (*see also above*) Obesity Renal disease Sickle-cell anaemia Smoking Superficial thrombophlebitis Varicose veins

administered concurrently have been reported (see BNF, Appendix 1); several of these interactions have important implications. A small risk of reduced contraceptive effect has been reported with administration of broad-spectrum antibacterials (e.g. ampicillin and tetracyclines). This risk arises at the start of antibacterial treatment, or upon changing long-term treatment. The decrease in contraceptive effectiveness is caused by a disturbance of the gastro-intestinal flora, which may impair absorption of the hormones. As the gastro-intestinal flora develop resistance to the antibacterial drug, the risk diminishes. This effect is, however, negligible, and is not thought to occur with narrow-spectrum antibacterials, with the long-term administration of broad-spectrum antibacterials, or with co-trimoxazole.

More serious interactions occur with the antituberculous drug, rifampicin, and with all antiepileptics except sodium valproate. These drugs induce microsomal hepatic enzymes, which enhance the metabolism of combined oral contraceptives. It is recommended that preparations containing 50 μg of oestrogen are used by women taking antiepileptics; alternative methods of contraception should be used for those prescribed rifampicin.

Combined oral contraceptives inhibit hepatic microsomal enzymes and may increase the effects of other drugs (e.g. prednisolone, diazepam, and alcohol).

Other interactions can be predicted on the basis of the adverse effects of combined oral contraceptives (Table 4.4). Among the most important are: impaired glucose tolerance, which antagonises the action of antidiabetic drugs; depression, which may counteract the intended effects of antidepressant drugs; and raised blood pressure, which antagonises the effects of antihypertensive therapy.

The excretion of theophylline is impaired by combined oral contraceptives and may lead to toxic effects because of the narrow therapeutic range of the bronchodilator.

Patients undergoing surgery

Oestrogen-containing oral contraceptives should be discontinued, four weeks before major elective surgery and all surgery to the legs. They should normally be recommended at the first menses occurring at least two weeks after the procedure. When discontinuation is not possible (e.g. after trauma or if, by oversight, a patient admitted for an elective procedure is still on an oestrogen-containing oral contraceptive), some consideration should be given to subcutaneous heparin prophylaxis. These recommendations do not apply to minor surgery with short duration anaesthesia (e.g.

laparoscopic sterilisation or tooth extraction, or to women taking oestrogen-free hormonal contraceptives).

Progestogen-only oral contraceptives

A complete list of the progestogen-only oral contraceptives available in the UK is given in BNF 7.3.2. They are mainly used by women over 35 years of age and by women of all ages in whom combined oral contraceptives are contra-indicated (Table 4.5).

The failure rate with progestogen-only oral contraceptives is estimated to be between 2 and 4 pregnancies per 100 woman years, and these rates are comparable with those quoted for intra-uterine devices (see Section 4.3) and diaphragms (see Section 4.4).

The choice of progestogen-only oral contraceptive for a first-time user is arbitrary because there are insufficient data to highlight any differences in effectiveness. It also appears that the adverse effects (see below) are dependent on the target tissue rather than the preparation. If the side-effects are unacceptable to the patient, another preparation should be chosen until a suitable one is found.

Mode of action

The primary mode of action of progestogen-only oral contraceptives is to alter the ease with which sperm can penetrate cervical mucus. Progestogen-only oral contraceptives do not generally prevent ovulation, and the continued production of ova accounts for the decreased effectiveness of progestogen-only contraceptives compared to combined oral contraceptives. Progestogen-only oral contraceptives provide 27 hours of protection.

Dosage and administration

Progestogen-only oral contraceptives are taken continuously for as long as contraception is desired, starting the first course on the first day of a cycle. The daily occurrence of the cyclical changes in cervical mucus highlights the importance of regular dosage, which should be at the same time each day. If a dose is taken as little as 12 hours late, the contraceptive effect on cervical mucus is lost. For the procedure for starting the first dose of the first course and the action to be taken in the event of a missed dose, see Fig. 4.2b.

Beneficial effects

Women taking progestogen-only oral contraceptives may experience improvement in the symptoms of premenstrual syndrome, dysmenorrhoea, and breast-tenderness.

Adverse effects

The most significant and common problem with progestogen-only oral contraceptives is a disturbance of normal menstruation patterns, which arises as a result of the effects of progestogen on ovarian function. Nevertheless, changes are not universal and some women may experience only minor deviations from their normal cyclical pattern, whereas others exhibit spotting and breakthrough bleeding. Amenorrhoea may occur and, once pregnancy has been excluded, is likely to indicate that ovulation has, in fact, been inhibited. Cycle irregularity tends to be worse during the early courses of progestogen-only contraceptives and gradually improves; it should not be taken as a sign of lack of contraceptive effectiveness. However, it may be sufficiently disruptive and persistent to lead women to seek other forms of contraception. Women can be reassured that previous patterns of menstrual regularity are normally resumed on stopping administration of progestogen-only contraceptives.

Functional ovarian cysts can develop, producing significant pain and discomfort. Cysts tend to arise because of accumulation of fluid within follicles following abnormal ovulation. There is also a greater risk that any failure of contraceptive effect may lead to an ectopic pregnancy.

The range of side-effects from progestogen-only oral contraceptives is similar to that observed with combined oral contraceptives. Breast-tenderness, headache, and nausea may occur, although these symptoms generally abate during the first 2 or 3 months of administration. However, unlike combined oral contraceptives, progestogen-only oral contraceptives have no demonstrable effect on the tendency for blood to coagulate and have not been associated with thrombosis or platelet aggregation. Similarly, effects on carbohydrate metabolism are minimal and therefore progestogen-only oral contraceptives may be used by insulin-dependent diabetics. Compliance may be enhanced by the administration of progestogen-only oral contraceptives at the same time as the evening dose of insulin.

Contra-indications

Some of the absolute and relative contra-indications to the administration of progestogen-only contraceptives are listed in Table 4.6.

Progestogen-only injectable contraceptives

Progestogens may be administered by intramuscular injection as long-acting contraceptives. They are effective, convenient, and easy to administer, and are suitable as a short-term measure while a couple are waiting for a vasectomy to become effective or after a woman has had a rubella vaccination.

Medroxyprogesterone acetate is given in a single dose of 150 mg during the first five days of the menstrual cycle and then repeated every 12 weeks; it is as effective as combined oral contraceptives. It may also be administered in the first six weeks following the birth of a baby, although heavy bleeding occurs in some women and it may be best to delay the first dose. It is also recommended to delay the dose until six weeks post partum if breast-feeding, to allow the infant's enzyme systems to develop fully; established lactation is not affected. Medroxyprogesterone acetate may be used as a long-term measure in women unsuited to any other method.

Norethisterone enanthate is given as a single dose of 200 mg during the first five days of the cycle or immediately after parturition, and may be repeated once

Table 4.6
Examples of absolute and relative contra-indications to the use of progestogen-only contraceptives

Absolute contra-indications	Relative contra-indications
Absolute contra-indications are conditions in which progestogen-only contraceptives should never be used.	Relative contra-indications are conditions in which progestogen-only contraceptives should not usually be used, or if they are, careful monitoring is required.
Breast cancer and other forms of sex hormone-dependent malignant diseases History of arterial disease, ischaemic heart disease, or a stroke History of ectopic pregnancy or a history of pelvic inflammatory disease in which there may be a high risk of ectopic pregnancy Hydatidiform mole (recent) Liver adenoma Pregnancy Vaginal bleeding (undiagnosed)	Active liver disorders Cardiovascular disorders Cholestatic jaundice (recurrent) Diabetes mellitus Functional ovarian cysts Hypertension Irregular menstrual bleeding at the menopause Malabsorption syndromes Migraine that is severe or focal, or began for the first time when taking combined oral contraceptives

eight weeks later. Norethisterone enanthate has not been reported to inhibit milk production. Traces of the hormone appear in the mother's milk but are not considered to be harmful to the healthy neonate. However, neonates with severe or persistent jaundice should not be breast-fed.

Full counselling is essential to anyone wishing to receive an injectable contraceptive because the effects cannot be reversed for the duration of the activity of the drug. Side-effects that may occur include:

- amenorrhoea in long-term use (more than one year)
- altered menstrual cycle, which may persist for some time after discontinuation of the method
- fluid retention
- infertility following discontinuation of the method, which may last up to two years or more
- menorrhagia
- weight gain.

Other progestogen-only devices

One of the methods nearing general availability is the vaginal ring. This is a soft compressible ring that can be inserted and removed by the woman herself. The ring provides continuous low-dosage progestogen-only contraception and can be left in place for up to 90 days.

Another slow-release device under development and containing levonorgestrel is called Norplant. It is a subdermal implant consisting of six matchstick-sized tubes, which are implanted in the upper arm and provide contraception for 5 to 7 years.

4.3 INTRA-UTERINE DEVICES

The main impetus for the development of intra-uterine devices (IUDs) (Fig. 4.3) was to provide women with contraceptive devices that had guaranteed effectiveness but demanded little or no attention after insertion. In addition to achieving this, other advantages to their use include: immediate effectiveness after fitting; non-interference with intercourse; and the high success rate in achieving reversibility of the contraceptive effect after removal. IUDs are also especially useful for women who have had children but do not wish to use hormonal contraceptives; those who find compliance with other contraceptive methods difficult; and older women who want an alternative to sterilisation. The use of IUDs in emergency contraception is discussed in Section 4.5.

It has been estimated that there are about 60 million women fitted with IUDs in the world, although 80% of

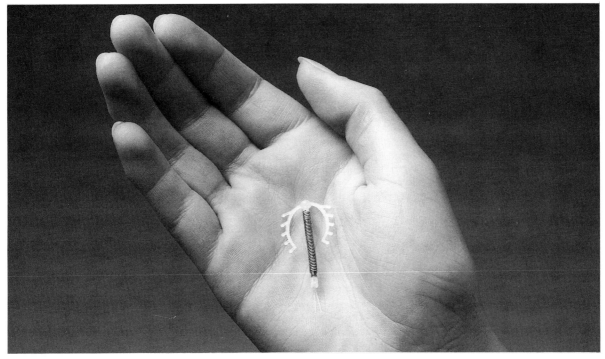

Fig. 4.3
Intra-uterine device.

them are in China alone. About 13% of women who attend family planning clinics in the UK use the IUD as a contraceptive.

The effectiveness of IUDs varies between types of device. Of 100 women using an IUD, the pregnancy rate is between 1 and 3 per year, with the lowest failure rate occurring in older women and after prolonged use.

Types of intra-uterine device

The development of IUDs began in the late 1920s with trials on the use of the Grafenberg ring, made of silver wire. Subsequently, the Ota ring was developed in the 1930s, and consisted of a metal or plastic ring with a central flattened disc. Neither of these is in use in the UK today.

Inert devices   Advances in polymer science during the 1960s led to the manufacture of plastic (silastic) IUDs. The most widely used of these was the Lippes loop, designed by, and named after, an American doctor. This plastic loop was formed in the shape of a double-S and, even when subjected to severe distortion (e.g. on insertion through an applicator), it resumed its original shape *in situ*. Another similar device that became available at the same period as the Lippes loop, and which was also commonly used, was the Saf-T-coil.

Inert devices are rendered visible on X-ray films by impregnating the plastic with barium sulphate. Although they are no longer available in the UK, the prolonged life of these inert devices makes it possible that some women may still be using them as a form of contraception, and may continue to do so until the menopause.

Bioactive devices   Bioactive devices were developed using the same basic structure as inert devices and are the most common form of IUD in use today. They were developed from the observation that adding copper to plastic IUDs significantly enhanced their contraceptive effect. Most of the currently used devices are shaped in the form of a letter T or a figure 7. One or more nylon threads attached to the lower end of the plastic facilitates self-examination to confirm that the device is in place; they also permit its removal.

The earliest bioactive IUDs consisted of copper wire of 200 μm thickness wound around a plastic stem. More recent modifications to the way in which copper is affixed include the use of copper collars or sleeves on the horizontal arms, or the presence of a copper wire with a central silver core on the vertical stem, which may reduce the risk of copper fragmentation that can occur after prolonged use. Thicker copper wires of 300 μm or 400 μm diameter are also used to reduce the risk of

fragmentation. The total surface area (not the thickness) of the copper in proprietary devices is often indicated by the number incorporated in its name (e.g. there is 250 mm^2 copper in the Multiload™ Cu250 device). Copper is leached from the wire at the rate of 38 μg each day. Because bioactive devices are more effective than inert devices they can be made narrower, less cumbersome, and less bulky. Consequently, the incidence of adverse effects caused by the physical presence of bioactive devices (*see below*) is less.

Further modifications to bioactive devices have been tried in attempts to improve contraceptive effectiveness by using IUDs as delivery devices for progestogens. The first of these incorporated progesterone into a T-shaped plastic frame, from which the hormone was released through a permeable polymer membrane at the rate of 65 μg per day. However, a high incidence of ectopic pregnancies associated with use of this device led to its withdrawal from the market. A second, more recently developed device (but not available in the UK) has a similar T-shape but releases the progestogen, levonorgestrel, at a rate of 20 μg each day. The much lower concentration of released progestogen produces a considerably lower incidence of ectopic pregnancies and reduces the likelihood of the occurrence of systemic side-effects from the drug.

Mode of action

The contraceptive efficacy of IUDs is thought to involve an alteration in the uterine environment as a result of a pronounced foreign body reaction. The changes in uterine and tubal fluid that occur, appear to impede the motility of sperm and transport of the ovum, and inhibit fertilisation. The release of copper ions from and IUD may potentiate these effects. IUDs may interfere with the implantation of a fertilised ovum, but this is no longer considered to be the prime mode of action.

Insertion and removal

Insertion   Most IUDs are inserted under aseptic conditions during the final days of menstruation or immediately after menstruation has terminated, although up to day 21 appears to be part of the normal guidelines offered by some authorities. Insertion at this time is preferred because the cervical canal is slightly dilated and the risk of insertion during an early, unconfirmed pregnancy is minimised. Nevertheless, it is also possible to insert devices at any time during the menstrual cycle.

After insertion of copper-coated devices, menstrual irregularities and dysmenorrhoea may occur. A watery, non-purulent vaginal discharge may be produced but this is usually considered as normal. However, changes to the colour and consistency of the discharge require referral, commonly for antibacterial drug treatment. Some women may report abdominal pain immediately after insertion and this can last for several days. Prolonged abdominal discomfort may necessitate removal of the device. Patients should be seen by the doctor 6 to 8 weeks after insertion, and then at yearly intervals.

Removal   The most common symptoms reported by women requesting removal of IUDs are pain and excessive bleeding (*see below*). These symptoms, which may occur together, are usually caused by incorrect positioning of the device or from the horizontal arms of the device becoming embedded in the walls of the uterus. Less frequently, pain and excessive bleeding may be caused by an infection.

Elective removal of IUDs may be carried out to permit attempts to become pregnant, at the menopause (normally 12 months after the last period), or when another method of contraception has been chosen. If there is no desire to become pregnant, the device should not be removed in mid-cycle unless an additional contraceptive was used for the previous seven days, or if intercourse has not occurred during the preceding seven days.

The length of time recommended for leaving bioactive IUDs in place varies between manufacturers from 3 to 5 years, although studies have shown that the most recent devices may be left in for 6 to 8 years. Ideally, devices should remain in place for as long as possible to reduce the risks of pelvic inflammatory disease and other complications that can occur after insertion.

Adverse effects

Pain and excessive bleeding   Lower abdominal pain may manifest as spasms and cramps, which can occur at any time during the menstrual cycle.

Inert and copper-containing devices commonly cause increased blood loss at menstruation. Menstrual blood losses of 70 to 80 mL are associated with inert devices and of 50 to 60 mL with copper devices. This compares to the average menstrual blood loss of 35 mL in women not fitted with an IUD. Bleeding and spotting may occur between each menses.

Ectopic pregnancy   There is an almost ten-fold increase in the risk of ectopic pregnancy in users of IUDs compared to women using no form of contraception.

Most ectopic pregnancies caused by IUDs occur in the Fallopian tubes, although they have been reported in other sites. The risk of ectopic pregnancy is also increased in women with a history of pelvic inflammatory disease, which may also be associated with the use of IUDs.

Pelvic inflammatory disease   There is an approximately four-fold increase in the risk of pelvic inflammatory disease in users of IUDs, particularly in young nulliparous women. The increased incidence is thought to be a direct consequence of the presence of a foreign body in the uterine cavity or may be associated with a sexually transmitted disease. One other factor has also been identified as an important cause of infection: the severe infections associated with use of the Dalkon Shield IUD in the early 1970s (which led to its withdrawal in 1974) were thought to be caused by the multifilament threads attached to the bottom of the device acting as a wick, drawing up bacteria.

Early detection of pelvic inflammatory disease is vital because, if untreated, it can cause infertility. Referral for treatment with broad-spectrum antibacterial drugs is essential; recurrent infection may necessitate removal of the IUD.

Perforation   There is an incidence of about one perforation of the uterine wall or cervix for every 1000 IUDs inserted; in extreme cases, the device may migrate over several weeks through the uterine wall and into the peritoneal cavity. Adhesions may develop with bioactive devices, or the IUD may perforate the wall of the bladder or gastro-intestinal tract. In the event of perforation, the device must be promptly removed by surgery.

Lost threads and expulsion   The thread or threads attached to the base of an IUD hang down through the neck of the uterus into the vagina. Their presence acts as reassurance that the device is in place and they also provide a means of removal. Causes of the absence of detectable threads include: their upward disappearance beyond the external os into the uterus; penetration of the IUD through the uterine wall; shifting of the device out of position; or the IUD has been expelled. It is essential that women adopt alternative forms of contraception if the threads are no longer detectable because, even if devices have not been completely expelled, their contraceptive effectiveness is likely to have been reduced.

Total expulsion is uncommon but the device may become sufficiently dislodged for the stem to protrude from the cervix. In such an the event, the device should be removed by a doctor and, if desired, replaced by another IUD.

TABLE 4.7

Examples of absolute and relative contra-indications to the use of intra-uterine devices

Absolute contra-indications	Relative contra-indications
Absolute contra-indications are conditions in which intra-uterine devices should never be used.	Relative contra-indications are conditions in which intra-uterine devices should not usually be used, or if they are, careful monitoring is required.
Active pelvic inflammatory disease Confirmed or suspected pregnancy History of ectopic pregnancy or tubal surgery Immunosuppressive therapy Malignancy of the genital tract Severe anaemia Undiagnosed abnormal vaginal bleeding	Fibroids History of pelvic inflammatory disease Severe dysmenorrhoea Women under 30 years of age, particularly if they have not had children Women of any age who have had a number of sexual partners and who may be at increased risk of sexually transmitted diseases Women who are not in mutually faithful relationships

Expulsion of IUDs is most likely to occur at menstruation during the first 3 months of use, and may occur undetected. Expulsion is more common in women who have not had children but the incidence decreases with age. Repeated expulsion is unlikely after insertion of a replacement device.

Contra-indications

Some of the absolute and relative contra-indications to the use of IUDs are listed in Table 4.7.

4.4 BARRIER METHODS AND SPERMICIDES

Condoms

Condoms (sheaths, French letters, or rubbers) are one of the oldest forms of contraception and are used all over the world. The condom is worn over the erect penis during coitus to prevent sperm from entering the woman's genital tract and to inhibit the exchange of sexually transmitted disease. Historically, condoms were formed of natural products or cloths, but standardisation of their production and their success as contraceptives was revolutionised by the large-scale production of rubber, initially for the pneumatic tyre industry. However, despite their widespread availability, historically there has existed an element of poor social acceptance for their use. Their 'social status' has, however, recently increased and use of condoms has witnessed a resurgence in popularity. This has been especially prominent among young people concerned about the risks of contracting HIV infection during unprotected casual sexual intercourse. Equally important, the use of condoms is one of the few methods of contraception in which the male partner can assume total responsibility. The condom acts as a contraceptive by collecting seminal fluid at its tip, thereby preventing the access of sperm to the female reproductive tract.

Condoms are commonly used as a sole form of contraception, although they may also be used as an additional measure in certain instances. Condoms should be used while a woman is learning to use a vaginal cap or diaphragm (*see below*). The use of condoms may promote greater reliability of contraceptive cover by counteracting the small risk of reduced effectiveness of combined oral contraceptives in women prescribed broad-spectrum antibacterials (*see* Section 4.2). Condoms are also suitable for contraceptive use immediately after the birth of a baby and before resumption of the contraceptive methods used before confinement.

The failure rate of condoms is about 2 to 15 pregnancies per 100 woman years, although their contraceptive effectiveness is better in older age groups. This increased effectiveness may be a result of reduced fertility and greater care in use.

A female condom is also under investigation. The device, known as Femidom, consists of a polyurethane tube with a flexible ring at either end. Once inserted, the ring at the closed end of the tube fits over the cervix while the other ring remains outside the vagina. It is intended for single use only. It is hoped that the device will provide protection against transmission of HIV infection and other sexually transmitted diseases.

Types of condom   The most common form of condom is made of fine, vulcanised latex rubber, hence its colloquial name. The thickness of the latex varies between 40 and 70 μm; the overall dimensions are 170 to 200 mm long and 50 mm wide. Condoms manufactured to British Standards Institution specification are tested as they come off the production line to ensure the absence of holes; samples are also tested for strength by inflation. Not all commercially available condoms are manufactured to these standards. Most good quality condoms have a capacity of up to 40 litres of air before they burst. Condoms made from latex rubber normally have a shelf-life of about five years when stored in a cool dry place, although more rapid deterioration may occur in hot and humid climates.

Condoms can also be made from lamb intestines. However, these natural products conform less readily to the shape of the penis than synthetic products and there is a greater tendency for them to slip off when the penis is retracted. Furthermore, the natural product is more expensive and it has not been conclusively demonstrated that it prevents the transmission of HIV infection.

Condoms are normally supplied in one size and are packaged flat by rolling onto the rim located at the open end. Variations of design and style, primarily to enhance the enjoyment of sexual intercourse, include the presence of ribbing and nodules over the surface; others may be coloured, perfumed, or flavoured.

Some condoms incorporate a spermicide (*see below*), lubricant, or both. The most commonly used spermicide is the nonionic surfactant, nonoxynol-9. The spermicide is coated over the inner and outer surfaces and is included as a precautionary measure against the accidental spillage of small amounts of seminal fluid. However, the concentration of spermicide used is not usually sufficient to be effective against the wholesale leakage of seminal fluid from a condom that has ruptured.

A lubricant (usually silicone based) may be included to minimise friction between the penis and vagina on penetration, which may be a particular problem if vaginal secretions are minimal. A lubricant may also reduce the friction on the condom thus lessening the chance of it slipping off. However, the Committee on Safety of Medicines (CSM) advise that oil-based vaginal and rectal preparations are likely to reduce the strength of condoms made from latex rubber, and may render them less effective as a barrier method of contraception and as a protection from sexually transmitted diseases (including AIDS).

In the UK, the majority of condoms are bought from pharmacies, and it has been suggested that most are bought by women. Supermarkets and vending machines provide the other main purchasing outlets. Free supplies can be obtained from family planning clinics (*see* Section 4.7), but doctors cannot prescribe them at NHS expense on prescription forms, unlike most other forms of contraception.

Method of use   To maximise effectiveness, a condom should be fitted before there is any contact between the penis and vagina. The small amount of seminal fluid that may be discharged from the penis before ejaculation contains sufficient sperm to cause pregnancy (*see* Section 4.1). There should be no contact between the penis and vagina after removal of the condom following intercourse; if further intercourse is to take place, a fresh condom should be used.

Great care should be taken in fitting and removal to prevent damage to the condom from sharp objects (e.g. fingernails or jewellery). The condom should be unrolled over the complete length of the erect penis, while keeping the closed end of the condom pinched between the forefinger and thumb; this allows an empty reservoir at the end of the condom to collect seminal fluid.

Ideally, the female partner should use a spermicide (*see below*), even if the condom has an integral coating of spermicide. If the condom does rupture, emergency contraception (*see* Section 4.5) should be arranged as soon as possible.

The condom should be held firmly by its rim at the base of the penis on withdrawal from the vagina, which should ideally take place as soon as possible after ejaculation. This helps to prevent the condom slipping off and reduces the risk of spillage of collected seminal fluid, which may occur particularly if the penis is withdrawn in a flaccid state.

Beneficial effects   The most important advantage that the use of condoms confers is protection against sexually transmitted diseases, and in particular against infection with HIV. The possible association between sexually transmitted diseases and genital cancer (e.g. cervical cancer) means that condoms may also reduce the risk of female malignancies.

Advantages can also occur in instances where greater, not less, fertility is desired. It has been estimated that about 1 in 5 women may produce antibodies to sperm; the regular use of a condom over 3 to 6 months reduces the antigenic challenge of the sperm and decreases the concentration of circulating antibodies.

Condoms can also prolong the period of erection before ejaculation; the rim at the base of the condom may enhance the degree of erection by constricting the base of the penis.

Adverse effects   The major drawback with the use of condoms is a perceived reduction in sensitivity, and hence enjoyment in the sexual act, that may be experienced. This may be partially overcome by using thinner (featherweight) condoms.

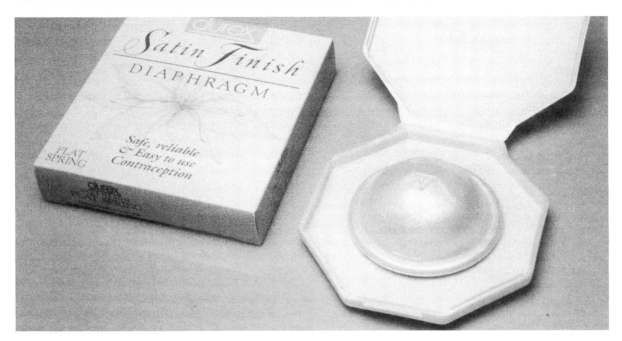

Fig. 4.4
Flat spring diaphragm.

Diaphragms

It has been estimated that between 1 and 2% of sexually active women in the UK use the diaphragm (vaginal cap or 'Dutch cap'). The effectiveness of diaphragms as a method of contraception increases with age, with greater motivation for preventing pregnancy, and with the length of time that the method has been used. Average failure rates during the first year of use are about 2 to 15 pregnancies per 100 woman years. The failure rate is less in older women, and in those experienced in use of this method.

Types of diaphragm   The diaphragm is a rubber dome mounted on a metal rim; it is held in place in the vagina by the spring located in the rim. The metal rim of the diaphragm can be formed of a flat spring, a spirally shaped coil spring, or an arcing spring. The most commonly used version is the flat spring (Fig. 4.4), which maintains a firmer shape than the coil spring and is relatively easy to manipulate when inserting. The coil spring is more flexible (and consequently more difficult to control on insertion) but may be used in women who find the flat spring diaphragm uncomfortable. The arcing spring diaphragm combines the properties of both the flat spring and coil spring versions. It may be used in women experiencing difficulty in fitting either the flat or coil spring types. The maximum recommended life of a diaphragm is two years.

Mode of action   The dome presents a physical barrier to the passage of sperm by lying across the cervical opening. Sperm cannot gain access to the alkaline cervical mucus but remain stranded and subsequently perish in the acidic environment of the vagina. Contraceptive action is improved by the concomitant use of a spermicide (*see below*).

Method of use   There are considerable variations in anatomical dimensions between women and this demands that the correct size of diaphragm be selected by careful measurement. The largest size that is comfortable is selected, as the upper portion of the vagina enlarges during intercourse. Measurement requires an internal examination and is carried out by a doctor or family planning nurse. The diameter of diaphragms available in the UK ranges from 55 to 95 mm in steps of 5 mm; if the internal measurement lies half-way between available sizes of the flat spring diaphragm, the reduced tension within the coil spring model will usually provide a comfortable fit. Women are usually issued with a temporary diaphragm for seven days to practise fitting and removal. Additional contraceptive cover (e.g. condoms) during this period is essential. After the initial measurement and fitting, subsequent size checks are made at one week and three months; thereafter, remeasurement is necessary every 12 months and after a birth, miscarriage or termination of pregnancy, or excessive changes in weight (greater than 3 kg).

The diaphragm does not provide a total seal around the neck of the cervix and it is therefore essential that two 5 cm strips of spermicide, in the form of a cream or gel, are coated onto both outer and inner surfaces immediately before insertion; spermicide may also be applied to the rim to facilitate insertion. Extra spermicide can also be used, and is essential if intercourse takes place more than three hours after insertion or is repeated. The CSM advise that oil-based vaginal and rectal preparations are likely to damage diaphragms made from latex rubber, and may render them less effective as a barrier method of contraception.

The diaphragm is inserted into the vagina before intercourse and should remain in position for at least six hours after intercourse. The diaphragm should be removed within 30 hours of fitting, washed in warm water, dried, and stored in a cool, dry place until next required.

Beneficial effects   Using a diaphragm can protect against some vaginal infections (e.g. chlamydia and gonorrhoea) but less effective protection is afforded to others (e.g. herpes and syphilis). The presence of a physical barrier may also act to reduce the incidence of pelvic inflammatory disease and cervical cancer.

Adverse effects   The intimate examination needed for sizing and fitting may be unacceptable to some women. Additionally, the need for this to be carried out by trained personnel in a clinical environment may be a further demotivating factor in their use.

Urinary frequency and urgency, and urinary-tract infections, are more common in diaphragm users. These adverse effects occur primarily as a result of the upward pressure from the device on the urethra and the base of the bladder and are often due to poor initial fitting. Attention to cleanliness in their use is essential to prevent the introduction of *Escherichia coli* and other coliform bacteria from the perianal region. Changing to a smaller device may help to reduce the incidence of infection. Local soreness and ulceration may occur because of the pressure of the diaphragm within the vagina. In the event of vaginal soreness, women should be referred to the doctor or family planning clinic for reassessment and resizing. Allergy to the rubber or added spermicide can occasionally occur.

Cervical caps

Cervical caps are used as alternatives to diaphragms in women who have poor muscle tone and in some women with uterovaginal prolapse; caps are also unlikely to produce urinary symptoms, and are unaffected by changes in body-weight. Compared to diaphragms, caps are less likely to reduce sensation in the vagina and may be more comfortable. However, because they are more difficult to fit than diaphragms, there is a greater tendency not to persist with the method.

Types of cervical caps   There are three types of cervical cap (Fig. 4.5): the cavity rim cervical cap, the vault cap, and the vimule cap. Each has a similar mode of action but they differ slightly in shape. Cervical caps differ from diaphragms in that the rim is not reinforced by metal. Moreover, cervical caps are held in place by suction, whereas diaphragms are retained by spring tension.

The cavity rim cervical cap is a thimble-shaped device with a thickened rim and fits tightly over the cervix; this is facilitated by a groove on the rim. It is available in four sizes, with internal diameters of 22 mm, 25 mm, 28 mm, and 31 mm.

The vault cap is a bowl-shaped flat-domed cap similar in appearance to a diaphragm, although its rim does not have a metal spring. It is available in five sizes, ranging from 55 to 75 mm in 5 mm steps; in the UK these five sizes are designated 1 to 5 and the numbering is moulded onto the rim.

The vimule cap has a bell-shaped dome and the open end is wider than its body. As a result, the cap covers the

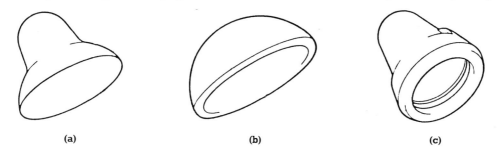

(a)   (b)   (c)

Fig. 4.5
Cervical caps: (a) Vimule cap. (b) Vault cap. (c) Cavity rim cervical cap.

outer walls of the vagina as well as the cervix. It is made in three sizes, which are size 1 (small; 45 mm), size 2 (medium; 48 mm), and size 3 (large; 51 mm).

Method of use   Spermicide must be placed inside the dome before fitting. The timings for insertion, reapplication of spermicide, and cleaning are the same as for diaphragms (*see above*). Spermicide must not be placed on the rim, as its presence may reduce suction. It is generally recommended that cervical caps should not be left in the vagina for longer than 30 hours. This timing allows for 24 hours of use, plus the six hours recommended before removal after last intercourse. If more than three hours elapse between insertion and sexual intercourse, further spermicide must be used.

Spermicides

Spermicides should not be recommended as a sole method of contraception. They are primarily agents to be used with other forms of contraception (e.g. diaphragms, condoms, and coitus interruptus). Their use may also help to reduce the incidence of sexually transmitted diseases, and they may increase lubrication in the genital tract.

Types of spermicide   Spermicides are formulated as aerosol foams, creams, gels, pessaries, soluble films, and in sponges. The creams and gels liquify at body temperature and are rapidly distributed throughout the vagina. The foams are released from the pressurised container into an applicator which is inserted into the vagina. Pessaries and films take longer to disperse and are possibly less effective than creams, gels, or aerosol foams. The most commonly used spermicide is nonoxynol-9 (used in varying concentrations); others include *p*-di-isobutylphenoxypolyethoxyethanol and octoxynol.

Mode of action   Spermicides are surfactants that inhibit the uptake of oxygen by the sperm, reduce cell-wall surface tension, and can alter the osmotic balance between sperm and their external environment. The viscosity of the inert basis may also prevent the progress of sperm.

Method of use   Products are normally inserted as high as possible into the vagina just before intercourse, although pessaries and foaming tablets should be inserted at least 10 minutes before.

The sponge   The vaginal contraceptive sponge (Fig. 4.6) is a more elegant presentation of a spermicide, and may be more acceptable to some women as it is less messy than other formulations. The sponge is about

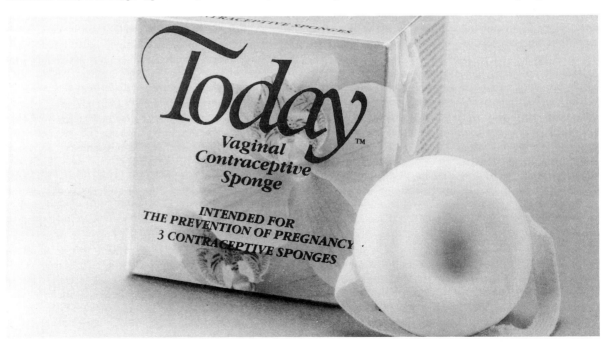

Fig. 4.6
Contraceptive sponge.

2.5 cm thick and 5.5 cm in diameter and is made of soft polyurethane foam impregnated with nonoxynol-9. There are widely varying estimates of contraceptive effectiveness from different studies although it is generally agreed that this is not a method to be used if prevention of pregnancy is absolutely essential. The sponge may be used by women who are spacing their pregnancies, during breast-feeding, around the menopause, or as an additional method.

One side of the sponge is shaped as a concave disc and this depression should be located over the cervix. Immediately before insertion into the vagina the spermicide should be activated by thoroughly wetting the sponge with water and then squeezing it until it foams. Intercourse can take place as often as desired during the 24 hours after insertion but the sponge must remain in position for at least six hours after the last act; the total time that it is in the vagina should not exceed 30 hours. After extraction by pulling by the integral loop, the sponge should be discarded. The sponge should not be used during menstruation because a small risk of toxic shock syndrome has been reported with its use.

4.5 EMERGENCY CONTRACEPTION

Most requests for emergency or post-coital contraception arise because intercourse has taken place without any form of contraceptive cover. This may include requests from women subjected to rape or from those undergoing treatment with potentially teratogenic agents (e.g. cytotoxic drugs and live vaccines) who have had unprotected intercourse. Other reasons for seeking emergency contraception include: loss of contraceptive cover caused by a damaged or displaced condom or diaphragm; failure of compliance with administration of oral contraceptives; or miscalculations in using natural family planning methods.

Historically, emergency contraception has consisted of attempts to flush out the contents of the vagina (e.g. using douches) to prevent sperm from reaching the cervix. However, this is invariably ineffective because sperm can reach the cervix in as little as 90 seconds; douching can even be harmful. More recently, two methods of emergency contraception have gained popularity: the hormonal or Yuzpe method and insertion of an IUD.

Emergency contraception is intended to prevent implantation of a fertilised ovum in the uterus. Conception can occur if sexual intercourse takes place any time between days 9 and 17 of a 28-day cycle (see Section 4.1). In theory, therefore, the use of emergency

contraception should only be necessary for a limited timespan each month. In practice, however, the irregularity of many menstrual cycles makes it impossible to give definitive statements about when emergency contraception may be required. If there is any doubt about dates within the cycle, emergency contraception should be used.

Following treatment with an emergency contraceptive, women are requested to return to the doctor or family planning clinic after three weeks, or earlier in the event of any untoward symptoms. Follow-up permits the absence of pregnancy to be confirmed as well as contraceptive counselling.

It has been estimated that there is about a 1 in 3 chance of conception if intercourse takes place immediately before ovulation, but of those ova that become fertilised, at least 1 in 3 will fail to implant naturally. Implantation is a continuous process that is usually completed by 7 to 10 days. Any agent administered after implantation for the purposes of preventing pregnancy is termed a medical abortifacient, not a contraceptive.

Hormonal method

Although oestrogen-only and progestogen-only regimens have previously been used, combinations of the two agents are now recommended. The failure rate of hormonal emergency contraception is low; pregnancy occurs in about 1 to 4% of women.

Mode of action The changes produced by the hormonal method depend upon the timing of administration during the menstrual cycle. If dosage is given sufficiently early in the cycle, ovulation may be prevented. Equally, however, ovulation may only be delayed and it is vital that a barrier contraceptive (see Section 4.4) is used during any future intercourse up to the time of the next menstrual period. Hormonal emergency contraception tends to cause an earlier than anticipated start to this subsequent menstruation.

Administration at the time of, or immediately after, ovulation produces local tissue changes and disturbs the phased changes in the endometrium. This renders the local environment inhospitable to the ovum should it become fertilised and prevents implantation. Specific mechanisms of this effect are uncertain but possible factors in preventing implantation include: blocking local oestrogen and progesterone receptors; disrupting the functions of the corpus luteum; interfering with the transportation of the ovum from the ovaries to the Fallopian tubes; and a direct action on the fertilised ovum.

Dosage and administration   Two tablets, each containing ethinyloestradiol 50 μg and levonorgestrel 250 μg, should be taken within 72 hours of having intercourse, followed by a further two tablets 12 hours later.

The high dose of oestrogen produces nausea in 2 out of 3 women and vomiting in one-third. If vomiting occurs within 2 to 3 hours of administration, the complete treatment regimen may have to be restarted. The addition of an anti-emetic to the regimen may help to prevent vomiting.

The most common reasons for failure of hormonal emergency contraception include: delayed start to dosage; repetition of unprotected sexual intercourse; failure to complete the course as a result of poor compliance; or a sub-therapeutic plasma concentration of the hormones caused by vomiting.

Adverse effects   The primary risk associated with hormonal emergency contraception is the potential for harmful effects on the fertilised ovum should contraception fail. There is a small, but statistically unproven, potential for high-dose oestrogens and progestogens to produce congenital malformations; ectopic pregnancy is also a possibility. However, such risks are normally thought to be considerably outweighed by the benefits of emergency contraception in preventing unwanted pregnancies. This method is not appropriate as a regular form of contraception.

Contra-indications   Contra-indications to the use of hormonal emergency contraception include pregnancy, unprotected intercourse on several occasions during the same cycle, and any condition for which oestrogen therapy is not recommended (e.g. thromboembolism).

Intra-uterine devices

The IUD method of emergency contraception should be used when: there is an absolute contra-indication to the use of oestrogens; intercourse occurred within five days previously; unprotected intercourse took place on several occasions during the same cycle; or tablets taken with the hormonal method have been vomited.

An IUD can be inserted to act as an emergency contraceptive up to five days after the expected date of ovulation (i.e. if intercourse occurs on day eight, an IUD may be inserted any time up to day 21 of a regular 28-day menstrual cycle). Bioactive IUDs are effective and the failure rate has been shown to be low. The mode of action and range of complications in the use of IUDs as emergency contraceptives are the same as in their more common use as regular contraceptives (*see* Section 4.3).

The main advantage of their use over hormonal emergency contraception is that, when in position, IUDs provide continued contraceptive cover.

Contra-indications to insertion of an IUD include: pregnancy; recent pelvic inflammatory disease; and a history of ectopic pregnancy.

4.6   ALTERNATIVE METHODS OF CONTRACEPTION

Coitus interruptus

Coitus interruptus (withdrawal method) is one of the oldest methods of contraception. It involves removing the penis from the vagina immediately before ejaculation. The method therefore requires considerable self-control and discipline at a time when sexual arousal is at its height. Despite considerable adverse criticism for many years, particularly about the lack of 'completeness' of the sexual experience that coitus interruptus is said to produce, it can be effective and its use is clearly without harmful adverse effects. The failure rate of the method has been estimated as between 5 and 20 pregnancies per 100 woman years.

Failure of the method may be particularly high in inexperienced couples. One of the major problems is the lack of recognition that only small quantities of seminal fluid can contain sufficient sperm for conception to take place (*see* Section 4.1), and that any delay in withdrawal of the penis may lead to the leakage of small amounts of seminal fluid immediately before the onset of ejaculation.

Greater confidence in the use of coitus interruptus may be possible if spermicides are also used. However, this may be unacceptable to people from certain ethnic and religious backgrounds.

Natural family planning

Natural family planning is a method for achieving or avoiding pregnancy by observation of the natural signs and symptoms of the fertile and infertile phases of the menstrual cycle.

Each of the methods of natural family planning is based upon the detection of changes in indicators that occur naturally during the course of the menstrual cycle.

Natural family planning may be regarded as the most acceptable form of contraception by couples who wish to feel in control of their own fertility. It may also be an advantageous method for those who are concerned about the use of appliances or drugs in controlling fertility, and for others who may not be allowed to use other forms of contraception for religious or ethical reasons. However, it must be clearly understood that a high degree of motivation and self-control is vital to ensure that intercourse is restricted to those times during each cycle when it is certain that there is no risk of conception. Women using this form of contraception must possess a reasonable understanding of the menstrual and ovarian cycles (*see* Section 4.1) and require adequate teaching.

Basal body temperature method   In this method, the body temperature is recorded throughout the menstrual cycle. Temperatures are measured with a fertility thermometer, which is calibrated between 35 and 39°C at 0.1°C intervals. Readings should be taken every day as soon as waking up, before getting out of bed, and before drinking any hot fluids. Temperatures can be taken via the oral, rectal, or vaginal routes, but whichever method is chosen it should be used consistently and the thermometer should remain in position for 3 to 5 minutes. Temperatures are recorded on specially designed charts, and a clear increase in temperature of between 0.2 and 0.4°C can usually be seen about 12 to 16 days before the next period. This rise corresponds to the increased release of progesterone occurring after ovulation. Users of this method should clearly understand, however, that the infertile phase does not begin until three raised temperatures have been recorded above six previous lower recordings (excluding days 1 to 4), and is maintained until the onset of the next menses. Following this peak, unprotected intercourse can take place until the next menses.

The main difficulty in using this method arises because of natural fluctuations in body temperature. Increased temperatures can occur as a result of a mild infection (e.g. the common cold) or from drinking alcohol the previous night; reduced temperatures may follow administration of aspirin. One further difficulty is that there is no sustained temperature rise (i.e. indicating the end of the fertile phase) in an anovulatory cycle, which is paradoxically an infertile cycle throughout.

The cervical mucus method   The cervical mucus method (Billings method or ovulation method) is based upon the physical changes that occur in the cervical mucus during the menstrual cycle. Immediately after menstruation, the mucus forms a viscid, thick plug in the cervix, and the opening of the vagina and vulva appear dry. The presence of continually increasing concentrations of oestrogen leading up to ovulation produces gradual and detectable changes in the consistency of cervical mucus. On its initial detection in the cycle, the mucus is thick, sticky, and opaque; further

gradual changes occur in which the mucus becomes more copious, more slippery, less viscous, and then almost clear immediately before ovulation; the vulva is moist and wet. After the mid-cycle point, the mucus rapidly becomes cloudy again and then completely disappears or is virtually undetectable.

Mucus is observed on toilet paper at micturition. The time when the maximum amount of mucus is detected closely correlates with peak plasma-oestrogen concentration. At this stage, the mucus is often described as stretchy and slippery. To be an effective contraceptive method, intercourse should be avoided on the days between initial detection of mucus and four days after the peak mucus day is detected.

As in the case of the basal body temperature method, unrelated factors may modify the accuracy of the cervical mucus method. Vaginal candidiasis and drugs used in its treatment may reduce cervical secretions at the mid-cycle point, which may make accurate assessment of the occurrence of ovulation difficult.

The calendar method   Terms formerly used to describe this method includes the 'rhythm' or 'safe period'. The infertile and fertile phases of the cycle have already been described (*see* Section 4.1). The length of the period between ovulation and the end of the menstrual cycle has been shown to be relatively constant at about 14 days (range 12 to 16 days), and this forms the basis of the calendar method. A high degree of motivation is necessary if this method is to be successful as it requires a record of the length of menstrual cycles to be kept over at least a six month period, and preferably over 12-months. The period of highest risk of conception for all subsequent cycles falls between 19 days from the end of the shortest cycle and ten days before the end of the longest cycle.

For the calendar method to be effective, intercourse should be avoided between these days. The calender method is not recommended as the sole indicator for predicting the infertile and fertile phases of the menstrual cycle.

Symptothermal method   This uses a combination of basal body temperature monitoring and assessment of cervical mucus, plus several other indices which, with practice, women can use to detect ovulation. The most important of these additional indices is the determination of the position and firmness of the cervix, and the extent to which it is open. During the days immediately before ovulation, the cervix becomes softer to the touch and higher in position, and the cervical opening becomes wider. After ovulation, it descends, becomes firmer to the touch, and the opening becomes smaller.

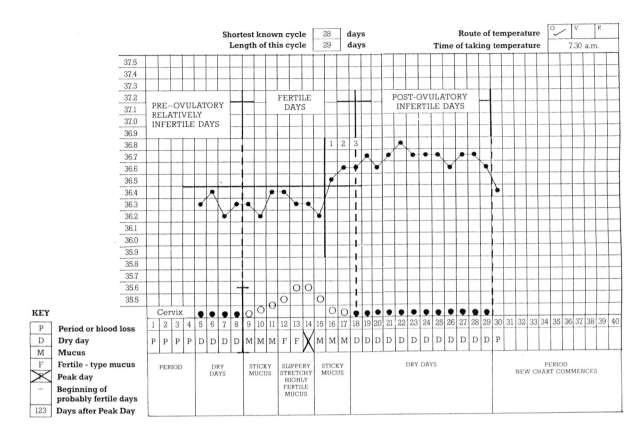

| | | Shortest known cycle | 28 | days | | | | Route of temperature | | O | ✓ | V | | R | |
| | | Length of this cycle | 29 | days | | | | Time of taking temperature | | | 7.30 a.m. | | | |

Fig. 4.7
Example of a symptothermal chart.

Charts are available to record the combination of characteristics used in this method (Fig. 4.7). Symptothermal methods must be taught by those who are experienced in their use, and interpretation of the indices must be carefully explained. If results from the different methods conflict, the results that indicate the latest date for the start of the infertile phase should be used.

Sterilisation

Sterilisation is one of the most effective methods of contraception and is usually irreversible. It is primarily selected by couples who have completed their family or, less commonly, for those who know that they will never want to have children. The average age at which sterilisation is selected as a means of contraception is falling. The number of vasectomy operations carried out has increased since they became available in the UK under the National Health Service in 1972.

Surgical male sterilisation is carried out to stop the passage of the sperm along the vas deferens. Female sterilisation by surgical techniques is carried out to stop the passage of the ovum along the Fallopian tubes. Normally, neither procedure affects the production of male and female hormones responsible for secondary sexual characteristics. The failure rate of vasectomy has been reported to be extremely low (0.02 pregnancies per 100 woman years, equivalent to 2 in 10 000). Failure rates of between 0.1 and 3 pregnancies per 100 woman years have been reported for female sterilisation although the true figure is likely to be nearer one pregnancy per 100 woman years. Some of the pregnancies that occur immediately after female sterilisation may be the result of a fertilised ovum present before the operation.

Male sterilisation is easy to carry out and involves minimal disruption to work or social activities. Female sterilisation takes longer to recover from, especially when carried out by laparotomy. However, female sterilisation is effective immediately, whereas it takes up to four months to confirm that male sterility has been achieved.

The importance to each partner of undergoing sterilisation must be discussed and stressed before surgery. Although the partner's consent is not required, it is clearly more desirable for both individuals to agree to the need for, and the objective of, sterilisation.

Male sterilisation   A vasectomy can be carried out under local or general anaesthetic. Surgery involves making a small incision in the upper portion of the scrotum and exposing the vas deferens, which carry sperm from the testes to the penis. Each vas deferens is cut and the cut ends ligated. Alternatively a small portion of each tube may be removed and the cut ends replaced in different planes of the scrotal fascial tissue.

After surgery, scrotal swelling, bruising, and discomfort will invariably occur. It is normally recommended that a scrotal support or tight-fitting underpants are worn during the day and at night for seven days after surgery, and heavy manual work should be avoided for up to three days. It is essential that men undergoing vasectomy are advised that the contraceptive effect does not develop immediately because of the presence of residual sperm in the distal portion of each vas deferens. Samples of seminal fluid are taken 12 weeks and 16 weeks after surgery to confirm the absence of sperm. Before confirmation of zero sperm counts, other forms of contraceptive cover must be maintained.

Various claims have been made for the reversibility of vasectomy. Although the surgical technique is relatively simple, fertility after vasectomy may be reduced in up to one-third of men because of the production of antibodies to sperm. Further reasons for lack of reversibility include: the formation of scar tissue around the anastomosed vas deferens, which may act as a physical barrier to the passage of sperm; and immunological reactions developing at the site of accumulation of sperm, leading to their gradual destruction.

Female sterilisation   Blockage of the Fallopian tubes can be performed by laparotomy or, more commonly, by the less invasive technique, laparoscopy.

Laparotomy is carried out under general anaesthetic and requires an incision of 5 to 8 cm in the abdominal wall. Subsequently, the Fallopian tubes may be tied and cut (tubal ligation); they may be occluded by using clips or bands; or they may be sealed by heat treatment (diathermy). Minilaparotomy involves a much smaller incision and permits a more rapid recovery, allowing

patients to return home within 1 to 2 days.

Laparoscopy is performed by inserting a fibre-optic tube, sometimes under local anaesthetic supplemented by analgesics, although general anaesthetic is more commonly used. The peritoneal cavity is inflated by gas and the tube is inserted through the abdominal wall to observe the Fallopian tubes. Occlusion of the tubes is carried out with clips or bands, or by diathermy. Recovery time is very short, with many women able to return home on the same day as surgery is carried out.

Rest is recommended for the first two days after surgery, with full activity resumed within one week for laparoscopy and within three weeks for minilaparotomy. A longer period of rest is usually required after laparotomy. The only after-effect sometimes reported is the development of menorrhagia. If sterilisation does fail as a method of contraception, there is a higher risk that the pregnancy will be ectopic.

4.7 CONTRACEPTIVE SERVICES

Pharmacists play an important part in providing contraceptive products and giving advice about contraception. However, this role must be considered within the context of the other family planning services. Widespread contraceptive services in the UK, even after the inception of the NHS in 1948, were primarily provided by voluntary organisations (e.g. the Family Planning Association). In the 1940s and 1950s, clinics run by voluntary organisations were predominantly used by married women. However, in the 1960s, changes in attitudes brought about by the development of hormonal contraception and the use of more effective IUDs led to increased demands for contraceptive services by both married and single women. Provision of free contraception for many women in the UK was first provided by the NHS (Family Planning) Act 1967. An expanded and completely free service was implemented following the NHS Reorganisation Act 1973. Since that time, free family planning has been available from hospitals, family planning clinics, and general practitioners from 1975. Further family planning needs that cannot be satisfied from these services are met by voluntary organisations, which are partially funded by government grants.

Primary contraceptive services

General practitioner family planning services   General practitioner family planning services attract most of the women seeking contraceptive products, advice on contraception, or both, and over 95% of doctors are registered to provide this service. (Those doctors who provide this service are denoted by a 'C' after their names in the Family Practitioner Service Authority lists.) However, not all general practitioners are trained to fit IUDs, diaphragms, or caps. Contraceptives that can be prescribed in the UK are exempt from prescription charges.

Family planning clinics   Family planning clinics usually provide a more comprehensive service than that provided by general practitioners, and tend to offer more alternatives to the supply of oral contraceptives. In addition to providing the contraceptive products described in this Chapter, other services available include well woman clinics and screening procedures, and advice on sex and relationships, menstrual problems, infertility, and sterilisation. Many of the staff in family planning clinics are specifically trained for their advisory role. Moreover, all contraceptive devices, including condoms, are supplied free of charge.

Referrals are made from general practitioner services and family planning clinics to NHS hospitals for male and female sterilisation. However, many of these operations are now carried out by voluntary or private organisations because of long waiting lists, although patients usually have to pay for these services.

Family Planning Association   Information on contraceptive methods and services in the UK can be obtained from the Family Planning Association (FPA). Pharmacists can also approach the local health education unit for information. The FPA produces literature, has an information and research centre, and operates a nationwide enquiry service for consumers and professionals.

The role of the pharmacist

For many years the medical profession disdained any association with contraception or contraceptive products, considering them to be a less than respectable form of medical treatment. The comprehensive involvement of the medical profession in contraception only resulted from the advent of prescription-only hormonal methods of contraception developed in the late 1950s and early 1960s (*see* Section 4.2).

In the late 19th century, condoms were obtained from pharmacies and surgical stores, and these outlets were particularly popular with members of the public who wanted easy access to effective birth control methods. This is still true today and pharmacists, with their associated professional image, are ideal suppliers of contraceptive products. The link between contraception and a respected profession helped to overcome many of the early objections to the use of contraceptives. Today, pharmacists provide a much needed complementary service for those who do not wish to use the comprehensive range of contraceptive services provided by the general practitioner family planning services and family planning clinics.

There are several reasons why those seeking contraceptive products or advice choose not to use the primary care services: some women may be reluctant to see a male doctor; clinics may not be used because women may lack awareness of their availability or location; there may be difficulties in transport to and from clinics; and frustration may occur at having to conform to an appointments system.

Advantages of pharmacists as suppliers of contraceptive products and a source of advice include: widespread locations allowing ease of accessibility to the majority of the population; availability for up to 6 days a week; anonymity of the pharmacist-client relationship; and no requirement for an appointment. Moreover, once contact has been established, the pharmacist can act as a source of information about the availability of local family planning services.

The pharmacy may also be an ideal place for helping men develop awareness of their responsibilities in contraception. The current non-availability of condoms on prescription means that men will not usually seek advice from their doctors about contraceptive methods. The display of leaflets and products in the non-threatening environment of the pharmacy may encourage inexperienced or shy men and women to seek advice. A display of family planning leaflets can be ideally complemented by a clear statement that contraceptive advice can be obtained from the pharmacist, the individual's doctor, or the local family planning clinic; the address of the local family planning clinic should also be displayed.

4.8 USEFUL ADDRESSES

BIRTH CONTROL TRUST
27–35 Mortimer Street
London W1N 7RJ
Tel: 071-580 9360

BRITISH PREGNANCY ADVISORY SERVICE (BPAS)
Austy Manor
Wootton Wawen
Solihull
West Midlands B95 6BX
Tel: (0564) 793225

BROOK ADVISORY CENTRES
153a East Street
London SE17 2SD
Tel: 071-708 1234

CATHOLIC MARRIAGE ADVISORY COUNCIL
Clitherow House
1 Blythe Mews
Blythe Road
London W14 0NW
Tel: 071-371 1341

FAMILY PLANNING ASSOCIATION
27–35 Mortimer Street
London W1N 7RJ
Tel: 071-636 7866

INTERNATIONAL PLANNED PARENTHOOD
FEDERATION (IPPF)
Regent's College
Inner Circle
Regent's Park
London NW1 4NS
Tel: 071-486 0741

IRISH FAMILY PLANNING ASSOCIATION (IFPA)
15 Mountjoy Square
Dublin 1
Ireland
Tel: (010 353 1) 740723

MARGARET PYKE CENTRE FOR STUDY AND
TRAINING IN FAMILY PLANNING (Bloomsbury and
Islington Health Authority)
15 Bateman's Buildings
Soho Square
London W1V 5TW
Tel: 071-734 9351

MARIE STOPES WOMEN'S HEALTH CLINICS
Marie Stopes House
108 Whitfield Street
London W1P 6BE
Tel: 071-388 0662/2585

PREGNANCY ADVISORY SERVICE
11–13 Charlotte Street
London W1P 1HD
Tel: 071-637 8962

SPOD
The Association to Aid the Sexual and Personal Relationships
of the Disabled
286 Camden Road
London N7 0BJ
Tel: 071-607 8851

4.9 FURTHER READING

Clubb E, Knight J. *Fertility. A comprehensive guide to natural family planning.* Newton Abbot: David & Charles, 1988.
DoH. *Handbook of contraceptive practice.* London: HMSO, 1990.
Drife JO. What proportion of pregnancies are spontaneously aborted? *Br Med J* 1983;286: 294.
Guillebaud J. *Contraception. Your questions answered.* Edinburgh: Churchill Livingstone, 1986.
Guillebaud J. *The pill.* 4th ed. Oxford: Oxford University Press, 1991.
Loudon N, ed. *Handbook of family planning.* 2nd ed. Edinburgh: Churchill Livingstone, 1991.
Robertson WH. *An illustrated history of contraception. A concise account of the quest for fertility control.* Carnforth: The Parthenon Publishing Group, 1990.
WHO. *Barrier contraceptives and spermicides. Their role in family planning care.* Geneva: WHO, 1988.
WHO. *Injectable contraceptives. Their role in family planning care.* Geneva: WHO, 1990.
WHO. Mechanism of action, safety and efficacy of intrauterine devices. *WHO Tech Rep Ser 753* 1987.

Chapter 5

SMOKING

5.1 INTRODUCTION

Tobacco smoking is the largest preventable cause of disease and premature death in Europe. Smoking was originally promoted as a recreational habit, which conferred pleasure and was associated with confidence, relaxation, and social acceptability. This has changed, and smoking is now considered to be a form of drug dependence, which is hazardous to health and anti-social. In the trend towards greater personal responsibility for health, giving up smoking or, more importantly, not starting to smoke, are among the most positive steps that can be taken towards improving or maintaining health. This attitude has become widespread primarily as a result of awareness of the adverse effects on personal health, the addictive properties of nicotine, and the implications of passive smoking.

This awareness has contributed to the growing trend towards establishing non-smoking as the social norm. Smoking is harmful whether 6 or 60 cigarettes are smoked a day and, ideally, the aim of all smokers should be to stop completely. This goal is unlike the aims of other forms of health education (e.g. alcohol use and dietary management), which recommend modifications to achieve a safe and enjoyable life-style.

Both smokers and non-smokers are becoming increasingly aware of the health risks associated with passive smoking. Non-smokers now view passive smoking as much more than a minor irritation and this has led to a greater demand for protection, especially in public places (e.g. on public transport, at work, and in restaurants).

In the UK, the annual cost of smoking to the health service has been estimated to be £500 million. Smoking-related diseases account for considerable morbidity and mortality, as illustrated by the following estimates of the consequences of smoking:

- 100 000 deaths annually (approximately 300 daily)
- 33% of deaths in middle-age
- 90% of deaths caused by bronchitis, chronic obstructive airways disease, and related illness
- 90% of deaths caused by lung cancer
- 20% of deaths caused by heart disease
- more than 30 million days lost at work annually.

The World Health Organization (WHO) Regional Office for Europe has estimated that between 1980 and the year 2000, 10 million people in its region are at risk of dying from smoking-related diseases. The WHO has encouraged member states to set a minimum target of non-smokers (e.g. 80% of the population) within a given time (e.g. by 1995).

Smoking tobacco was found to be a habit of natives of North and South America by European explorers in the late 1400s, with methods of use including cigar smoking (leaves rolled-up), in pipes, and snuff (powdered leaves). Tobacco was subsequently introduced into mainland Europe in 1519. It was claimed to have powerful healing properties and was used in the treatment of many diseases (e.g. asthma, gout, scabies, and even cancer).

Tobacco was introduced into England in 1565 by colonists from Virginia; the dubious distinction for its popularisation in court circles is credited to Sir Walter Raleigh. The preferred method of use in England was in pipes. The first well known person to warn against the dangers of tobacco was King James I, but he fought a losing battle against its use. Despite harsh penalties for its use in some countries (e.g. smokers were beheaded in Turkey whereas in Russia they were flogged and exiled to Siberia), tobacco use continued to spread. It was quickly realised by many countries that substantial revenue could be obtained from taxation. In England, tobacco revenue financed the English merchant navy and played a major part in the development of English colonies in North America. During the 18th century tobacco use spread world-wide.

Americans were known to smoke tobacco wrapped in paper tubes. These forerunners of the first cigarettes were introduced into England in 1854, and made smoking easier, cheaper, and widely available. The first cigarette-making machine, patented in America in 1881, was capable of making 200 cigarettes a minute (this compares with machines today that can make more than 5000 cigarettes a minute). This marked the beginning of the mass proliferation of smoking.

The USA is the largest producer of tobacco products; Brazil, India, and Malawi are also producers. In some countries the tobacco industry provides agricultural advice, credit, and a guaranteed price for the product, whereas; equivalent support for other agricultural products is usually absent. The world-wide supply of tobacco products is dominated by a small number of large, integrated multinational companies who are involved in all aspects of production (leaf purchasing, manufacture, and sale of products).

5.2 SMOKING PREVALENCE, TRENDS, AND BEHAVIOUR

The steady decline in smoking prevalence in the early 1980s means that smokers are now in a minority in all groups (e.g. by age, occupation, and social status). However, the rate of decline in cigarette smoking appears to have lessened. There are numerous factors that could account for this apparent slowing in the rate of decline, including a lack of appropriate information or the information is targeted at the wrong groups. However, one of the most important reasons for the reduced rate of decline in prevalence is that tobacco possesses potent psychoactive properties. Moreover, smokers generally have less regard for health issues than non-smokers and are less responsive to all forms of health education. Hence, some smokers continue to smoke despite all efforts to inform and educate, often citing irrational and illogical reasons for continuing (e.g. 'my father smoked until 80 years of age' or 'I could be run over by a bus tomorrow'). These hardened smokers will probably never abstain from smoking. There are others who are severely addicted, or who have been smoking heavily for many years, and who find it extremely difficult to give up. The predominant social and occupational environment of smokers is also important in achieving effective education. If smoking is widely accepted at home and at work, the responsiveness to health education and the motivation to give up smoking will be low.

The prevalence of cigarette smoking is much higher in manual occupational groups compared to non-manual occupational groups. This difference indicates that cigarette smoking may be influenced by educational standards and that people in non-manual occupations may generally be more responsive to health education. Differences are also seen between the numbers of men and women in each of these groups of smokers. There is little difference in cigarette smoking between men and women in the non-manual group but a larger difference in the manual group, in which more men smoke.

Prevalence of smoking among children

In England and Wales, there is a disturbing prevalence of cigarette smoking among schoolchildren. Studies have revealed that most current adult smokers began the habit before 18 years of age. It has been estimated that 14% of children of 11 years of age have experimented with cigarettes. From 13 years of age, more girls than boys smoke, although boys smoke a greater number of cigarettes than girls. To obtain such information, however, it should be recognised that there may be substantial under-reporting or failure to supply saliva samples for analysis. The actual prevalence of smoking among schoolchildren may, therefore, be higher.

Legislation governing the sale of cigarettes to children exists in the UK. It is illegal under the Protection of Children (Tobacco) Act 1986, to supply any tobacco product to children under 16 years of age. However, a survey in England showed that in 1988 only 27% of children attempting to purchase cigarettes were unsuccessful. Retailers were more likely to refuse sale to younger children (11 to 12 years of age) than to older children (15 years of age).

The reasons why children start to smoke and, more importantly, continue to smoke are discussed under Smoking behaviour, below.

External influences on the prevalence of smoking

The prevalence of smoking is influenced externally by tobacco taxation (and hence price), personal disposable income, and tobacco advertising. Cigarettes are heavily taxed and the impact of taxation on the prevalence of smoking has been clearly demonstrated. Over 70% of the cost of cigarettes is direct taxation. Following a price increase of 10% through increased taxation, a reduction of about 5% in the prevalence of smoking can be expected. A high price for cigarettes will therefore reduce the prevalence of smoking and, more importantly, will deter children from starting an expensive habit.

However, this method of reducing the prevalence of smoking has not been fully utilised. In the UK, the price of cigarettes has not kept pace with the increased personal disposable income and purchasing power, and generally a lower proportion of income is required to sustain the smoking habit. The reasons cited against imposing high taxes on tobacco are not compelling, despite the powerful business and political interests of the tobacco industry. Arguments and their counter arguments include: there will be loss of government revenue in the short term, but this should be compensated by increased spending on other goods using the money saved from not buying cigarettes; there may be loss of jobs in the tobacco industry, but as tobacco industries are already diversifying into other products and services, job losses should be minimal.

The role of tobacco advertising in influencing the prevalence of smoking is debatable. Tobacco manufacturers claim that advertising establishes brand loyalty and does not influence the prevalence of smoking. Manufacturers in the UK spend an estimated £100 million annually on advertising and sponsorship.

Health experts claim that this influences the prevalence of smoking through indirect mechanisms. All forms of advertising and sponsorship maintain the social acceptability of smoking, counteract the effects of health education, and encourage smokers to increase their tobacco use. Advertising takes many forms, including sports sponsorship, travel sponsorship, advertising posters, branded clothing, magazine advertising, and leisure promotions.

Advertising may be one of the reinforcing factors involved in the continuation of smoking by young people. It has, therefore, been widely stated that advertising of tobacco products needs to be more tightly controlled or banned altogether.

Smoking behaviour

Smoking is generally started in childhood. It is clear that children do not start smoking for its psychological effects and perhaps do not even know what they are. It is only once they are addicted that the psychological benefits (e.g. arousal and mood control) become apparent, especially when trying to give up. Children who begin smoking are almost invariably exposed to the habit in their home or leisure environment. Commonly their parents, older siblings, or relatives are smokers. The influence and pressure from peer groups is also critical.

The effects of starting smoking are extremely unpleasant and include nausea and dizziness. However, despite these unpleasant effects, people continue to smoke, primarily as a result of reinforcing factors (Table 5.1). Nicotine addiction quickly develops and the pleasurable and psychological benefits aid the rapid establishment of smoking.

Table 5.1
Reinforcing factors influencing the continuation of smoking

Reinforcing factor	Mechanism
Nicotine addiction	alleviation of nicotine withdrawal symptoms
Pleasure	pleasure of smoking or the enhancement of other pleasure activities (e.g. alcohol consumption)
Psychological	lowers the levels of anxiety, emotional disturbances, and aggression
Stimulation	improvement in concentration, attention, and memory; increased confidence and improved long-term memory
Weight control	appetite suppression and loss of weight; avoidance of weight gain

The plasma-nicotine concentration in smokers is critical. Over-smoking will result in unacceptable toxic effects; too low a concentration will not achieve the desired pleasurable effects and withdrawal symptoms may also develop. The act of smoking is manipulated to achieve the desired concentration of nicotine by altering parameters that influence its intake and absorption. These include:

- concentration of smoke/air (dilution)
- inhalation depth
- number of cigarettes smoked
- puffing intensity
- puffing rate
- volume of inhaled smoke.

The nicotine content of the tobacco within a cigarette or the nicotine yield of a complete cigarette is not a reliable measure of the nicotine intake by a smoker. This also applies to the other tobacco constituents. To achieve a higher nicotine dose from a low nicotine yield cigarette, some of the above factors can be manipulated by the smoker (e.g. increase in puffing rate or the number of cigarettes smoked). This is referred to as compensatory smoking. Hence smoking fewer cigarettes does not necessarily mean a reduction in the dose of nicotine or other constituents as compensatory smoking may increase these to previous levels.

5.3   TOBACCO

Tobacco is manufactured in many forms and quality grades from the tobacco plants, *Nicotiana tabacum* and *N. rustica*. The leaves are cured (dried) using a range of methods (e.g. air-curing, flue-curing, and sun-curing), each producing a specific grade and quality of tobacco. Air-curing consists of drying the tobacco leaves by exposure only to air; flue-curing consists of the application of hot air. Following curing, tobacco leaves are further conditioned, resulting in tobacco that yields smoke mild enough to inhale. All grades of tobacco have different properties and the grades are selectively used to make different tobacco products (e.g. pipe tobacco, cigars, or cigarettes).

All tobacco products are designed to facilitate nicotine absorption. Cigarette smoke is acidic and contains nicotine in its ionised form, resulting in its rapid absorption from the lungs. There is negligible, if any, buccal absorption. Cigar and pipe smoke is alkaline and contains nicotine in an unionised form, resulting in good buccal absorption. Nicotine inhaled from cigar and pipe smoke is also rapidly absorbed from the lungs.

Tobacco that is chewed, snuff, and nicotine chewing gum are all buffered to an alkaline pH to facilitate absorption of nicotine.

Oral snuff was used in a small sachet held between the gum and cheek (snuff dipping). Its use was linked to oral and malignant disease, especially cancer of the mouth, and the sale of such products is banned in the UK.

Cigarettes

Cigarette tobacco consists of a blend of different grades of tobacco to ensure consistency of the product. A large number of additives are permitted and are selectively added to the tobacco and the paper to modify cigarette characteristics (e.g. flavour, smell, and burning profile). Most cigarettes also incorporate a filter. Filters were initially introduced to reduce tobacco wastage in the unsmoked portion and to improve appeal to women who were thought not to like soggy cigarette ends. Improved filter technology has made the largest contribution towards lowering the amount of tar inhaled during smoking (*see below*). The tar content per cigarette, which is the quantity inhaled by the smoker, is graded and printed on the cigarette pack (Table 5.2).

'Safer' cigarettes are those with a low tar grading. There has been a gradual decline in the yield of tobacco constituents, especially tar, from cigarettes. Although the quantity of inhaled tar has been reduced there has been no change in the tobacco itself. Factors that have led to greater use of reduced tar products include:

- greater public awareness of the health risks of smoking (especially from higher tar cigarettes)
- improved manufacturing methods
- introduction of filters
- introduction of ventilation holes in filters (certain low tar brands)
- legislation requiring the labelling of tar content on cigarette packs, thereby providing manufacturers with an incentive to reduce tar content to appeal to smokers wishing to switch to low tar brands.

Generally, low tar cigarettes pose a reduced health risk compared to high tar cigarettes. They may also help smokers to eventually give up after changing from high

Table 5.2
Tar yield bands for cigarettes (from 1 January 1985)

Low tar	less than 10 mg/cigarette
Low to middle tar	above 10 mg but less than 15 mg
Middle tar	above 15 mg but less than 18 mg
High tar	18 mg and over

tar to low tar brands. Nevertheless, it should be emphasised that low tar cigarettes are still hazardous to health, despite some smokers considering them to be completely safe. A further danger is that children may find it easier to start smoking these brands as a result of the diminution of the initial, extremely unpleasant, effects of first cigarettes (*see above*) and the false perception that these cigarettes are relatively harmless.

Tobacco smoke

There are more than 4000 compounds in tobacco smoke contained in two phases, the gaseous and particulate phases. Some of the constituents of tobacco smoke are listed in Table 5.3; the most important constituents are tar, carbon monoxide, and nicotine. The concentration of constituents inhaled by smokers from a cigarette depends on:

- brand of cigarette (e.g. low tar or high tar brand)
- cigarette length
- filter characteristics (efficiency of tar removal)
- paper characteristics (e.g. degree of porosity)
- packing density of tobacco
- smoking behaviour (*see* Section 5.2)
- temperature (rapid and prolonged drawing on the cigarette increases the temperature).

There are two types of smoke generated during tobacco use:

- Mainstream smoke

  This is smoke inhaled by the smoker. It is usually filtered and the lungs retain 85 to 99% of the particulate matter and approximately 55% of carbon monoxide.

- Sidestream smoke (environmental tobacco smoke)

  This is smoke emitted from smouldering tobacco that is produced from the burning end of a cigarette. It is greatly diluted by air but is unfiltered and contains a much higher concentration of all tobacco constituents. The particulate phase (containing tar and nicotine) is deposited primarily at the apex and central regions of the lungs.

The pattern of penetration into the lungs of the two phases of tobacco smoke may be different, although few studies have been performed to investigate this aspect further. The gaseous phase (containing carbon

Table 5.3
Some constituents of tobacco smoke

Gaseous phase	Particulate phase
Alcohols	Nicotine
Aldehydes	Tar
Ammonia	Water
Carbon monoxide	
Carbon dioxide	
Hydrocarbons	
Hydrogen cyanide	
Ketones	
Nitrogen oxides	
Nitrosamines	
Sulphur compounds	

monoxide) penetrates easily into the lungs (including the alveoli), allowing rapid absorption of constituents.

Carbon monoxide   Carbon monoxide is present in the gaseous phase of tobacco smoke. It is rapidly absorbed into the bloodstream and its high affinity for haemoglobin results in the formation of carboxyhaemoglobin. The oxygen-carrying capacity of haemoglobin is greatly reduced in the presence of carbon monoxide. The gradual accumulation leads to an increased plasma-carbon monoxide concentration in smokers throughout the day with each cigarette smoked. The maximum concentration is reached before bedtime; subsequently during the night, there is a gradual decline, but a residue often persists the following morning.

The precise consequences of inhaling carbon monoxide are difficult to determine. In healthy people there are apparently no noticeable effects because compensatory mechanisms operate to meet oxygen demands. However, in the presence of heart disease, these mechanisms may be insufficient to prevent myocardial hypoxia.

Tar   The particulate phase of tobacco smoke is composed almost entirely of tar droplets. Tar droplets consist of polycyclic hydrocarbons, of which over 1000 have been identified. The nicotine content of tobacco smoke is concentrated, with some moisture, in the tar droplets. The particle size of the tar droplets (0.1 to 1.0 μm) is small enough to penetrate to the alveoli, allowing rapid absorption of the nicotine within the droplets. Most of the remaining particulate matter (85 to 99%) is retained in the lungs.

Nicotine   Nicotine is the major constituent of the particulate phase of tobacco smoke and is rapidly absorbed following inhalation. It binds to acetylcholine receptors and readily crosses the blood-brain barrier. It undergoes rapid distribution throughout the brain,

Table 5.4
General effects of nicotine on body systems

Cardiovascular system	increased cardiac output
	increased cardiac stroke
	  volume
	increased coronary blood
	  flow
	increased heart rate
	peripheral vasoconstriction

Central nervous system	altered EEG pattern dizziness

Endocrine system	decreased oestrogen
	  concentration
	increased release of the
	  hormones:
	  adrenocorticotrophin
	  beta-endorphin
	  growth hormone
	  cortisol
	  prolactin
	  vasopressin

Musculoskeletal system	skeletal muscle relaxation

although concentrations in brain tissues decline quickly as distribution to other body tissues occurs. Nicotine also crosses the placenta freely and can be found in amniotic fluid and the umbilical cord. Low concentrations are found in breast milk, which may be a cause of infantile colic in some instances. The effects of nicotine on body systems (Table 5.4) are mediated predominantly through the central and peripheral nervous systems. Dopamine release is stimulated in the brain, together with adrenaline and noradrenaline release from the adrenal medulla. Catecholamine release is also stimulated from sympathetic nerves in blood vessels.

Nicotine undergoes rapid metabolism primarily in the liver. The main metabolic products are cotinine and nicotine-*N*-oxide, both of which are inactive. Cotinine is used as a marker to determine nicotine intake and hence smoking behaviour. Cotinine has a long half-life (10 to 20 hours) and can be measured in saliva, urine, and blood; it has also been detected in cervical mucus secretions. Some of the constituents of tobacco smoke can cause induction of microsomal liver enzymes, which enhance the metabolism of nicotine and its metabolites.

Smoking behaviour (*see* Section 5.2) is related to plasma-nicotine concentrations and cigarettes are smoked as necessary to produce the effects required by the smoker. However, smoking usually occurs intermittently throughout the day, causing frequent fluctuations in plasma-nicotine concentrations. Nicotine accumulates during the day and gradually declines during the night. There is often a residual plasma concentration in the morning.

5.4 SMOKING-RELATED DISEASES

The influence of smoking on disease and mortality is well established. Cigarettes constitute the most widespread form of tobacco use, and cigarette smoking is therefore the greatest cause of smoking-related diseases. The range and diversity of smoking-related diseases is constantly expanding as more evidence is gathered. A summary of diseases caused by, or exacerbated by, smoking is shown in Table 5.5. Precisely defined mechanisms responsible for smoking-related diseases are difficult to determine,

Table 5.5
Summary of diseases caused or exacerbated by smoking

Cardiovascular system disorders	Aortic aneurysm
	Arrhythmias
	Atherosclerosis
	Cerebrovascular disease
	  cerebral aneurysm
	  stroke
	  subarachnoid haemorrhage
	Hypertension
	Ischaemic heart disease
	  angina pectoris
	  myocardial infarction
	Migraine
	Peripheral vascular disease
	Thrombosis
	Transient ischaemic attacks

Eye disorders	Cataract Irritation and infection (contact lens wearers)
Gastro-intestinal disorders	Dyspepsia Peptic ulceration
Malignant disease	Cancer of the pharynx Cervical cancer Leukaemias Lung cancer Oesophageal cancer Oral cancer Pancreatic cancer Renal cell carcinoma
Obstetric disorders and effects on the foetus	Low birth-weight Pre-term delivery Spontaneous abortion Placental malfunction
Oral diseases	Aphthous stomatitis Gingivitis Glossitis Oral leucoplakia
Respiratory system disorders	Bronchiectasis Bronchitis (acute and chronic) Chronic obstructive airways disease Emphysema Pharyngitis Respiratory-tract infections Smoker's cough

usually as a result of the insidious development of the disease. However, many possible mechanisms have been proposed.

Data relating to the chronic health risks of modern, low tar cigarettes is limited, primarily because smoking-related diseases usually appear in the long-term (over 10 to 20 years). However, there is evidence that modern, low tar brands pose a reduced health risk when compared to traditional high tar (plain and unfiltered) cigarettes. Although the risks are still considerably higher than those of non-smokers, the risks of malignant disease (e.g. lung cancer, and cancer of the bladder, oesophagus, or pharynx) is reduced compared to smokers of high tar brands. There may also be a small reduced risk of respiratory system disorders, although there appears to be no similar beneficial effect on ischaemic heart disease and myocardial infarction.

Cardiovascular system disorders

Smoking is associated with a range of cardiovascular system disorders (see Table 5.5), which may be caused by the effects on haemostatic mechanisms. Nicotine and carbon monoxide are primarily involved in the mechanisms causing cardiovascular disease. Haemostasis may be disturbed by the following changes produced by nicotine and carbon monoxide, which have been observed in smokers:

- decreased prostacyclin concentration
- increased carboxyhaemoglobin concentration
- increased fibrinogen concentration
- increased concentration of free fatty acids
- increased plasma cell volume
- increased tendency towards platelet aggregation.

Nicotine has also been reported to damage blood-vessel endothelium directly. Reduced prostacyclin concentrations cause vasoconstriction and increased platelet aggregation.

Ischaemic heart disease   Ischaemic heart disease is the most important smoking-related disease. Other risk factors besides smoking (e.g. poor diet) also need to be taken into consideration in assessing overall risk of developing ischaemic heart disease. In pre-existing ischaemic heart disease, the role of smoking is more clearly established. Smoking causes an increase in the demands of heart muscle for oxygen, and this occurs in combination with a reduced oxygen-carrying capacity of the blood caused by the presence of carbon monoxide and the formation of carboxyhaemoglobin. Coronary blood-flow increases to meet this extra demand and, in

healthy people, this is a satisfactory compensatory mechanism. However, in the presence of ischaemic heart disease, this demand is not met and ischaemia leads to angina pectoris or myocardial infarction. Exercise tolerance in angina pectoris is reduced in smokers.

There are more deaths caused by smoking-related ischaemic heart disease than from any other smoking-related disease, including lung cancer. The increased risk of developing ischaemic heart disease reverts to almost normal within five years of giving up smoking. It has been estimated that mortality from myocardial infarction would be reduced by 25% if all smokers gave up. It is essential to give up smoking following myocardial infarction, and cessation is regarded as the most effective treatment and reduces the risk of further infarction. Smokers who do not give up carry a high risk of further myocardial infarction.

There is an age-related correlation between the risk of developing ischaemic heart disease and mortality rates from it; middle-aged smokers are at greatest risk. The difference in smoking prevalence between social and occupational groups (see Section 5.2) also reflects the risk of ischaemic heart disease within these groups. There is a substantially increased risk of ischaemic heart disease in manual workers compared to non-manual workers.

Hypertension   There is little difference in blood pressure between smokers and non-smokers, despite nicotine evoking an increase in blood pressure after smoking a single cigarette or following administration of test doses of nicotine to healthy non-smokers. In chronic smokers (who are also usually lean), the development of compensatory mechanisms stabilise these blood pressure increases.

In the presence of chronic hypertension, smoking increases the risk of its progression to malignant (accelerated) hypertension. Smoking may also exacerbate diseases associated with hypertension (e.g. in phaeochromocytoma, paroxysmal hypertensive attacks may be precipitated by smoking).

Atherosclerosis   The development of atherosclerosis is related to smoking and other factors (e.g. poor diet, see Chapter 2). There appears to be a dose-dependent relationship between smoking and the development of atherosclerosis, which is probably mediated through the effects of smoking on haemostasis (see above) and the damage to blood-vessel endothelium caused by nicotine.

Thrombosis   Blood coagulates more easily because of the effects of smoking on haemostasis. Haemostatic disturbances are thought to be linked to the development of atherosclerosis and ischaemic heart disease. The risk of developing thrombosis is increased when combined with other risk factors (e.g. use of combined oral contraceptives, *see* Section 4.2). Smoking may also be responsible for the failure of certain types of cardiovascular surgery. Smoking is associated with failure of arteriovenous shunts for haemodialysis as a result of thrombosis.

Cerebrovascular disease   Smoking is a risk factor in the development of cerebral aneurysm, stroke, and subarachnoid haemorrhage. Mechanisms by which smoking causes cerebrovascular disease, and especially stroke, include the increased risk and development of atherosclerosis and thrombosis, the effects of smoking on haemostasis, and reduced cerebral blood flow. Giving up smoking reduces the risk gradually.

Peripheral vascular disease   At least 95% of patients presenting with peripheral vascular disease are smokers. The risk is cumulative in the presence of other factors (e.g. diabetes mellitus) that are associated with peripheral vascular disease. Mechanisms causing this effect are probably mediated through the effects of smoking on haemostasis and peripheral vasoconstriction. Intermittent claudication, occurring as a result of peripheral vascular disease, is thought to be caused by carbon monoxide leading to the formation of carboxy-haemoglobin; giving up smoking is the most important element of treatment. Surgical treatment of peripheral vascular disease is also influenced by smoking with increased failure of grafts in smokers.

Respiratory system disorders

Smoking is causally related to many respiratory system disorders (Table 5.5). Mechanisms causing these respiratory system disorders are primarily mediated through the effects of the particulate phase of tobacco smoke (*see* Section 5.3). Irritants are deposited in the lungs, resulting in the reflex narrowing of bronchioles. Continued smoking causes chronic obstruction of the airways and decreased lung function. Cilia lining the respiratory tree cease to operate effectively to remove particulate matter. This reduced function occurs because the bronchial mucus secretion is increased in response to irritants and damage. Inflammatory responses are also evident in the lungs, and the earliest sign of smoking-related damage is decreased lung function, which is invariably followed by chronic cough ('smoker's cough').

Chronic obstructive airways disease   Chronic obstructive airways disease is the main group of

respiratory system disorders caused by smoking and is rarely seen in non-smokers. Chronic bronchitis is almost always caused by smoking because of the increased bronchial mucus secretion, although other causes have also seen implicated (e.g. prolonged exposure to environmental pollutants). Emphysema has been linked to smoking because of the disturbance caused to the protease-antiprotease enzymes in the lungs. Smoking increases the activity of the proteases indirectly by decreasing the actions of the antiprotease enzyme, alpha-1-antitrypsin. Both chronic bronchitis and emphysema are progressive but if smoking is stopped before severe disability develops, lung function may improve towards normal. Giving up smoking before the early development of chronic obstructive airways disease reduces the risk towards normal levels.

Respiratory-tract infections   Respiratory-tract infections (e.g. acute bronchitis) are more common in smokers than non-smokers, and many are recurrent. Infections probably occur as a result of the decreased ability of the lungs to remove foreign material, together with compromised lung function and capacity.

Malignant disease

Smoking has been established as the most important risk factor in the development of many malignant diseases and the list of smoking-related malignant diseases is growing. Nicotine itself is not carcinogenic but there are other carcinogens in tobacco smoke (e.g. nitrosated derivatives of nicotine formed during the curing process or during smoking).

Lung cancer   Lung cancer is causally related to smoking; cigarette smoking is associated with the highest incidence of lung cancer. However, cigarettes represent the most prevalent form of tobacco use, which may account for this increased incidence, although lung cancer can occur with all forms of smoking. The most common forms of lung cancer associated with smoking are epidermoid (squamous) cell and small (oat) cell carcinoma. Other factors have been linked to the susceptibility to develop lung cancer (e.g. genetic predisposition) but smoking represents the largest risk factor. The relationship of smoking to lung cancer appears to be related to:

- duration of smoking (number of years)
- depth of inhalation
- number of cigarettes smoked daily
- number of puffs
- starting age of the smoker.

Giving up smoking reduces the relative risk of developing lung cancer when other risks are taken into consideration. Other malignant diseases linked to smoking are listed in Table 5.5.

Gastro-intestinal system disorders

Smoking has been linked to the development and delayed healing of peptic ulceration. Following successful drug treatment of peptic ulceration the relapse rates are considerably higher in smokers. The precise mechanisms are unknown, although studies on the chronic effects of smoking on gastro-intestinal physiology suggest the following mechanisms:

- increased gastric acid secretion
- increased reflux of bile into the stomach
- reduced synthesis and concentration of prostaglandin E_2 in the gastric mucosa.

Oral diseases

There is a reduced blood-flow to the gums in smokers, which is implicated in the association between smoking and gingivitis and other oral inflammatory diseases. Aphthous stomatitis and glossitis are also frequently seen. Oral diseases are thought to be caused by irritants in tobacco smoke and its high temperatures. Oral leucoplakia is also associated with smoking, and may lead to malignancy.

The effects of smoking on the aesthetic appearance of teeth are dramatic. Teeth develop a yellow stain, which is extremely difficult to remove. Staining is often accompanied by characteristic breath odour. Dental caries (see Chapter 3) occurs more frequently in smokers than non-smokers, but this may reflect poor dental health-care exhibited by smokers generally.

Obstetric disorders and effects on the foetus

Smoking leads to a decrease in maternal uterine perfusion primarily as a result of increased maternal and lactate caused by nicotine. Nicotine and carbon monoxide cross the placenta freely, and the effects on the foetus include:

- central nervous system dysfunction caused by increased foetal-lactate concentration
- increased heart rate caused by release of catecholamines
- hypoxia caused by the formation of carboxy-haemoglobin in the presence of carbon monoxide
- vasoconstriction caused by nicotine and catecholamines.

The resultant effect on the foetus of both nicotine and carbon monoxide is foetal hypoxia.

Birth-weight and perinatal mortality Babies born to mothers who smoke often have a lower birth-weight compared to those born to non-smokers. The presence of hydrogen cyanide is also implicated in the reduction in birth-weight. Hydrogen cyanide is converted to thiocyanate, thereby increasing maternal thiocyanate concentrations and reducing maternal concentrations of vitamin B_{12}, which is utilised in the conversion.

The incidence of perinatal mortality is also increased in smokers. It is thought to occur as a result of the rapid placental ageing and premature rupture of the membranes, which is more common in smokers.

Pre-term delivery There is an increased incidence of pre-term delivery of the order of 1 to 3 days among smokers. It is thought to occur as a result of foetal hypoxia and increased myometrial stimulation. There may also be foetal initiation of labour mediated through stimulation of the foetal adrenal glands.

Spontaneous abortion Spontaneous abortion is more common in smokers, and the risk may be double that of non-smokers. It usually occurs in late pregnancy, thereby precluding other causes (e.g. congenital abnormalities).

Placental malfunction Placental malfunction is caused by pathological changes in the placenta and occurs as a result of smoking and hypoxia. It is thought to be responsible for the increased incidence of major antepartum haemorrhage, minor antepartum haemorrhage, and premature membrane rupture.

Pre-eclampsia and eclampsia Pre-eclampsia and eclampsia appear to have a lower incidence in smokers compared to non-smokers. This may be a consequence of:

- increased early abortion in smokers, reducing the numbers of smokers at risk
- nicotine producing capillary dilatation in muscles
- the tendency of smokers to be lean and less likely to gain weight
- the presence of increased concentrations of thiocyanate, which has antihypertensive properties.

However, in those smokers in whom pre-eclampsia and eclampsia do occur, smoking is associated with an increased risk to the foetus.

Postnatal development There may be a reduction in the rate of intellectual development until puberty, although adult performance remains unaffected. Smokers also tend to discontinue breast-feeding as a result of insufficient milk. Infantile colic may be related to maternal smoking, as the incidence is higher in breast-fed babies of smoking mothers whereas bottle-fed babies of smokers appear not to be affected.

5.5   Passive smoking

Passive smoking is defined as the unwanted and involuntary exposure to, and inhalation of, tobacco smoke. It is also sometimes defined as exposure to environmental tobacco smoke, although this definition fails to convey the message of unwanted and involuntary inhalation. It is now generally accepted that passive smoking has harmful health implications, although the extent and magnitude of any increased risk remains to be quantified. Assessment is often difficult as passive smoking is generally impossible to quantify on a widespread scale, although the level of passive smoking for specific environments (e.g. home and work) may be easier to determine.

Both smokers and non-smokers are changing their attitudes to passive smoking. Many smokers now consider it unacceptable to expose non-smokers to tobacco smoke. However, this concern tends to apply more to friends and family rather than to all non-smokers, which is illustrated by the extent of smoking and levels of tobacco smoke in public places (e.g. bars and clubs). However, the general trend is towards eliminating passive smoking. This can be attributed to:

• no-smoking policies at work and in public places
• increased public awareness of the health risks
• legislation prohibiting smoking in certain public places
• recognition by smokers of the risk of passive smoking
• social unacceptability.

Some non-smokers detest the smell of tobacco smoke and find even low atmospheric concentrations extremely irritating. The smell of ashtrays, in the absence of tobacco smoke, is also irritating to some non-smokers.

Exposure levels in passive smoking

The volume and concentration of sidestream smoke (see Section 5.3) determines the exposure levels in passive smoking. Sidestream smoke also affects smokers who are consequently exposed to a double risk from smoking and passive smoking.

The extent of passive smoking can be assessed in non-smokers by measuring plasma-carboxyhaemoglobin concentration; carbon monoxide concentration in expired air; or cotinine concentrations in blood, saliva, or urine.

Factors which determine the extent of passive smoking include those that influence the atmospheric concentration of tobacco smoke. Generally, the extent of passive smoking is dependent upon the distance from smokers, duration of exposure, number of cigarettes smoked, size of the room, and ventilation efficiency.

The health risks of passive smoking are thought to be caused by constituents other than nicotine. The concentrations of nicotine found in non-smokers exposed to passive smoking is usually in the order of 1 to 5% of that in smokers. This concentration is accepted as being extremely small and insignificant in terms of the pharmacological effects of nicotine and relative health risk.

The ideal atmospheric concentration of tobacco smoke is zero. Concentrations that pose a health risk to non-smokers have not yet been quantified. It has been suggested that low concentrations of atmospheric tobacco smoke, or a short duration of exposure, may be an irritation to non-smokers rather than a health hazard. However, until exposure levels have been quantified, passive smoking should be regarded as a health risk to non-smokers and atmospheric concentrations of tobacco smoke should be actively reduced.

Effects of passive smoking on health

Children and adults may present to pharmacists with ailments, especially respiratory conditions, which could be related to tobacco smoke. Therefore, questioning about passive smoking, where applicable, should now form part of pharmacists' key questions.

Acute effects of passive smoking   Passive smoking produces acute effects on non-smokers in a dose-dependent fashion. At low concentrations, non-smokers may experience irritation of the eyes and nose, but at higher concentrations effects may include chest tightness, coughing, headache, nausea, and wheezing. There is considerable variation between individuals; some people are more susceptible to the acute effects of passive smoking than others.

In the presence of underlying disease in non-smokers, susceptibility to the acute effects of passive smoking is increased. Non-smokers with ischaemic heart disease may show a reduction in exercise tolerance and asthmatic patients are generally sensitive to all the acute effects of passive smoking and attacks may be

Table 5.6
Increased incidence of conditions in children subjected to passive smoking

Asthma	Laryngitis
Bronchitis	Middle-ear effusion
Cough	Pneumonia
Decreased height and growth	Respiratory illnesses
Decreased lung function	Snoring
Infantile colic	Tracheitis

precipitated. People who wear contact lenses (*see* Section 10.3) are more susceptible to eye irritation and eye infection as a result of passive smoking.

Chronic effects of passive smoking   It is the chronic effects of passive smoking on the health of non-smokers, and especially children, that cause the most concern. There appears to be a dose-dependent relationship in the development of chronic effects, although data for many disorders is limited.

Cardiovascular system disorders have been associated with passive smoking. There may be an increased risk of heart disease, particularly in women who have never smoked. Respiratory system disorders are related to chronic passive smoking and include respiratory-tract infections, asthma, and emphysema. The forced expiratory volume in one second (FEV_1) is significantly lower, indicating decreased lung function. Children generally are more susceptible than adults to the chronic effects of passive smoking on the respiratory system. The development of lung cancer is related to dose and length of exposure. The risk of developing other forms of malignant disease (e.g. breast and cervical cancer) may also be increased.

Passive smoking by children

In the presence of additional members of the household (e.g. parents or relatives) who smoke, the extent of passive smoking in children may be high. The link between passive smoking and a wide range of childhood illnesses (Table 5.6) is now clearly established. There is a higher incidence of acute and chronic respiratory-tract disorders in children exposed to passive smoking compared to those that are not. Passive smoking in children has also been implicated in delayed development (e.g. height and growth).

Passive smoking is particularly hazardous to children for a variety of reasons:

- the higher respiratory rate in children causes increased inhalation of atmospheric tobacco smoke

- children, especially babies, cannot move away from smokers
- children, especially babies and infants, may be subjected to prolonged exposure if they are in the vicinity of smokers throughout the day.

5.6   PREVENTION OF SMOKING

Primary prevention

Primary prevention programmes and campaigns aim to influence people through education and promotion of non-smoking as socially acceptable behaviour. Their main aim is to discourage people from starting to smoke, although in some cases primary prevention programmes directed at specific groups (e.g. pregnant women) include advice to give up smoking. Children are the largest and most important target group of primary prevention programmes.

The Health Education Authority and the Department of Health instituted a five-year programme in 1989 to reduce the prevalence of cigarette smoking in children and teenagers. The target group identified for this programme was children between 11 and 15 years of age, with greatest emphasis placed upon children between 11 and 13 years of age. The programme, which aims to achieve its objectives by promoting non-smoking uses the following methods:

- no-smoking policies in all schools for staff and children
- promotion of non-smoking as attractive, fashionable, and stylish behaviour by the use of the media (e.g. cinema, television, and youth press)
- school-based activities to reduce smoking (e.g. projects to determine the prevalence of smoking, supplemented by educational support).

Other popular and successful methods include the formation of non-smoker clubs. Action on Smoking and Health (ASH) has organised, on a nation-wide scale, many such clubs called Smoke Busters. Their aim is to prevent children from starting to smoke by highlighting positive incentives for them to remain non-smokers.

No-smoking policies at work are generally well received if implemented with understanding and provision of work-based programmes to help people give up smoking. In the long-term, the number of smokers can be reduced with active no-smoking policies. Smoking cannot be eliminated overnight as it is a form of drug dependence and the initial provision of designated smoking areas is desirable. Setting up a working-party on smoking within work-places would

Table 5.7
Reasons for giving up smoking

Health	long-term health risk
	onset of major illness
	pregnancy
Passive smoking	health risk to others
Price	financial cost of smoking
Social	smell on the breath and clothes
	social unacceptability

Table 5.8
Nicotine withdrawal symptoms

Anxiety	Irritability
Bradycardia	Nausea
Confusion	Poor concentration
Craving	Restlessness
Depression	Sleep disturbances
Gastro-intestinal disturbances	Sweating
Hypotension	Tremor
Increased appetite	Weight gain

enable investigation into all aspects of smoking, and is one way of gaining more support for a no-smoking policy.

Secondary prevention

Secondary prevention is the term applied to preventing smoking-related diseases by encouraging smokers to give up. A large proportion of smokers regard smoking as anti-social, unacceptable, and a risk to health, and want to give up. Nevertheless, although many try, only a few succeed. The reasons why smokers want to give up are summarised in Table 5.7.

Smoking is now recognised as drug dependence on nicotine, characterised by both physiological and psychological dependence. Tolerance to the effects of nicotine is also exhibited. On withdrawal, characteristic symptoms appear (Table 5.8), which usually begin within 24 hours and reach a peak at about one week. This is followed by gradual subsidence, which may be prolonged in some cases. The main symptom that causes failure in people trying to give up smoking is craving which, in some cases, may be intense for over one year. It is characteristically intermittent and can be triggered by environmental effects (e.g. other people smoking) or at a time when a cigarette was habitually smoked (e.g. after a meal). Nicotine substitution therapy (*see below*) will not completely eliminate craving, although other withdrawal symptoms are relieved, which implies that mechanisms other than nicotine addiction may influence the degree of craving.

Methods of giving up smoking

Smokers have to proceed through three stages to give up successfully: initial cessation, short-term maintenance, and long-term maintenance. Nicotine withdrawal symptoms are evident following initial cessation and during short-term maintenance, and constitute the main reason for failure. During long-term maintenance, nicotine withdrawal symptoms are non-existent, indicating that other poorly understood factors are responsible for an individual's return to smoking.

All methods and aids for successful cessation of smoking are recommended only when successive attempts to give up smoking without artificial support have failed. Most smokers who achieve successful cessation do so without the use of any of the following methods.

Aversion therapy   Aversion therapy involves the development of a conditioned aversion to tobacco smoke and is available at smoking clinics. Therapy consists of smoking cigarettes in rapid succession (usually inhaling at six-second intervals), which results in the appearance of toxic effects of nicotine and irritant effects of tobacco smoke including burning mouth and throat, dizziness, nausea, numbness, and tachycardia.

Aversion therapy claims to have good success rates for initial cessation and short-term maintenance. Long-term maintenance is influenced by a sense of achievement, overcoming craving, and apparent health benefits (e.g. improved exercise tolerance and loss of smoker's cough).

Group therapy   Group therapy involves training smokers to cope with nicotine withdrawal symptoms and is available at smoking clinics. Group therapy provides mutual support, which may be important for some smokers in achieving successful cessation. Training is given in techniques that improve awareness and recognition of the effects of smoking, and in coping with nicotine withdrawal symptoms. Methods employed include relaxation techniques, stress management, and methods to cope with craving (e.g. distracting activities). Group therapy claims to achieve good results for initial cessation and short-term maintenance, although results for long-term maintenance appear to be poor. This may be a consequence of the tendency for smokers to forget the techniques once the course is over.

Nicotine replacement   Nicotine replacement is generally regarded as the most effective aid to help smokers give up. The preferred dosage form is nicotine chewing gum and is available in strengths of 2 and 4 mg. The lower strength gum can be purchased over-the-counter from pharmacies,   but   the   higher   strength

> Chew one piece of gum when you want to smoke.
>
> Chew the gum slowly a few times − not like normal chewing gum.
>
> When the taste becomes strong, 'park' the chewing gum between your gum and the inside of your cheek.
>
> Chew the gum again when the taste has faded, then 'park' it again.
>
> Chew like this for about half an hour.

Fig. 5.1
Chewing instructions for Nicorette™ chewing gum.

preparation is only available on private prescription. It is important that the patient understands how to use the chewing gum. The correct chewing technique is described in Fig. 5.1. When the gum is chewed, nicotine is released and absorbed via the oral mucosa. If the chewing gum is chewed too quickly, nicotine is released at a faster rate, which increases salivation and results in some of the nicotine being swallowed. It has been suggested that food and drinks that markedly reduce the pH of the saliva may impair absorption of nicotine. Minor side-effects have been reported including a bitter taste, hiccups, sore throat, headache, dizziness, sickness, and mild indigestion. The manufacturers advise that the chewing gum should be used for about three months before gradually withdrawing treatment. Patients who smoke more than 20 cigarettes a day and have their first cigarette within 20 minutes of waking may require the higher strength preparation. Nicotine chewing gum does not produce any of the positive effects of smoking (e.g. improved concentration) but does relieve nicotine withdrawal symptoms. However, it has little, if any, effect on craving.

Hypnosis and acupuncture   Although high success rates are claimed, hypnosis and acupuncture appear to be ineffective. Results are difficult to assess because of a lack of study data.

Other products   Other products used as aids to giving up smoking are claimed to have good success rates and are widely advertised. Products include a chewing gum containing silver nitrate, which produces an unpleasant taste when a cigarette is smoked. Lobeline is marketed as a nicotine substitute and is taken orally. A preparation containing quinine and menthyl valerate is marketed to reduce craving. However, all the claims of good success rates of non-prescription products are largely unsubstantiated and there is no evidence that they are effective.

The role of the pharmacist

The pharmacist is in an ideal position to develop a counselling role and assist in preventing smoking-related diseases. Pharmacists can participate in primary prevention programmes and assist in secondary prevention by identifying smokers and helping them to give up. Health education material in the form of leaflets and booklets, which can be read and studied at leisure, constitutes the most suitable form of information to reinforce professional advice.

The pharmacist can play an important role in primary prevention programmes by disseminating relevant information. The pharmacist can influence parents to develop a positive no-smoking attitude in their children, even if they themselves are smokers. This is best performed by using constructive arguments against smoking and by recommending primary prevention programmes (e.g. Smoke Busters). Pharmacies in the UK already take an active part in promoting the National No-Smoking Days organised annually in March by the Health Education Authority. On the No-Smoking Day held in March 1988, it was estimated that more than two million people abstained for the day and that 50 000 may have done so permanently. These positive results should encourage pharmacists to become more involved.

Pharmacists should also be able to advise by example and, ideally, those who smoke should give up. No-smoking policies should be instituted in all pharmacies, combined with the necessary understanding and help for employees who are smokers. The Council of the Pharmaceutical Society decided at its meeting in March 1987 that pharmacies should not sell tobacco or tobacco products, including cigarettes containing tobacco. Pharmacists should not sell non-smoked tobacco, and to do so would constitute professional misconduct.

The pharmacist also needs to be aware of the possible effects of smoking on drug response. Cigarette smoking can affect the pharmacodynamic and pharmacokinetic properties of drugs. Nicotine has pharmacological actions that can alter the net therapeutic effect of a drug, and the polyaromatic hydrocarbons in cigarette smoke can induce microsomal liver enzymes responsible for the metabolism of some drugs. This is important in smokers who may be receiving drugs with a narrow therapeutic index (e.g. theophylline). Theophylline metabolism is enhanced in smokers, necessitating increased dosage requirements. However, if patients give up smoking, the dose may need to be reduced to avoid toxic concentrations.

Heparin metabolism is elevated in smokers, which may necessitate increases in dosage. Warfarin clearance is enhanced, but has not been associated with changes in prothrombin time. It has also been reported that histamine H$_2$-receptor antagonists (e.g. cimetidine, ranitidine) exhibit a lower healing rate in smokers; patients also show an increased relapse rate following successful treatment. Benzodiazepines produce significantly less drowsiness in smokers, which this may be important in the treatment of insomnia.

Successfully stopping smoking   Pharmacists recognise that giving up smoking is not easy and that many smokers will have had one or more unsuccessful attempts. Health education can provide the initial motivation. Pharmacists should emphasise all the benefits of not smoking, including those other than health (e.g. financial benefits).

It is beneficial to have a structured programme to adhere to when giving up, and the following practical steps can be recommended:

- it is not advisable to cut down, you must stop completely
- choose a day to stop
- list the benefits of giving up smoking
- motivate yourself
- obtain the support of family and friends
- avoid situations where smoking is likely (e.g. public houses)
- discard all smoking-related materials (e.g. cigarettes, lighters, and ashtrays) the day before
- try and give up with a friend.

Self-motivation of smokers is one of the most important aspects of successful cessation. It can be improved by pharmacists emphasising the benefits of stopping smoking (e.g. improved health and reduced future health risks, increased exercise capacity, improved taste of food, and an improved personal tobacco-free odour). Most smokers tend to underestimate the cost of smoking and the financial benefits of giving up. Removal of the staining effect of tobacco smoke may significantly enhance smoker self-motivation; the appearance of the mouth (*see* Section 5.4) may also improve. Smoking also stains the fingers and clothes and virtually anything with which it comes into contact (e.g. paintwork, furniture, and interior of cars). The pharmacist should also consider smokers' other risk factors (e.g. lack of exercise). The effects of passive smoking, especially on children, should also be emphasised.

Initial cessation and short-term maintenance will be successful if withdrawal symptoms and craving can be controlled. Smokers cough may initially get worse, as the cilia begin to function again, but it usually subsides within a few days; sometimes, however, it may persist for weeks.

Maintaining long-term cessation is difficult, whereas smokers often think that the first few weeks will be the worst. The pharmacist can compliment ex-smokers in their achievement. Ex-smokers should be encouraged to resist any form of temptation, particularly 'just one puff' during social occasions, and they should tell their friends never to give them a cigarette.

Weight gain is common, and smokers, especially women, are often anxious about its likely magnitude. It is an accepted finding that smokers are generally leaner. However, when this is related to mortality, it is found that there is an increased mortality among lean men who are smokers compared to obese non-smokers. This can only be attributed to smoking and associated illnesses. The benefits from giving up smoking overwhelmingly outweigh the risks associated with the weight gain in smokers who give up. Smokers should be advised that weight gain is usually not substantial and lasts for only a short time, after which their weight will stabilise. If weight gain is unacceptable, measures can be recommended for its reduction. However, these measures should only be recommended after successful cessation of smoking has been achieved, and the ex-smoker's confidence regained.

Less hazardous smoking is often mentioned and smokers may be convinced that modern cigarettes, especially low tar brands, are safe. Pharmacists may also be asked if switching to other forms of tobacco will reduce or eliminate health risks. Switching to a pipe or cigars will not reduce health risks, and perhaps even increase them as smokers accustomed to inhaling cigarette smoke usually, on switching, inhale pipe and cigar smoke. It is claimed that life-long pipe and cigar smokers do not inhale, and this therefore reduces their risks. However, the overall health risks remain unchanged, which when compared to non-smokers are much higher. The use of herbal cigarettes should also be discouraged because the smoke from the burning herbs contains tar and carbon monoxide, although not nicotine.

5.7   USEFUL ADDRESSES

ACTION ON SMOKING AND HEALTH (ASH)
5–11 Mortimer Street
London W1N 7RN
Tel: 071-637 9843

SMOKER'S QUITLINE
Latimer House
40–48 Hanson Street
London W1P 7DE
Tel: 071-323 0505

QUIT
Latimer House
40–48 Hanson Street
London W1P 7DE
Tel: 071-636 9103

5.8 FURTHER READING

Ashton H, Stepney R. *Smoking. Psychology and pharmacology*. London: Tavistock Publications, 1982.

Ney T, Gale A, eds. *Smoking and human behaviour*. Chichester: John Wiley & Sons, 1989.

Royal College of Physicians. *Health or smoking?* Edinburgh: Churchill Livingstone, 1986.

Chapter 6

EXCESSIVE ALCOHOL CONSUMPTION

6.1 ALCOHOL CONSUMPTION

The use of alcohol is widely accepted in many different cultures, and is commonly at the centre of social and business interactions. It is seen as providing a common, relaxing, and enjoyable dimension, with the encouragement to drink being realised as welcoming and friendly. Regular but low alcohol consumption has even been tentatively linked to a reduced risk of developing certain diseases, especially ischaemic heart disease, when compared to the incidence in non-drinkers. However, the available data do not conclusively support this finding; one of the reasons may be that investigative studies usually only categorise people into non-drinkers and drinkers, and overlook the fact that some non-drinkers may in fact be ex-drinkers. Alcohol is more likely to have harmful than beneficial effects, particularly when consumed to excess, and has been associated with the development of both health and social problems.

The range of alcohol-related health and social problems is diverse and involves many parts of the social and medical framework. Alcohol is responsible for causing a wide range of diseases, and alcohol-related premature deaths in Great Britain have been estimated to be between 25 000 and 40 000 each year. Social problems that may be attributed wholly or in part to alcohol consumption include road traffic accidents, violence, criminal offences, marital problems, and occupational problems.

The costs of excessive alcohol consumption cannot be quantified accurately but rational calculations and estimates indicate an annual total cost of approximately £2 billion at 1987 prices. This figure can be broken down into component costs:

- cost to industry of approximately £1.7 billion
- cost to the NHS of approximately £120 million
- cost of material damage (e.g. road traffic accidents) of approximately £112 million
- cost of police and judicial system of approximately £41 million.

The World Health Organization (WHO) has concluded that there is no threshold below which alcohol consumption can be considered safe. However, to aim for total abstinence would prove to be an impossible goal to attain, and the promotion of sensible drinking has been advocated as a more realistic target. Limits for safe alcohol consumption are difficult, if not impossible, to define accurately. Limits are therefore estimated (*see below*) and take into consideration the paucity of information and the marked individual variation in the response to alcohol.

The terms 'alcoholism' and 'alcoholic' are widely used in everyday language to refer to alcohol abuse with or without dependence. As a result of this ambiguity, and also because these terms have derogatory connotations with implications of an incurable and permanent state, it has been suggested by some authorities that they should not be used. A preferred term is excessive alcohol consumption, which indicates a level of alcohol consumption that may cause alcohol-related health and social problems. It may be related to the limits and habits of alcohol consumption discussed below, and includes all levels of alcohol intake considered to be above sensible limits. Excessive alcohol consumption on a frequent and regular basis can induce dependence (*see* Section 6.4), and the term alcohol dependence syndrome has been put forward by the WHO to describe this state.

Awareness of the effects of excessive alcohol consumption is necessary to recognise and manage the health and social problems that may occur as a result, and to promote sensible drinking. However, there is widespread ignorance regarding the role of alcohol in health and social problems. Alcohol consumption is seldom viewed as harmful, except in alcohol dependence (*see* Section 6.4), and this perpetuates the popular belief that alcohol-related problems only occur in people who become dependent. The influence of alcohol is governed by the amount and frequency of consumption, the rate of consumption, and the reasons for consumption (e.g. social drinking or drinking to relieve depression). The precise levels responsible for causing problems are impossible to determine because of the marked individual variation in response to alcohol and the lack of available data. Alcohol-related morbidity and mortality are frequently unrecognised and therefore not recorded.

Alcohol consumption varies between men and women, and among different age groups. On average, men drink more alcohol on a regular basis than women, although in recent years, the gap has narrowed as women's consumption has increased. For both sexes, alcohol consumption is highest among those between 18 and 24 years of age, decreasing among the older age groups.

The number of deaths from cirrhosis of the liver (*see* Section 6.2.2) is a good indicator of the prevalence of excessive alcohol consumption. The increase in *per capita* alcohol consumption between 1965 and 1987 ran in parallel with an increase in deaths from cirrhosis of the liver within the same period.

Causes of excessive alcohol consumption

The causes of excessive alcohol consumption appear to be multifactorial and closely integrated. It is therefore difficult to determine the precise aetiology, although some contributory factors have been suggested.

The availability and accessibility of alcohol are determinants of the *per capita* consumption of alcohol, which in turn influences the extent of alcohol-related health and social problems within a population. In some communities (e.g. Jews and Muslims), drinking alcohol is not socially or culturally acceptable, and this results in a lower incidence of excessive consumption.

It has been demonstrated that the tendency to excessive alcohol consumption, and in particular to becoming dependent, may be inherited, although the mechanisms and magnitude of a genetic contribution have not yet been identified. People with a family history of alcohol dependence are liable to develop the condition at an earlier age than those who do not have such a genetic disposition; it is also likely to be more severe and chronic. The data that support this finding are more conclusive in men than women. It is, however, possible that the children of parents who abuse alcohol may follow this example in later life simply as a result of learned behaviour; they may equally become non-drinkers. The effects of parental excessive alcohol consumption on their children are discussed in Section 6.3. Personality disorders may also lead to alcohol abuse, although they are not associated with all cases and cannot, therefore, be used as a reliable indicator.

Measurement of alcohol consumption

The term alcohol is used in this Chapter to refer to the consumption of ethanol, which is the constituent alcohol of all alcoholic beverages. Methods available to quantify alcohol consumption include:

- conventional measures (e.g. pint of beer, bar measure of spirits, or glass of wine)
- quantity of alcohol contained in beverages (in grams or percentage alcohol by volume)
- units of alcohol.

Conventional measures are frequently used to assess alcohol consumption. However, they do not provide a reliable indicator of the amount of alcohol consumed because of the wide variation in the alcohol content of different beverages. The quantity of alcohol expressed in grams or as the percentage alcohol by volume is the most accurate way of quantifying intake. However, this may only be applicable to health-care personnel familiar with their use; the general public find both conventional measures and quantity of alcohol difficult to use. For this reason, the unit system was developed. One unit is defined as 8 g or 10 mL of alcohol. It is the amount of alcohol contained in an average standard drink, and is equivalent to:

- half a pint of ordinary beer or lager
- one glass of wine
- one small glass of fortified wine (e.g. sherry or port)
- one single bar measure of spirits*
- one bar measure of vermouth.

The unit system for determining alcohol consumption is the simplest and most widely accepted method. It is easily related to conventional measures by the use of the defined standard drinks and enables quick and reliable estimation of alcohol consumption, especially when a number of different alcoholic drinks are consumed. Table 6.1 indicates the approximate alcohol content of different beverages, the corresponding value in units, and their relationship to conventional measures. It should be emphasised, however, that the unit system only allows for estimated values of alcohol consumption. There is a wide variation in alcohol content between brands of the same type of beverage and considerable variation in the size of measures (e.g. wine glasses vary considerably in size); home measures are generally larger than those in licensed public places (e.g. measures of spirits at home may be the equivalent of 3 to 4 units of alcohol). The labelling of low-alcohol and alcohol-free drinks creates much confusion, and it is more difficult to estimate the number of units consumed. This problem is discussed in Section 6.5. The easier unit system has led to a campaign to label all alcoholic drinks with the number of units.

*One single bar measure of spirits is 1/6 gill (1 unit) in England and Wales but in some parts of Scotland it is 1/5 gill (1.25 units), and in other parts of Scotland and Northern Ireland it is 1/4 gill (1.5 units). (1 gill = 142 mL)

Table 6.1

Approximate alcohol content of various beverages†

Type of beverage	Measure	Alcohol content (%)	Alcohol content (grams)	Alcohol content (units)
Beer or lager				
Ordinary strength	pint	3	16	2
	half pint	3	8	1
Export beer	pint	4	20	2.5
	half pint	4	10	1.25
Strong beer or lager	pint	5.5	32	4
	half pint	5.5	16	2
Extra strong beer or lager	pint	7	40	5
	half pint	7	20	2.5
Cider				
Ordinary strength	pint	4	24	3
	half pint	4	12	1.5
Strong cider	pint	6	32	4
	half pint	6	16	2
Spirits (e.g. whisky, gin, brandy)				
in England and Wales	single bar measure (1/6 gill)	32	8	1
in some parts of Scotland	single bar measure (1/5 gill)	32	10	1.25
in N. Ireland and some parts of Scotland	single bar measure (1/4 gill)	32	12	1.5
Wine				
Table wine	glass	8 to 10	8	1
Fortified wine (e.g. port and sherry)	standard small measure	13 to 16	8	1
Vermouth	single bar measure	13 to 16	8	1
Liqueurs				
	standard small measure	15 to 30	8	1

†The average is quoted and some beverages will have a higher alcohol content (and some a lower one), although the majority satisfy the average criteria.

Limits and habits of alcohol consumption

An estimate of weekly alcohol intake provides people who drink on a regular basis a means of assessing their risk of developing alcohol-related health and social problems.

Limits of alcohol consumption applicable to adult men and women are defined as:

• Sensible limits

Sensible limits of alcohol consumption are up to 21 units/week for men and up to 14 units/week for women. Consumption should be spaced out over the week rather than in 1 or 2 sessions of heavy drinking. There should also be occasional drink-free days. Within these sensible limits, the risk of developing alcohol-related health and social problems is low.

• Hazardous limits

Hazardous limits of alcohol consumption are between 21 to 49 units/week for men and 14 to 34 units/week for women. The risk of alcohol-related problems increases as consumption rises. Drinking within these limits is associated with a moderate or intermediate risk of developing alcohol-related health and social problems.

• Dangerous limits

Dangerous limits of alcohol consumption are above 49 units/week for men and above 34 units/week for women. These levels of alcohol consumption carry a high risk of alcohol-related health and social problems. It is rare for consumption to reach these levels without incurring alcohol-related health or social problems.

The limits of alcohol consumption represent a general guide for people to assess their level of intake. However, people generally have a range of drinking habits, and the response to alcohol is additionally governed by individual variation. Social drinking is within sensible limits; it is less than 2 to 3 units/day and does not cause intoxication. Heavy drinking falls within hazardous limits, and includes consumption of more than six units/day but without immediate alcohol-related problems. Problem drinking describes alcohol consumption that has caused alcohol-related problems (e.g drink-driving offences) and may occur at any level of alcohol consumption. There is considerable overlap between these categories with people moving from one category to another (e.g. from social drinking to heavy drinking or problem drinking). Heavy drinkers or problem drinkers are not necessarily dependent on alcohol but may progress to dependence.

Metabolism of alcohol

Alcohol is rapidly absorbed from the gastro-intestinal tract, mainly from the stomach and small intestine. Alcohol is eliminated primarily by oxidation to acetaldehyde catalysed by the enzyme, alcohol dehydrogenase; a small proportion is metabolised to acetaldehyde by the microsomal ethanol-oxidising system in the liver. The latter pathway is enhanced in heavy drinkers and is thought to account for the substantial tolerance (*see below*) that commonly develops. The acetaldehyde is further oxidised to acetate, which is a good source of energy for a number of tissues. However, metabolism of acetate utilises members of the vitamin-B group, which may result in deficiency if there is inadequate dietary intake. Vitamin-B deficiency, particularly thiamine deficiency, has been implicated in the aetiology of some alcohol-related diseases (*see* Section 6.2.2).

Generally, for equivalent consumption of alcohol, women attain higher blood-alcohol concentrations than men, particularly at the time of ovulation or just before menstruation. The bioavailability differences of alcohol in women are thought to be caused by the higher fat content and therefore lower water content in women compared to men. Alcohol is water soluble and a lower water content therefore reduces the volume of distribution of alcohol, resulting in higher blood-alcohol concentrations. However, following intravenous administration of alcohol, blood-alcohol concentrations are similar in both men and women, indicating the possibility that other mechanisms may be responsible for, or contributing to, the higher blood-alcohol concentrations in women following oral intake. Cyclical variations are probably caused by hormonal fluctuations.

In both men and women, alcohol is metabolised primarily in the liver. However, there is also some initial oxidation in the gastric mucosa involving the enzyme, gastric alcohol dehydrogenase, which may be responsible for reducing the amount of alcohol absorbed into the blood circulation. Differences in the degree of gastric metabolism of alcohol may account for, or contribute to, higher blood-alcohol concentrations in women. In men, there is greater gastric metabolism of alcohol, although it is reduced in alcohol dependence. In women, the gastric metabolism of alcohol is much lower and is almost negligible in alcohol dependence.

The maximum blood-alcohol concentration that may be attained is affected by the rate of absorption, which is in turn affected by several other factors. The rate of absorption of alcohol from the stomach is reduced by the presence of food, particularly fatty foods. Absorption rate increases as the concentration of alcohol in a drink increases, and the most rapid absorption occurs at about 20% alcohol by volume. However, when the concentration of alcohol exceeds 20%, the absorption rate starts to slow down again, and undiluted spirits are not absorbed as quickly as when diluted with water or mixer drinks. Carbonated drinks are absorbed more quickly than non-carbonated drinks.

Heavier people have a higher body water content than lighter people, and therefore are more likely to attain a lower blood-alcohol concentration for a given amount of alcohol ingested. However, if the extra weight is fat, then the proportion of body water may be less and the comparison becomes more complex (see above). The faster a drink is consumed, the higher the blood-alcohol concentration achieved.

Small quantities of alcohol are excreted unchanged in the urine and from the lungs in expired air, and can also be detected in the saliva. There is a correlation between blood-alcohol concentrations and concentrations present in the saliva, urine, and expired air. This fact is exploited in the estimation of blood-alcohol concentrations from small samples, particularly in suspected cases of drinking and driving.

At high blood-alcohol concentrations (above 100 mg/100 mL), the rate of elimination is constant and not dependent on the blood-alcohol concentration (zero-order kinetics). Blood-alcohol concentrations will, therefore, decline at a constant rate, which is usually in the region of 6 to 40 mg/100 mL per hour (the typical average is 15 mg/100 mL per hour). In relation to the number of units consumed it can be crudely estimated that it will take about one hour for the body to remove one unit of alcohol. This can also be usefully translated into the time required for the body to eliminate a given quantity of alcohol (e.g. eight hours for eight units).

Acute effects of alcohol consumption

The acute effects of alcohol (acute intoxication) are caused by its depressant action on the central nervous system, although the precise mechanisms are complex. The clinical features of acute alcohol intoxication (Table 6.2) are related to the blood-alcohol and brain-alcohol

Table 6.2

Acute effects of alcohol consumption in relation to the blood-alcohol concentration

Blood-alcohol concentration (mg/100 mL)	Acute effects
below 50	altered mood increased confidence relaxation sense of well being talkativeness
50 to 100 (inebriation)	impaired judgement incoordination loss of sensory perception loss of some social inhibitions slurred speech
100 to 300 (intoxication)	ataxia blurred vision loss of self-control slow reactions
300 to 500 (severe intoxication)	severe ataxia diplopia convulsions coma
above 500 (very severe intoxication)	loss of tendon reflexes hypothermia respiratory depression coma death

concentrations. The risk of accidental injury also increases with rising blood-alcohol concentrations.

It must be emphasised that there is a wide variation in the response to alcohol between individuals. Factors responsible for this variation include:

• Tolerance to the effects of alcohol

Tolerance develops with continued and regular consumption. Heavy drinkers who have developed substantial tolerance may show little sign of intoxication at blood-alcohol concentrations that would cause severe intoxication in people who usually drink less (e.g. occasional drinkers).

• Presence of food in the stomach

The presence of food in the stomach reduces the rate of absorption of alcohol.

- Blood-alcohol concentration

  The effects of alcohol and the severity of intoxication are greatest when the blood-alcohol concentration is rising to its peak level compared to when it is falling. This may be caused by the development of tolerance within this short period of time. A rapid rise in blood-alcohol concentration will enhance the effects of alcohol to a greater extent than a slow rise.

- Gender

  The acute effects of equivalent alcohol intake are enhanced in women compared to men.

- Other medication

  Other CNS depressants considerably enhance the effects of alcohol.

6.2   ALCOHOL-RELATED PROBLEMS

It is difficult to assess the amount of alcohol that may be responsible for producing alcohol-related health and social problems because many of these problems only occur after long-term alcohol abuse. Retrospective estimates of alcohol consumption are bound to be inaccurate, particularly as people who consume excessive amounts are often evasive about their intakes.

Some people appear to be relatively unaffected by consumption of inordinate amounts of alcohol whereas others readily develop problems. This suggests that there may be additional factors (e.g. nutritional deficiency, underlying disease, or genetic susceptibility), which must be also considered.

6.2.1   Alcohol-related social problems

Social problems may arise as a result of alcohol abuse or, alternatively, excessive alcohol consumption may be caused by social problems. It is likely, however, that alcohol is not solely responsible for the development of social problems, and other factors (e.g. personality disorders) may play an important role.

Social problems attributable to alcohol (e.g. violence between football fans, and drinking and driving) are being increasingly recognised, although measures to reduce their incidence have had little effect.

Family problems, particularly marital difficulties, are commonly encountered in association with unrestrained drinking; alcohol is a contributory factor to violence within the family. Children are likely to be severely affected by parental excessive alcohol consumption (see Section 6.3), with neglect being the predominant feature. The expense of maintaining drinking habits contributes to poverty and debt, which may accentuate alcohol-related family problems.

Difficulties at work may arise as a result of drink problems and include absenteeism, accidents, and inefficiency. Alcohol-related occupational problems can arise at any level, and managerial and leadership qualities may be diminished resulting in poor overall performance of the company. Time spent away from work as a result of alcohol-related disorders contributes substantially to industrial costs.

Alcohol consumption and aggressive behaviour are often encountered together, although the association is complex and other factors may be involved. Perceived threat and provocation may contribute to aggression in a particular situation. Alcohol consumption may even cause a paranoid state (see Section 6.2.2), which in some cases can be dangerous.

Drinking and driving increases the risk of accidents if the blood-alcohol concentration rises above 50 mg/100 mL; this threshold is lower for learners, inexperienced drivers, and occasional drinkers. The blood-alcohol concentration above which it is illegal to drive is 80 mg/100 mL, although it is generally accepted that this limit should be lowered, perhaps to 50 mg/100 mL or, ideally, to zero. However, evidence suggests that altering limits will not in itself affect the prevalence of drinking and driving. It is the increased likelihood of being caught that will have a more pronounced effect, and this may be achieved by random breath testing of drivers.

It has been estimated that drinking one unit of alcohol (see Section 6.1) raises the blood-alcohol concentration by about 15 mg/100 mL in men, and about 20 mg/100 mL in women. However, it is not possible to accurately determine the blood-alcohol concentration from the number of drinks a person has had because the actual amount of alcohol absorbed and the rate of absorption is subject to wide individual variation (see Section 6.1). The only advice that can safely be given is not to drink at all before driving. It should also be pointed out that, on average, it takes one hour to eliminate one unit of alcohol from the body, and someone who has indulged in a heavy drinking session late into the night may still be over the legal limit for driving the following morning.

6.2.2   Alcohol-related diseases

The relationship between alcohol consumption and development of disease is difficult to determine accurately because most of the available data are derived from studies of alcohol-dependent people who regularly drink alcohol at a level above the sensible limits. Although the majority of serious alcohol-related diseases do occur in alcohol-dependent people, they are not exclusive to this group and may equally arise in non-dependent heavy drinkers. Alcohol may not be the sole cause of a disease and other contributory factors (e.g. smoking or nutritional deficiencies) must be taken into consideration. There is a tendency for one major alcohol-related disease to dominate in the absence of any other sign of disease. Women are more vulnerable to the toxic effects of alcohol (see Section 6.1), and are at greater risk of developing alcohol-related diseases than men.

Anaemias

Anaemias are common in long-term heavy drinkers, and result from the interaction of several factors including poor diet, chronic blood loss, liver disease, and a direct toxic effect of alcohol on bone marrow. Megaloblastic anaemia may arise, and is commonly seen in alcohol dependence associated with nutritional deficiency. It is caused by folate deficiency and a direct toxic effect of alcohol. Sideroblastic anaemia is associated with reduced serum-folate and erythrocyte-folate concentrations; a mixed macrocytic and microcytic anaemia, and liver disease may also be present. Iron-deficiency anaemia is frequently seen in alcohol-dependent patients. Haemorrhage (e.g. from oesophageal varices or gastritis, see below) or poor diet may also cause, or contribute to, iron-deficiency anaemia.

Cardiac disorders

A session of binge drinking may produce acute effects on the heart. These include ectopic beats, paroxysmal atrial fibrillation, reduced myocardial contractility, or ventricular tachycardia, and occur as a result of a direct toxic effect on cardiac tissue. In non-drinkers or occasional drinkers, acute effects usually occur at lower intakes than in people who have developed tolerance to alcohol as a result of regular drinking; susceptibility is also increased in the presence of established heart disease.

Alcohol-related dilated cardiomyopathy occurs as a result of sustained heavy drinking. The mechanism is thought be a direct toxic effect on cardiac muscle. A dose-effect relationship between the amount of alcohol ingested and the development of dilated cardiomyopathy appears to exist, although the relationship is with the total lifetime alcohol consumption and not the present level.

Coagulation defects

Chronic alcohol abuse may impair platelet production, survival, and function, producing thrombocytopenia. This resolves when alcohol is withdrawn although, initially, the platelet count may rise above the normal value.

Alcohol has no direct toxic effect on coagulation factors. However, severe alcohol-related liver disease (e.g. cirrhosis of the liver or alcoholic hepatitis) suppresses vitamin-K dependent coagulation factors thus reducing the synthesis of prothrombin. Associated features include increased fibrinolysis and disseminated intravascular coagulation. This disturbance of haemostasis is not completely reversed by the administration of vitamin K.

Coagulation defects predispose the patient to life-threatening haemorrhage.

Endocrine disorders

Hypoglycaemia may occur between 6 and 36 hours after a session of heavy drinking. The risk of developing alcohol-related hypoglycaemia is increased if alcohol is consumed on an empty stomach, following heavy exercise, or in the presence of nutritional deficiency, and in diabetics on oral hypoglycaemics or insulin. In some cases, it may be severe and lead to hypoglycaemic coma. In patients with cirrhosis of the liver (see below), alcohol-related hypoglycaemia represents a severe deterioration in liver function.

Excessive alcohol consumption is causally linked to the development of diabetes mellitus, usually Type II (non-insulin dependent) diabetes mellitus. Alcohol-related diabetes mellitus may be caused by chronic pancreatitis (see below) if extensive damage occurs. It may also arise as a result of cirrhosis of the liver.

Alcohol may cause a deterioration in sexual function, and these effects are thought to be mediated by impaired hypothalamic function, impaired metabolism of oestrogens by the liver, or a direct toxic effect of alcohol on the testes or ovaries. There is a reduction in plasma-testosterone concentration in men and plasma-oestrogen concentration in women. Some disorders (e.g. temporary impotence or loss of libido) may be associated with a single session of heavy drinking whereas chronic alcohol abuse may produce permanent impairment. The disorders that may occur in men include gynaecomastia, impotence, loss of libido, loss of pubic hair, low sperm count, scrotal wrinkling, and testicular atrophy. In women, alcohol-related sexual disorders include atrophy of the breasts and external genitalia, diminished flow of vaginal secretions, menstrual disorders, and progressive masculinisation.

Alcohol causes an increase in the release of cortisol from the adrenal cortex. This is thought to be the mechanism responsible for causing pseudo-Cushing's syndrome in alcohol dependence. The clinical features resemble Cushing's syndrome proper, and resolve completely on abstinence.

A clinical syndrome resembling hyperthyroidism may arise in the presence of long-term alcohol abuse. The precise mechanism responsible is not known, although alcohol does not appear to have a direct effect on the thyroid gland. It is essential to distinguish this condition from true hyperthyroidism.

Gastro-intestinal disorders

Alcohol is a common cause of gastro-oesophageal reflux, which often leads to reflux oesophagitis; a characteristic symptom is heartburn. Alcohol also frequently causes acute gastritis, which may result in retching and vomiting, particularly in the morning after a night of heavy drinking; erosion of the gastric mucosa may produce haematemesis.

Oesophageal bleeding may occur as a result of reflux oesophagitis or ruptured varices; laceration of the oesophageal mucous membrane (Mallory-Weiss syndrome) during retching and vomiting may also be a cause. Spontaneous rupture of the oesophagus (Boerhaave's syndrome) is an uncommon but life-threatening condition that may occur as a result of binge drinking.

Alcohol has been implicated as a cause of peptic ulceration, although there is no evidence to support this conclusion, or that moderate alcohol consumption may delay ulcer healing.

Excessive consumption of alcohol may cause diarrhoea as a result of increased intestinal motility and disturbed intestinal microflora.

Long-term abuse of alcohol is a major cause of chronic pancreatitis, and complications of extensive pancreatic damage include malabsorption and diabetes mellitus. A heavy drinking session may produce acute pancreatitis, and life-threatening complications include hypovolaemic shock, renal failure, liver failure, and respiratory failure. Various authorities disagree about the definitions of alcohol-related acute and chronic pancreatitis. It is thought by some that acute episodes are superimposed on an underlying chronic condition whereas others believe that repeated attacks of acute pancreatitis eventually produce chronic pancreatitis.

Gout

Historically, alcohol consumption has been implicated in the development of gout and, while this still holds true today, the exact role of alcohol in the aetiology has not been conclusively demonstrated. Gout is caused by hyperuricaemia, which may arise as a result of increased uric acid production or decreased uric acid excretion. Studies have shown that alcohol may play a part in both of these pathways.

Hypertension

Alcohol causes an immediate rise in blood pressure, and thus may exacerbate underlying hypertension or even be a primary cause; hypertension is commonly seen in heavy drinkers.

The precise mechanism of alcohol-related hypertension is not known, although increases in plasma concentrations of cortisol, renin, aldosterone, and vasopressin have been demonstrated following alcohol consumption; the increased sympathetic activity produced by alcohol may also contribute. However, these pressor effects are seen after the increase in blood pressure has occurred and therefore do not account for the immediate rise.

Blood pressure returns to normal when alcohol consumption ceases, although it may not be necessary to stop drinking completely in all cases; reduction to sensible limits may be all that is required.

Liver disease

Varying degrees of liver disease are commonly associated with excessive alcohol consumption although the precise mechanism is unknown. There is little evidence to suggest that alcohol has a direct toxic effect on liver cells. However, acetaldehyde, a metabolite of alcohol, may be involved, and nutritional deficiency may be a contributory factor. Alcohol-related liver disease in women tends to occur following a shorter period of alcohol abuse compared to men, even when lower quantities of alcohol are consumed, and is often more severe with a poor prognosis.

Fatty degeneration is characterised by the presence of large fat droplets within liver cells, producing an enlarged liver. It is common in heavy drinkers and is probably dose-related. It is not necessarily harmful, and is usually reversed if alcohol consumption is stopped or reduced to sensible limits.

Acute alcoholic hepatitis is associated with sustained excessive consumption and is more serious than fatty degeneration, although it does not develop in all heavy drinkers. Features include hepatomegaly with necrosis and fibrosis to varying degrees; it is thought to precede cirrhosis of the liver. However, it can remain unchanged for years or, in some cases, recovery may occur despite continued drinking. Chronic active hepatitis may also occur as a result of chronic alcohol consumption.

Cirrhosis of the liver is a serious disorder caused by chronic excessive alcohol consumption, although it occurs in only 10 to 30% of heavy drinkers. The first clinical signs usually present between 50 to 70 years of age. It is characterised by the destruction of parenchymal cells, loss of their normal lobular structure with widespread fibrosis, and regeneration of the remaining cells to form nodules. Complications may arise as a result of portal hypertension and include ascites, jaundice, oesophageal varices, renal failure, and hepatic encephalopathy. Some patients develop hepatocellular carcinoma (*see below*), which has a poor prognosis. Alcohol-related cirrhosis of the liver may be accompanied by varying degrees of fatty degeneration, or acute alcoholic hepatitis, or both in patients who continue drinking.

Cirrhosis of the liver is a progressive disorder, although it can be arrested if alcohol consumption is stopped. The liver is able to compensate for lost function and some patients can lead relatively normal lives.

Malignant disease

Alcohol consumption and development of malignant disease have been tentatively linked but, as data is limited, the precise role of alcohol has not yet been identified. Alcohol itself is probably not carcinogenic but may act by accelerating the development of malignancy. However, some alcoholic drinks do contain carcinogens (e.g. nitrosamines and polycyclic hydrocarbons); acetaldehyde, a metabolite of alcohol, is carcinogenic. The risk of developing alcohol-related cancer appears to be dose-related.

Malignant diseases that may be associated with excessive alcohol consumption include breast cancer, oropharyngeal cancer, and malignancies of the gastro-intestinal system, particularly oesophageal cancer. Hepatocellular carcinoma (primary liver cell cancer) is linked to alcohol consumption because about 80% of cases develop in the presence of cirrhosis of the liver (*see above*). It has a higher incidence in men and a poor prognosis.

Nervous system disorders

Long-term consumption of alcohol above sensible limits is associated with a wide range of nervous system disorders, which are thought to be mediated by nutritional deficiency, or a direct toxic effect of alcohol on nervous system tissue, or both.

Memory loss   Memory loss is characterised by the loss of short-term memory ('black outs') and is commonly seen following a bout of heavy drinking. Memory of the events that occurred during the binge is usually affected, despite full consciousness and awareness being maintained at the time.

Chronic alcohol abuse is associated with regular episodes of memory loss, which may last several hours or even days. Awareness, consciousness, and relatively normal behaviour may be maintained during this time. In some cases, patients travel long distances but are unable to recall the experience later.

Wernicke's encephalopathy   Wernicke's encephalopathy is caused by alcohol-related thiamine deficiency, although the aetiology may be multifactorial with other contributory factors. The predominant symptoms are ataxia, confusion, and paralysis of the eye muscles; peripheral neuropathy (*see below*) may also be present and there is often some degree of memory impairment. Stupor and coma may occur in the late stages before death. In many cases, symptoms are non-specific, and the condition is not diagnosed until post-mortem.

There is an association between Wernicke's encephalopathy and Korsakoff's syndrome (*see below*), and the two are sometimes referred to as Wernicke-Korsakoff's syndrome. Wernicke's encephalopathy may also be considered as the acute phase and Korsakoff's syndrome as the chronic phase. Parenteral administration of thiamine elicits a rapid response and arrests progression of the disease, although some abnormalities may persist.

Korsakoff's syndrome   Korsakoff's syndrome is caused mainly by alcohol-related thiamine deficiency and is thought to be the chronic form of Wernicke's encephalopathy (*see above*). It is sometimes referred to as Wernicke-Korsakoff's syndrome as a result of this association.

Short-term memory is grossly impaired and patients are unable to recall events for longer than a few seconds or minutes after they have occurred. General intellectual ability remains relatively unaffected although there is a disordered sense of time and place. Patients remain alert and often fabricate very plausible but inaccurate details of incidents to fill in the memory gaps (confabulation); they are not overtly lying and believe their accounts to be true. Memory of past events usually remains intact.

Cerebellar degeneration   Cerebellar degeneration may occur after prolonged alcohol abuse and is characterised by progressive ataxia. The main manifestation is an unsteady gait with little or no effect on the arms. The cause is not known, although nutritional deficiency, especially of thiamine, has been suggested. Wernicke's encephalopathy (*see above*) with peripheral neuropathy (*see below*) is also commonly present. There is some improvement with abstinence and administration of thiamine.

Peripheral neuropathy   Peripheral neuropathy is commonly encountered with chronic abuse of alcohol, and is most likely to be caused by deficiency of members of the vitamin-B group, especially thiamine; there may be a direct toxic effect of alcohol. It is characterised by distal axonal degeneration, producing paraesthesia and pain in the feet; subsequently, the hands may also become affected. Muscle weakness and wasting may eventually develop distally in the arms and legs, and tendon reflexes are lost.

Cerebrovascular disorders   Alcohol has been implicated as the cause of strokes in young men following alcoholic binges; the mechanism may be either the hypertensive effects of alcohol or disturbed haemostasis. Subarachnoid haemorrhage has also been associated with excessive alcohol consumption.

Nutritional deficiency

Nutritional deficiency and excessive alcohol consumption are inextricably linked (especially in alcohol dependence), and factors that may be responsible include:

- utilisation of alcohol as an energy source
- dietary neglect
- financial constraints
- impaired storage of nutrients
- impaired utilisation of nutrients
- increased excretion of nutrients
- increased nutritional requirements
- malabsorption.

Alcohol is a source of energy but it does not contain any nutrients and, as a consequence, its calorific value is referred to as 'empty calories'. One gram of alcohol yields 0.029 MJ (7.0 kcal) of energy and therefore one unit provides 0.232 MJ (56.0 kcal) of energy. This extra source of energy in addition to a normal diet will contribute to the development of obesity. If dietary sources of energy are gradually replaced by alcohol, body-weight remains static as long as the total energy requirements are being met. If the diet is further reduced, the total intake of energy may be insufficient with resultant weight loss and more severe nutritional deficiency.

Chronic excessive alcohol consumption is commonly associated with an inadequate and irregular intake of food and an unbalanced diet; people who live alone are at increased risk. Heavy drinking also results in loss of appetite because the immediate energy demands are being met by the alcohol and, in the case of beer drinking, the stomach feels bloated. Drinking alcohol on a regular basis is an expensive habit to maintain, and financial constraints may mean that priority is given to alcohol over food. Alcohol may also cause malabsorption, and nutrients affected include folic acid, pyridoxine, thiamine, and vitamin B_{12}. Members of the vitamin-B group are used as coenzymes in the metabolism of alcohol (*see* Section 6.1) and, in the presence of an inadequate intake, there may be insufficient amounts to meet normal metabolic requirements.

Psychiatric disorders

Alcohol abuse is associated with psychiatric disorders or emotional disturbances, although it may be difficult to determine which is the cause and which is the effect. Behaviour disorders commonly arise as a result of chronic problem drinking, with irresponsible and unreliable behaviour being particularly evident.

Sustained drinking may induce depressive disorders, although it is not known what role alcohol plays in the aetiology. Alternatively, people may start drinking because of low self-esteem, lack of confidence, or feelings of guilt or worthlessness, which are all symptoms of depression. Alcohol-related depressive disorders represent a high risk of suicide. There is an association between manic-depressive illness and alcohol consumption, although the relationship is unclear and complex. The manic phase may contribute to excessive drinking as a result of elation and hyperactivity whereas alcohol may be used during the depressive phase to help improve mood. Excessive consumption is therefore frequent and regular and may lead to alcohol dependence.

Paranoid states, especially pathological jealousy, are commonly associated with alcohol abuse. Sexual jealousy and an unfounded belief in a partner's infidelity may arise. A common state of paranoia, which often occurs following a session of heavy drinking, is the belief that other people (usually passers-by) are making derogatory and insulting remarks.

Skeletal myopathy

Acute skeletal myopathy commonly arises after a session of heavy drinking, particularly in alcohol-dependent patients. It is probably caused by hypokalaemia as a result of vomiting, diarrhoea, and aldosteronism. The muscles of the thigh and the upper arm are most usually affected, and symptoms include pain, swelling, and weakness. In severe cases, there may be extensive destruction of muscle fibre, which may lead to renal failure.

Chronic skeletal myopathy is associated with long-term alcohol consumption, the relationship being with the total lifetime alcohol consumption rather than the current level. Atrophy of proximal muscles produces weakness and flaccidity; other symptoms may include low back pain and leg cramps.

6.3 ALCOHOL AND SPECIFIC GROUPS

The effects of alcohol vary considerably with age and sex, and influences the development of alcohol-related health and social problems. Groups that require special consideration are children, the elderly, and pregnant and breast-feeding women.

Children

Alcohol consumption by children

The effects of alcohol on children arise from their own alcohol consumption and that of their parents. At this stage, the dangers of alcohol consumption by children arise from acute intoxication rather than alcohol dependence.

Compared to adults, the capacity of alcohol metabolism is relatively limited in children, and the symptoms of acute intoxication (see Section 6.1) are more severe. Hypothermia is commonly encountered and is thought to arise as a result of impairment of temperature regulation systems. Respiratory depression may also occur in severe intoxication and requires close supervision and, in some cases, respiratory support. Hypoglycaemia is a serious effect of acute alcohol intoxication in children and is most likely to occur when alcohol is consumed in the morning before eating.

Infants and young children are particularly at risk of accidental poisoning as a result of their inquisitive natures. In the home, alcohol is generally considered to be relatively harmless and, unlike other potentially dangerous substances (e.g. bleach, weed-killer, and medicines), bottles of alcoholic drinks are often kept within sight and easy reach. Young children also imitate their parents behaviour and are likely to drink what they have seen their parents drinking. Accidental poisoning may occur when they consume alcohol in the morning

following a social event held in the home by their parents the night before. There may be remnants of alcoholic beverages in glasses or bottles left within reach. Older children, especially those approaching their teenage years, are usually familiar with alcohol, its effects, and use in social situations. To a smaller extent, they may also be aware of its intoxicating effects. However, they are normally unaware of alcohol-related diseases and the potency of alcohol.

Adolescents are invariably aware of alcohol. Experimentation is one of the most important causes of severe acute intoxication in teenagers. Regular alcohol consumption may start at a young age and, although long-term alcohol-related diseases may not be a problem, social and psychological effects may become apparent. Violence, crime, and other behavioural problems are commonly caused by alcohol. Factors that influence regular alcohol consumption in teenagers include:

- peer influence
- social pressures
- the desire to appear grown up
- wide availability.

The prevalence of regular alcohol consumption is higher among boys, although girls are narrowing the gap.

Excessive alcohol consumption by parents

Excessive alcohol consumption by parents has serious implications on the development of their children; the effects may be emotional and psychological in nature. The home environment is frequently tense and children develop feelings of uncertainty, neglect, rejection, and isolation, as a result of which, they may become socially and emotionally labile. Children may be blamed by their parents as the cause of their own drink problem, and are likely to believe this to be true because of their lack of knowledge and understanding. It should be emphasised, however, that children respond to parental excessive alcohol consumption in a variety of ways and whereas some children develop social and psychological problems, others remain unaffected.

Children may find it difficult to cope with parental alcohol-related health and social problems, and are often put under enormous pressure. In some cases, older children may have to take responsibility for younger siblings. Children often hide their own emotional and psychological problems, and those of their parents, from outsiders and pretend that home life is normal. They may have learning difficulties at school, and their childhood days are generally less happy. Parental alcohol abuse may lead to delinquency in their children;

these children are also liable to consume alcohol regularly, and drug misuse may be an additional feature.

The effects of parental excessive alcohol consumption on the health of their children are wide ranging. Infants may develop feeding difficulties, incessant crying, and vomiting. As they grow up psychiatric disorders may arise, and hyperactivity is frequently seen, although it may be a direct result of maternal excessive alcohol consumption during pregnancy.

The elderly

Elderly people are more vulnerable to the toxic effects of alcohol compared to younger people, which may be because for equivalent consumption of alcohol, elderly people attain higher blood-alcohol concentrations. This effect can be attributed to the ageing process, which results in a reduction of lean body mass, lower water content, and increased proportion of fat, compared to younger people. Delirium tremens (see Section 6.4) is associated with a higher mortality in the elderly; alcohol is also commonly involved in suicide attempts. Causes of excessive alcohol consumption in the elderly are numerous and include bereavement, boredom, loneliness, social isolation, and age-related disorders.

The elderly have a greater tendency to hide drink problems than younger people, and are more likely to consume alcohol throughout the day rather than indulge in sessions of heavy drinking. Non-specific alcohol-related disorders are commonly caused or exacerbated by excessive alcohol consumption in the elderly and include:

- hyperlipidaemia
- hyperuricaemia and gout
- hypoglycaemia
- hypothermia
- musculoskeletal disorders (especially skeletal myopathy)
- poor hygiene.

The elderly may have started drinking heavily at an early age, in which case chronic alcohol-related diseases (e.g. cirrhosis of the liver, cerebellar degeneration, and peripheral neuropathy) may already be present. The effects of alcohol on drug response are more important in the elderly as a result of the frequent use of one or more drugs. The dosage of all concurrent medication should be carefully assessed if excessive alcohol consumption is a problem.

Pregnant and breast-feeding women

Foetal alcohol syndrome

Alcohol freely crosses the placenta and similar blood-alcohol concentrations are seen in the foetus as in the mother. There is evidence that alcohol consumption during early pregnancy adversely affects foetal development. The condition is referred to as the foetal alcohol syndrome (FAS) and varies in severity depending on the level of alcohol consumption. Mild FAS may occur at levels greater than ten units/week and is characterised by prematurity, short body length, small head circumference, and low birth-weight; the risk of spontaneous abortion during the second trimester is also increased. Heavy drinking (e.g. more than 4 to 5 units/day) increases the risk of development of the complete FAS. This syndrome is characterised by developmental defects producing facial abnormalities, mental retardation, and central nervous system disorders (e.g. epilepsy, spasticity, and lack of coordination). There is also growth deficiency both *in utero* and following birth. Other disorders that may arise include cardiac disorders, urogenital disorders, musculoskeletal defects, and haemangiomas. Not all symptoms are apparent at birth, and the extent and severity of FAS may not be realised for some years. Late manifestations include behaviour disorders.

The development of FAS cannot be predicted from alcohol consumption alone because not all women who drink heavily during pregnancy give birth to infants exhibiting signs of developmental abnormalities. The role of alcohol in the aetiology of FAS is unknown and women at risk cannot yet be identified. Similarly, a safe level of alcohol consumption during pregnancy has not been established. The damaging effects may occur as early as conception, and alcohol should therefore be avoided by all women planning to become pregnant. Complete abstinence until delivery would be the ideal but it is considered by some authorities that such restrictive advice may be too severe to be heeded. A more realistic recommendation is that an occasional drink (up to a maximum of eight units/week) after the first few weeks of pregnancy is unlikely to harm the foetus; it is, however, important that this weekly amount is not consumed in one binge. It has also been suggested that heavy beer drinking carries a greater risk than excessive consumption of wine or spirits. Reduction of alcohol consumption late in pregnancy from excessive levels to sensible limits may not reverse some of the adverse effects, particularly growth retardation.

Alcohol in breast milk

The consumption of alcohol before breast-feeding may result in adverse effects in the infant, although these are rare and only likely to occur at high maternal blood-alcohol concentrations. Alcohol in breast milk is thought to cause a slight decrease in motor development of breast-fed infants, although this appears to be clinically insignificant. The concentration of alcohol in breast milk closely parallels maternal blood-alcohol concentration, but the resultant blood-alcohol concentration in the infant is usually low. Maternal blood-alcohol concentrations would have to be very high (e.g. 300 mg/100 mL) to result in mild sedation in the infant. Hence, an occasional drink during breast-feeding is not thought to be of any clinical significance to the infant.

6.4 ALCOHOL DEPENDENCE SYNDROME

Continued excessive alcohol consumption may eventually result in the alcohol dependence syndrome, which is most often seen in men in their mid-forties, although it can occur earlier. In women, alcohol dependence is associated with the early onset of nervous system disorders, which tend to occur following a shorter period of dependence and at lower levels of consumption than in men, and with an increased risk of death. There is also a greater tendency for permanent nervous system abnormalities in women following successful treatment of dependence and abstention from further alcohol consumption.

Tolerance to the acute effects of alcohol is substantial in alcohol dependence, and can occur up to a point where the dependent person may be able to tolerate blood-alcohol concentrations that would be associated with severe intoxication in the average person (*see* Section 6.1). A common misconception held by alcohol-dependent people is that since the amount of alcohol consumed does not result in acute intoxication, it is not having a detrimental effect. In the late stages of dependence tolerance may be reduced to the point where the acute effects of alcohol consumption return to those seen in the average person.

The alcohol dependence syndrome is characterised by the manifestation of withdrawal symptoms when the blood-alcohol concentration falls. Other features include:

- consumption of alcohol to relieve alcohol withdrawal symptoms (relief drinking)
- consumption of alcohol on a daily basis

- development of substantial tolerance to the effects of alcohol
- inability to stop consumption
- priority given to alcohol consumption above all else (e.g. social interaction, work, and health).

Alcohol withdrawal symptoms

Alcohol withdrawal symptoms characteristically appear on waking and are relieved by drinking. The severity and intensity of alcohol withdrawal symptoms are variable and may be classed, for clinical purposes, as minor withdrawal, intermediate withdrawal, and delirium tremens (major withdrawal).

Minor withdrawal   Minor withdrawal occurs within a few hours of the blood-alcohol concentration reaching zero and peaks between 24 and 36 hours. Symptoms may also appear as the blood-alcohol concentration is falling, especially if the decline is rapid. The characteristic symptoms of minor alcohol withdrawal are apprehension, raised blood pressure, insomnia, irritability, nausea and retching, sweating, tremor, and weakness.

Intermediate withdrawal   Intermediate withdrawal usually lasts for 5 to 7 days and is characterised by similar symptoms as seen in minor withdrawal (*see above*) but to a more severe degree. Additionally, hallucinations may occur, usually within 48 hours of stopping alcohol; they are generally visual in nature, although auditory hallucinations may also be experienced. Convulsions may occur in a small proportion of patients after 7 to 48 hours of stopping alcohol, and are usually generalised tonic-clonic (grand mal) convulsions. In rare cases, status epilepticus may occur, although other causes (e.g. hypoglycaemia, subdural haemorrhage, or CNS infection) must be considered. Arrhythmias may occasionally be associated with intermediate alcohol withdrawal although they may be caused by other alcohol-related disorders (e.g. hypokalaemia and acid-base imbalance). Heart failure may be precipitated, particularly if alcohol-related cardiomyopathy is present.

Delirium tremens   Delirium tremens is a serious and life-threatening manifestation of alcohol withdrawal, and begins within 4 days of stopping or reducing alcohol consumption; it may last for 3 to 7 days. It is not common, and occurs in only about 5% of patients. It is characterised by severe agitation and irritability, confusion, disorientation, impaired perception, insomnia and nightmares, delusions, nausea and vomiting, fever, profuse sweating, dehydration, electrolyte imbalance, gross tremor, hypertension, and arrhythmias. Hallucinations in delirium tremens are commonly visual in nature, although auditory hallucinations may also occur. Feelings of extreme fear and apprehension arising from the hallucinations may lead to aggressive or suicidal behaviour. Most deaths are caused by fever, arrhythmias, or coexisting illness (e.g. infection); the elderly are at increased risk of fatal delirium tremens.

Management of the alcohol dependence syndrome

Recognising alcohol dependence early can lead to successful treatment before any alcohol-related diseases develop. However, alcohol dependence is not always easy to detect even by health-care professionals. Persuading the patient that he may be dependent on alcohol and require treatment may be even more difficult.

Alcohol-dependent patients are usually secretive about their drinking behaviour even when they know it is dependence. They will deny being dependent on alcohol and may even believe that they can stop whenever they want to. Patients may want to stop drinking alcohol but are unable to, and asking for help is often a difficult first step for them. This may arise as a result of the social stigma associated with alcohol dependence.

Alcohol dependence can be identified in two ways. Firstly, patients may present with alcohol withdrawal symptoms (*see above*). Secondly, patients may present with signs and symptoms of alcohol-related health and social problems. However, presentation may not be clearly apparent and clues to the presence of alcohol dependence may be obtained from some of the following features:

- emotional and psychiatric disturbances (e.g. anxiety, depressive disorders, or insomnia)
- facial appearance (e.g. bloated face, facial flushing, and blood-shot eyes)
- family history of excessive alcohol consumption
- frequent requests for medical assistance (e.g. for gastro-intestinal disorders)
- gynaecomastia
- hand tremor and red palms
- obesity (e.g. 'pot belly')
- social problems (e.g. marital problems and work problems, especially Monday morning absences and inefficiency)
- tachycardia

- trouble with the police (e.g. drinking and driving, assault, and drunkenness)
- untidy appearance and smelling of alcohol.

Alcohol-dependent patients are commonly affected by anger, frustration, guilt, and isolation. Anger is often directed towards members of the family, and patients frequently blame them for the alcohol dependence. Family members often try not to antagonise the patient and, in some cases, may believe that the problem is not serious. These, and other social, emotional, and psychological problems (e.g. financial difficulties, bereavement, marital problems, and social isolation) that may contribute to excessive alcohol consumption must be identified and addressed in association with the management of alcohol dependence.

The management of alcohol dependence involves the short-term phase during which alcohol consumption must be stopped, and the more difficult long-term modification of drinking behaviour.

Short-term phase   The short-term phase involves alcohol withdrawal and control of the resultant symptoms.

The management of alcohol withdrawal (sometimes referred to as detoxification) is based on the extent and severity of the withdrawal symptoms, which are subject to marked individual variation. Communication with patients who are intoxicated or experiencing severe symptoms may be difficult, and details about alcohol consumption is often more reliably obtained from relatives or friends.

The drinking habits of the patient are first identified and the degree of tolerance assessed. If the patient appears to be only mildly intoxicated despite evidence of a large intake, substantial tolerance is likely and withdrawal may be severe. The extent and severity of previous episodes of alcohol withdrawal are also a reliable guide to predict the outcome on the present occasion, although successive episodes of withdrawal may increase in severity each time. Misuse of drugs must be identified as their withdrawal effects may occur in conjunction with, or follow, alcohol withdrawal. It is also important to determine the presence of any coexisting medical condition (alcohol-related or otherwise).

Alcohol withdrawal in all its forms is associated with considerable psychological distress for the patient, and management should be directed towards optimising comfort and safety. The environment should be well-illuminated and designed to be supportive, calm, and non-threatening. Patients may also require assistance with walking, bathroom functions, changing their clothing, and adjusting their bedclothes. Disorientation is a common feature of alcohol withdrawal and support is necessary to overcome it.

In the absence of complications (e.g. presence of coexisting disease), minor withdrawal symptoms are usually transient and self-limiting, and specialist supervision is not necessary. The patient may be managed at home or as an out-patient provided that there is adequate support from family or friends; recovery is usual within a few days. Drug administration in minor withdrawal is not usually necessary, although thiamine is commonly given to all patients to restore depleted reserves (see Section 6.2.2); multivitamin preparations may also be used. Other disorders (e.g. diarrhoea, and nausea and vomiting) are treated symptomatically. Fluid intake should be encouraged and food readily available on request.

The management of minor withdrawal in the presence of complications (e.g. coexisting medical conditions, dehydration, or fever) or if there is a history of intermediate withdrawal or delirium tremens requires specialist care. Patients presenting with symptoms of intermediate withdrawal or delirium tremens should always be managed under specialist care. In most cases, drug treatment is necessary to control the symptoms, and trained counsellors and nurses are also required to assist the patient and provide reassurance. Recovery can occur in the absence of drug therapy but the level of patient supervision that is required is extremely time-consuming and not practicable in most hospitals.

The benzodiazepines are commonly used in the management of alcohol withdrawal to suppress autonomic hyperactivity. They also have an anticonvulsant action, and their sedative properties confer a further advantage. Diazepam and chlordiazepoxide are widely used and large doses are usually necessary; lorazepam is used in the presence of advanced liver disease. Chlormethiazole is also used in the management of alcohol withdrawal. All patients should be given thiamine during the withdrawal period, which is also necessary before the administration of glucose because thiamine is necessary for glucose metabolism. Dehydration caused by sweating, fever, or increased muscular activity must also be corrected. Electrolyte imbalance (e.g. of potassium, magnesium, and phosphate) and coexisting infection also require treatment.

Although total abstinence during withdrawal is an ideal situation, some authorities believe that controlled drinking (i.e. modifying alcohol consumption to bring it within the sensible limits) may be sufficient. It may be a realistic target for alcohol-dependent patients under 40 years of age if alcohol dependence is detected early and in the absence of severe dependence or alcohol-related disease. However, total abstinence is necessary for patients above 40 years of age, if severe dependence or alcohol-related disease is present at any age, or if controlled drinking has been attempted without success. Some authorities advocate total abstinence for all patients as they believe even one drink will cause relapse and progress to alcohol dependence very quickly.

Long-term phase   The long-term phase involves helping the patient to establish modified drinking behaviour, and concentrates on rehabilitation with appropriate management of any contributory factors (e.g. anxiety). Coping with everyday problems without alcohol plays an important part in the rehabilitation process.

Drugs may also be used in some cases to help patients abstain from alcohol. Disulfiram is used to discourage alcohol consumption by producing unpleasant reactions (e.g. facial flushing, tachycardia, and nausea and vomiting) if alcohol is consumed concurrently. However, its use must be supervised, usually by relatives, and its mode of action explained in full. Even the small amounts of alcohol included in many oral medicines may be sufficient to precipitate a reaction.

The aim of the long-term phase is to help patients achieve life-style modifications that will allow them to cope with, or eliminate, the pressures responsible for their former drinking problem. Recreational activities, particularly those not related to alcohol consumption, are useful during the long-term phase to establish the changed drinking behaviour.

It should be emphasised to patients and their families that relapses and setbacks, although sometimes frequent, do not imply an incurable state. Encouragement is essential for patients to have another attempt at stopping or reducing alcohol consumption. In some cases, specialist care may be necessary following several failed attempts, or if the risk of alcohol-related disease is increasing or social problems become more evident.

Self-help groups and organisations (see Section 6.6) concerned with the problems of excessive alcohol consumption are of value in helping patients modify their drinking behaviour. They are staffed by people with extensive knowledge of the problems associated with excessive alcohol consumption who, in some cases, may formerly have had drinking problems themselves. Self-help groups should be recommended at an early stage to all people with suspected or identified alcohol dependence.

6.5 PROMOTION OF SENSIBLE ALCOHOL CONSUMPTION

The prevention and control of excessive alcohol consumption by advocating total abstinence would not be acceptable to the majority of people and, in most cases, is not necessary. Promotion of sensible alcohol consumption is a more realistic goal. Health education should aim to make clear the relationship between alcohol consumption and the development of health and social problems, although it is recognised that this may not be sufficient in itself to reduce levels of consumption and additional methods may be necessary.

Factors influencing alcohol consumption and, more importantly, excessive alcohol consumption are wide-ranging and diverse in nature (*see* Section 6.1). The WHO has identified the following areas that could be targeted to promote sensible alcohol consumption:

- availability of low-alcohol and alcohol-free drinks
- modifications in life-style
- health education (of both the public and the professions)
- pricing policies to increase the 'real' price (i.e. the price in relation to disposable income) of alcoholic drinks
- regulation of production
- reducing the availability (e.g. restrictive licensing laws)
- restrictions on advertising
- treatment and counselling.

Campaigns should be coordinated between all relevant agencies (e.g. government departments, the medical profession, voluntary organisations, and health education authorities). There is wide regional variation in the services available; some authorities do not have a policy on alcohol consumption, and the burden is allowed to fall on voluntary organisations. In the UK, government involvement in the promotion of sensible alcohol consumption is directed by the Ministerial Group on Alcohol Misuse, which recommends policy measures. Initiatives recommended by this group include:

- alcohol education to form part of the national school curriculum
- the appointment of regional alcohol coordinators
- the exclusion of anyone who looks under 25 years of age from alcohol advertisements
- funding Alcohol Concern to aid local organisations dealing with excessive alcohol consumption
- reducing the ease with which convicted drink-drive offenders may regain their licences

- making the sale of alcohol to under-age children illegal, even if done unwittingly, combined with increased fines
- National 'Drinkwise' days to promote sensible drinking
- enquiries about alcohol consumption to form part of the general life-style enquiries made by health-care personnel.

Low-alcohol and alcohol-free drinks

The image of non-drinkers as being 'antisocial' is one of the main reasons for regular alcohol consumption (especially in young people). However, this stigma is gradually disappearing with the development and marketing of low-alcohol and alcohol-free drinks, which present a sophisticated profile resembling that of alcohol rather than soft drinks. As yet, these alternative products are not necessarily any cheaper than alcoholic drinks and are not always widely available or encouraged. It is important that the current position is reversed, especially with respect to the young who are particularly vulnerable to social pressures. Adolescents, especially schoolchildren, may not go out specifically to drink, but rather to meet friends, and, if alcohol is available in these situations, then it is likely to be consumed. A change in environment may have a greater influence on the drinking habits of children than campaigns warning of health risks, and centres where food and alternative drinks to alcohol are available should be promoted to them. Similarly, widespread promotion of low-alcohol and alcohol-free drinks to drivers could have a significant impact in reducing the number of alcohol-related road traffic offences and accidents.

Selecting appropriate drinks to avoid consuming excessive amounts of alcohol can be difficult because the labelling of low-alcohol and alcohol-free drinks is frequently confusing. There are, as yet, no rules or guidelines on product labelling; government proposals to limit the use of the term low-alcohol to beverages containing less than 1.2% alcohol by volume have been dropped in anticipation of proposed European Commission guidelines. It is important to emphasise, therefore, that the label on all such products should be studied carefully to determine the alcohol content, which is usually stated as percentage alcohol by volume. However, in certain situations (e.g. in licensed premises or at parties) this may be difficult.

Drinks labelled as alcohol-free would be expected to have no alcohol in them. However, they may contain a small quantity of alcohol (less than 0.05% by volume) and would therefore not be suitable for people who avoid alcohol on religious, dietary, or cultural grounds. De-alcoholised beverages would also be expected to contain no alcohol. However, not all the alcohol may be removed and quantities approaching 0.5% alcohol by volume may be found.

Drinks labelled as low-alcohol represent the most confusing area. The term 'low' is taken to mean that the alcohol content is lower than in regular beverages. Generally, low-alcohol beers and lagers have an alcohol content of less than one-fifth of the regular beers or lagers, and therefore may have an alcohol content below 1% by volume. Wines of normal strength contain 8 to 10% alcohol by volume and low-alcohol wines may, in some cases, contain up to 5% alcohol by volume. This concentration of alcohol is higher than many regular beers and lagers, and if several glasses are consumed, may increase blood-alcohol concentrations above the legal limit for driving.

The terms 'reduced alcohol' and 'greatly reduced alcohol', have no specific relationship to the content of alcohol in the drink, and these beverages may contain substantial quantities of alcohol. The term light (or 'lite') commonly mean the same as low-alcohol. However, these terms are also used to mean a low-calorie drink, which may have the same alcohol content as a regular alcoholic beverage.

The role of the pharmacist

Pharmacists can make an impact on reducing excessive alcohol consumption by becoming actively involved in the promotion of sensible drinking, and national and local campaigns would benefit from their involvement. 'Drinkwise' is one such regular campaign, which aims to promote sensible drinking and to educate people about the dangers of alcohol. The pharmacist can have an even greater impact at an individual level by giving advice, where appropriate, about sensible alcohol consumption. Use of available health education material is essential to complement the professional advice.

Questioning a patient or customer about their level of alcohol consumption has not been part of a pharmacist's routine enquiries, and may at first be difficult. It should be regarded in the same light as any other enquiry about life-style (e.g. smoking) and will soon become an established routine. To assess the individual risk attached to alcohol consumption (see Section 6.1) it is important to estimate a person's average weekly consumption. However, alcohol consumption is frequently underestimated, particularly by those who consume excessive amounts. It may be helpful to suggest that the patient keeps an 'alcohol diary' to record each

alcoholic drink, noting the amount, time, place, and situation (e.g. business, social, or alone).

The pharmacist should, where possible, encourage people who drink at hazardous or dangerous levels to reduce their consumption to sensible limits, and non-drinkers or people who drink moderate amounts should be made aware of the risks associated with starting or increasing consumption. An explanation of the unit system to calculate alcohol consumption (see Section 6.1) should form the basis of alcohol education, and the importance of assessing individual weekly intakes stressed. Low-alcohol and alcohol-free drinks should be highlighted, although appropriate advice should be given about the alcohol content of these drinks and the importance of studying the labels carefully (see above). If the alcohol dependence syndrome is suspected, the patient should be referred to their doctor, a specialist unit, or to a self-help group (see Section 6.6). It should be remembered that there is little to be achieved from talking to people who are intoxicated, and it may be necessary to wait until a more appropriate time when the person is responsive.

The pharmacist should pay particular attention to special groups who may be at increased risk from alcohol-related health and social problems (see Section 6.3). Parents with young children should be aware of the dangers of alcohol, and should not introduce their children to alcohol, even at special occasions. The elderly are also at increased risk, and the pharmacist can influence alcohol consumption levels by improving their awareness of the effects of alcohol. In addition, the pharmacist should be alert to the possibility of non-specific symptoms in the elderly indicating excessive alcohol consumption. Women require specific advice on alcohol consumption as a result of their increased susceptibility to alcohol-related problems (see Section 6.1), and the rationale behind the lower limits for women compared to those for men should be explained. Pregnancy and breast-feeding are particular areas where the pharmacist can advise about alcohol consumption.

Drinking and driving (see Section 6.2.1) is a particularly serious social consequence of alcohol consumption. It should be emphasised that driving ability is significantly reduced by lower blood-alcohol concentrations than that set as the legal limit for driving (see Section 6.2.1). It is important to stress that alcohol should not be consumed at all if driving and this should be the message that the pharmacist must try and convey. It is also important to mention that low-alcohol drinks (see above) contain a substantial amount of alcohol, and may in themselves cause a reduction in driving ability if sufficient is consumed; in some cases, they may even result in increasing the blood-alcohol concentration above the legal limit for driving. However, there will be a demand for information about what levels of alcohol consumption put people over the legal limit for driving. To this end, the most useful advice the pharmacist can provide concerns the acute effects of alcohol (*see* Section 6.1), how alcohol behaves in the body, and the numerous factors governing its effects. The pharmacist should inform people of the wide variation in the response to alcohol and that blood-alcohol concentrations cannot be accurately predicted from intake. General advice on the excretion patterns of alcohol may, however, be useful in helping people realise the time that the body needs to completely eliminate alcohol.

The pharmacist is familiar with interactions between medicines and alcohol, and this area should be included in counselling on the appropriate use of medicines. A summary of potential drug-alcohol interactions is included in the BNF (Appendix 1) for quick and easy reference. In addition to alcohol, the pharmacist should also be alert to the fact that people who consume excessive amounts of alcohol may also be drug misusers. The presence of alcohol-related disease (e.g. liver disease) should also be borne in mind when considering drug contra-indications.

6.6 USEFUL ADDRESSES

ACCEPT
200 Seagrave Road
London SW6 1RQ
Tel: 071-381 2112/3155

AL-ANON FAMILY GROUPS UK & EIRE
(including Alateen)
61 Great Dover Street
London SE1 4YF
Tel: 071-403 0888

ALCOHOL CONCERN
305 Gray's Inn Road
London WC1X 8QF
Tel: 081-833 3471

ALCOHOL COUNSELLING SERVICE
34 Electric Lane
London SW9 8JT
Tel: 071-737 3570/3579

ALCOHOLICS ANONYMOUS (AA)
General Service Office
PO Box 1
Stonebow House
Stonebow
York YO1 2NJ
Tel: (0904) 644026/7/8/9
Tel: 071-352 3001

DAWN (Drugs, Alcohol, Women, Now)
Omnibus Workspace
39–41 North Road
London N7 9DP
Tel: 071-700 4653

TACADE
1 Hulme Place
The Crescent
Salford M5 4QA
Tel: 061-745 8925
The advisory council on alcohol and drug education.

TURNING POINT
CAP House
4th Floor
9–12 Long Lane
London EC1A 9HA
Tel: 071-606 3947

6.7 FURTHER READING

Gelder M, *et al.,* eds. The Abuse of Alcohol and Drugs. In: *Oxford textbook of psychiatry.* 2nd ed. Oxford: Oxford University Press, 1989: 507–55.
The Royal College of Physicians. *A great and growing evil. The medical consequences of alcohol abuse.* London: Tavistock Publications, 1987.
Thorley AP. Alcohol. In: Tyrer PJ, ed. *Drugs in psychiatric practice.* London: Butterworths, 1982: 352–366.

Chapter 7

DRUG MISUSE

7.1 INTRODUCTION

The misuse of both prescribed and illicit drugs is a major national problem. In 1990, almost 18 000 people were registered as drug addicts, representing a 20% increase compared to the previous year. The cost of drug misuse to society is difficult to determine because of the paucity of adequate data, but there can be little doubt that, in terms of serious health and social problems, the costs are substantial. The need to prevent and control drug misuse has been accentuated by the risk of spread of diseases such as AIDS and hepatitis B by the misuse of intravenous drugs. In some countries, the majority of cases of HIV infection have occurred as a result of drug users using shared syringes and needles.

There is no definitive description of drug misuse that will cover all of the issues and criteria associated with drug use and misuse; such definitions are generally subjective and arbitrary. The Royal College of Psychiatrists define drug misuse as 'any taking of a drug which harms or threatens to harm the physical or mental health or social well-being of an individual, of other individuals, or of society at large, or which is illegal'.

The concept of problem drug use perhaps provides a better working definition. A problem drug user has been defined by the Advisory Council on the Misuse of Drugs as 'a person who has physical, psychological, social or legal problems associated with drug abuse'. Problem drug use encompasses all levels and stages of drug use, and not only that which has resulted in drug dependence; it covers experimental use through to uncontrolled use of many drugs. However, the definition of a 'problem' is subjective and what constitutes a 'problem' to one person may well be 'no problem' to another.

The problems associated with the use of the recreational drugs tobacco and alcohol are covered in Chapters 5 and 6 respectively. The illicit use of ergogenic drugs by athletes is discussed in Section 8.5.

Drug misuse may be linked to the relief of unpleasant feelings and experiences, which include anxiety, depressive disorders, lack of self-identity, frustration, diminished self-esteem, and boredom; drugs may be used in these instances to provide pleasure and happiness. Increased availability is also associated with increased misuse; this is reflected by certain over-prescribed medicines and illicit drugs on the black market. Peer pressure, personality traits, and social deprivation may also be contributing factors to drug misuse. An unstable family life may be associated with drug misuse whereas a stable family background is commonly, but not always, associated with a reduced likelihood of drug misuse.

Factors contributing to drug misuse are wide-ranging, and no single cause can be identified as the most important. Drug misuse was considered to be associated with younger people, and although experimentation does commonly occur at a young age, in general, drug misuse covers all age groups. Drug misuse is also more frequent in males than females, although the number of females misusing drugs is increasing.

Drug misusers often have a stigma attached to them, and may try to conceal their habits from family and friends because of social unacceptability. Disclosure of drug-related problems can lead to difficulties in relationships and alienation.

The many consequences of drug misuse include suicide, accidents, absenteeism, crime, delinquency, marital problems, unemployment, homelessness, and the spread of HIV infection.

The Misuse of Drugs Act was passed in 1971 to provide control over drug misuse of all kinds. The Misuse of Drugs Regulations 1985 and the Misuse of Drugs (Notifications and Supply to Addicts) Regulations 1973 were also introduced under the Act. The legislation is detailed in *Medicines, Ethics and Practice: a Guide for Pharmacists*, which is issued regularly to all members of the profession. The Advisory Council on the Misuse of Drugs was set up under the Act, and its function is to advise the government on measures to prevent and deal with problems arising from the misuse of drugs.

7.2   DRUG DEPENDENCE

The World Health Organization (WHO) recommended use of the term 'drug dependence' and offered the following definition: 'a state, psychic and sometimes also physical, resulting from the interaction between a living organism and a drug, characterised by behavioural and other responses that always include the compulsion to take the drug on a continuous or periodic basis in order to experience its psychic effects, and sometimes to avoid the discomfort of its absence. Tolerance may or may not be present. A person may be dependent on more than one drug'. This definition attempts to cover all aspects of drug dependence and to remove the use of the terms 'drug addiction' and 'drug habituation', which are thought by some authorities to have derogatory connotations.

Physical dependence   Drug misuse, especially of drugs that exert their effects on the central nervous system, can lead to a state of physical dependence, which is generally characterised by the development of tolerance, neuroadaptation, and withdrawal symptoms

on stopping use. The use of a drug that produces physical dependence may also confer cross-dependence to other related drugs.

Drug tolerance may be defined as a state of decreased responsiveness to the pharmacological actions of a drug as a result of previous use of that drug or a related drug. The central nervous system responds by reducing the effects of repeated drug administration; higher doses are then required to produce the same effect. In some cases, the use of one drug may produce cross-tolerance to other related drugs, which may be complete or partial. Tolerance can range from a small reduction to complete absence of the pharmacological effects of the drug. It can develop slowly or rapidly; rapid development of tolerance is sometimes called acute tolerance or tachyphylaxis.

Neuroadaptation is the ability of the central nervous system to adapt at a cellular level to the presence of a drug; it is thought to be at least partly responsible for the development of tolerance and characteristic withdrawal symptoms on stopping drug use.

Withdrawal symptoms (also called the abstinence syndrome) occur when drug use is stopped following the development of dependence. Generally, withdrawal symptoms are characteristic physiological reactions to the type of drug used; they also tend to be opposite to the effects produced by the drug (e.g. stimulants will produce depressant withdrawal symptoms and depressant drugs will produce excitatory withdrawal symptoms). Withdrawal symptoms can be terminated by the administration of the drug or another drug to which cross-dependence has developed.

The relationship between tolerance, neuroadaptation, withdrawal symptoms, and physical dependence is complex and not fully understood. Physical dependence can occur in the presence of little, if any, tolerance; conversely, profound tolerance can occur in the absence of physical dependence. Tolerance may also occur in the absence of withdrawal symptoms when drug use is stopped; dependence can also occur without the development of physical withdrawal symptoms. These differences are related to the pharmacological effects of the various classes of drugs.

Psychological dependence   Learned behaviour and personality characteristics are two of a wide range of psychological factors that contribute to the development and maintenance of drug dependence. Learned behaviour influences the further use of a drug for its effects following initial use; this process is termed reinforcement, where the consequences (or effects) increase the frequency of drug use. Other reinforcing factors include the development of withdrawal symptoms. Learned behaviour can also be related to the environment; triggers which initiate craving or withdrawal symptoms (e.g. the sight of injecting equipment, other methods of using drugs, or friends who use drugs) act as environmental reminders of drug use, and thus as reinforcers.

Personality characteristics are involved in the development and maintenance of drug dependence, although there is not an identifiable 'dependence personality'; some individuals appear to use drugs experimentally, for stimulation, or as a response to adverse circumstances, although there is wide variation.

Social factors   The sense of personal identity associated with being an 'addict' or 'junkie' may be rewarding for some individuals; such roles may also contribute to acceptance and identification as part of the 'drug scene'. The self-image of users is also an important aspect; a person who views their own drug misuse as dependence and a life-long, intractable condition is more likely to maintain the habit.

Peer group pressure may partly be responsible for the initiation and acceptance of drug misuse by an individual. Drug dependence may also be reinforced further as a result of common experiences and a shared way of life. The daily acquisition of drugs and their misuse may become meaningful and a part of everyday life.

Drug dependence syndrome   Multiple criteria are necessary for the assessment of the drug dependence syndrome and in 1981 the WHO defined the main criteria:

- a subjective awareness of compulsion to use a drug or drugs, usually during attempts to stop or moderate drug use
- a desire to stop drug use in the face of continued use
- a relatively stereotyped drug-taking habit, i.e. a narrowing in the repertoire of drug-taking behaviour
- evidence of neuroadaptation (tolerance and withdrawal symptoms)
- use of the drug to relieve or avoid withdrawal symptoms
- the salience of drug-seeking behaviour relative to other important priorities
- a rapid reinstatement of the syndrome after a period of abstinence.

The most important feature of the dependence syndrome is the compulsion to use drugs. However, it is important not to assess drug dependence using only a single criterion; the whole list should be considered.

Management of drug dependence   One of the main aspects in the management of drug dependence is drug withdrawal (detoxification) and the consequent management of withdrawal symptoms. The management of drug withdrawal symptoms is described, as appropriate, under each drug or group of drugs, in Section 7.4.

Supportive therapy, counselling, and psychotherapy are essential at all stages of drug withdrawal, and should be introduced as early as possible. They are of prime importance following drug withdrawal to assist individuals in maintaining a drug-free way of life. Self-help and community groups may provide useful assistance and advice in the management of drug dependence; some of these are included in Section 7.6.

7.3   ROUTES OF ADMINISTRATION AND ASSOCIATED ADVERSE EFFECTS

Drugs may be misused by various routes, including oral ingestion, inhalation, injection, and intranasal administration. The route of administration can determine the type and severity of medical complications associated with drug misuse, which may also be related to the presence of adulterants or contaminants. The route of administration may also influence the risk of dependence.

Inhalation of a drug enables absorption from the lungs, which can be almost as rapid as that from intravenous injection. Inhalation of a drug may be linked to the development of inflammation of the lung tissue and reduced lung function, which is caused by the inhalation of drug particles, impurities, or excipients. Forced inhalation of drugs is associated with the development of pneumothorax, pneumomediastinum, and pneumopericardium. In the case of volatile substance misuse (*see* Section 7.4), asphyxiation may be caused by the plastic bag that is, in some cases, placed over the head in order to inhale the substance.

Parenteral administration of a drug may be by the intravenous route ('mainlining'), subcutaneous injection ('skin popping'), or intramuscular injection. Intravenous injection enables rapid plasma-drug concentrations to be achieved and is the preferred route for the opioids.

Drug misuse by injection is associated with a wide range of adverse effects. Subcutaneous administration may cause chronic suppurating skin infections at the injection sites, which can lead to amyloidosis and nephropathy. A failed attempt at an intravenous injection may result in an abscess, particularly following injection of ground tablets. Infected (hot) abscesses may also occur following injection using unsterile techniques (e.g. use of tap water to dissolve drugs or dirty injecting equipment). If a vein is missed, tissue reactions may arise as a result of the drug excipients used in tablet and capsule manufacture or the drug itself.

Local irritation and trauma on intravenous injection can lead to thrombophlebitis, which again may be caused by the irritant effects of the drug or the presence of contaminants or adulterants. Barbiturates, for example, are highly irritant and cause the skin above the injection site to slough off, which is referred to as a 'barb burn'. Inadvertent injection into an artery can cause vasospasm and lead to gangrene of the tissues supplied by the artery (e.g. the fingers are commonly affected or gangrene of the leg may arise if the femoral artery is involved). Unintentional injection into nerves can cause paraesthesia or hyperaesthesia; paralysis may also occur.

Injection of adulterants or contaminants may cause adverse reactions, including cellulitis and granulomatous lesions in organs such as the lungs, liver, and kidneys. Quinine and strychnine may be found as adulterants; quinine can cause cinchonism and amblyopia if sufficient is injected, and strychnine can cause opisthotonos and life-threatening seizures.

Infection is the most serious health risk that is encountered by drug misusers, particularly those who inject drugs. Micro-organisms may be introduced into the body as a result of using contaminated needles and syringes, poor injection technique, or from the drug itself. Endocarditis, septic arthritis, and osteomyelitis may occur, and rarely, tetanus and wound botulism. However, hepatitis (hepatitis B and non-A non-B hepatitis) and HIV infection are the most serious infections associated with injection of drugs, particularly as a result of sharing injection equipment.

Intranasal administration ('snorting' or 'sniffing') may cause irritation of the highly vascular nasal mucosa. Hyperaemia, rhinorrhoea, and sinusitis may also occur. Prolonged intranasal administration may cause necrosis and perforation of the nasal septum, which is commonly associated with cocaine misuse.

7.4 DRUGS OF MISUSE

The range of drugs that are subject to misuse, or have a misuse potential, is extensive. It is impossible to discuss in detail all the drugs that are misused, and only those commonly encountered or those causing the most public concern are discussed in detail.

Amphetamines and related stimulants

The drugs referred to in this section include the amphetamines (amphetamine, dexamphetamine, and methylamphetamine), methylphenidate, and pemoline. The appetite suppressants diethylpropion, mazindol, and phentermine are also CNS stimulants. Fenfluramine, another appetite suppressant, is also related to amphetamine, but has a sedative effect at standard doses, and has a lower potential for misuse. Tranylcypromine, a monoamine-oxidase inhibitor, is structurally similar to the amphetamines and is subject to misuse.

Amphetamine, a synthetic compound, was first available for medicinal use in the 1930s as a nasal vasoconstrictor. Its stimulant and appetite suppressant properties were realised, and amphetamine was used for a range of disorders (e.g. depressive disorders, obesity, impotence, and migraine). During the 1960s, use of amphetamines became restricted to obesity and depressive disorders. Medicinal use is now restricted to narcolepsy and hyperactivity in children, under specialist care only.

As a result of the extensive availability of amphetamines, misuse became inevitable and widespread. Amphetamines became accepted and were used supposedly to enhance energy, concentration, and mental and physical performance. Sportsmen and sportswomen began to use amphetamines to improve athletic performance, although this is now prohibited (*see* Section 8.5).

In the late 1960s, there was widespread misuse of intravenous methylamphetamine. Voluntary restrictions were imposed by prescribers, and supplies of methylamphetamine were withdrawn by manufacturers, but misuse was diverted to amphetamine sulphate. The Pharmaceutical Society of Great Britain advised pharmacists not to supply amphetamine sulphate as some doctors, wittingly or otherwise, were still writing prescriptions. This action was widely approved and helped stem misuse of amphetamine sulphate. As the awareness of the misuse of amphetamines grew, voluntary restrictions were placed on prescribing, and the availability of amphetamines was drastically reduced.

There are many street names to describe the amphetamines; these include 'pep pills', 'speed', and 'uppers'; dexamphetamine tablets are often referred to as 'dexies'; and methylamphetamine is known as 'crank', 'crystal', or 'ice'.

The only amphetamine currently available on prescription is dexamphetamine sulphate. Methylamphetamine is occasionally encountered in a form used for smoking, sometimes called 'ice'. Methylphenidate was formerly used for the treatment of narcolepsy and hyperactivity in children, but was withdrawn from the market in 1985; it is, however, still occasionally encountered. Pemoline is a mild CNS stimulant also used under specialist supervision for hyperactivity in children, and is subject to misuse.

Actions and methods of administration

Amphetamines and related stimulants are sympathomimetics and have similar effects; they differ only in their potency. For this reason the effects of amphetamines will be discussed and those of related stimulants can be taken to be largely the same, although they may be less intense.

Amphetamines stimulate the central and peripheral nervous systems; stimulation of the CNS is responsible for their misuse potential. Amphetamines produce CNS stimulation by promoting the release of the neurotransmitters, dopamine and noradrenaline. In addition, amphetamines inhibit neuronal re-uptake of these neurotransmitters and may exert a direct agonistic effect on catecholamine receptors. The amphetamines and cocaine have almost identical mechanisms of stimulant action, although amphetamines have a longer duration of action and no local anaesthetic effect.

At low doses, amphetamines cause increased alertness, prevention or reduction of fatigue, mood elevation (including increased self-confidence, initiative, and concentration), elation, and euphoria; there is also increased activity and talkativeness. The need for food and sleep is postponed until use is discontinued. Physical performance is improved as a result of decreased fatigue, which may be exploited by athletes (see Section 8.5).

Amphetamines are not popular as enhancers of sexual activity. Although the intravenous use of amphetamines has been associated with an 'orgasm-like' effect, high doses result in a loss of coordination and restlessness, which interferes with sexual response. Long-term use of amphetamines has been associated with loss of libido.

High doses of amphetamines result in toxicity. An amphetamine psychosis has been described, which may be difficult to distinguish from acute paranoid schizophrenia. Auditory and visual hallucinations may occur and feelings of persecution may be present. Recovery is usually attained within a few days following intake, although occasionally a chronic condition develops. Other symptoms include restlessness, dizziness, tremor, irritability, insomnia, fever, confusion, panic attacks, and anxiety. There is also a risk of violent behaviour. These effects are almost invariably followed by profound depression and fatigue. The doses that induce toxic symptoms are not predictable.

Toxic effects on the cardiovascular system include headache, pallor or flushing, palpitations, cardiac arrhythmias, anginal pain, hypotension or hypertension, and circulatory collapse. Effects on the gastro-intestinal system include dry mouth, anorexia, nausea and vomiting, diarrhoea, and abdominal cramps. Excessive doses produce convulsions and coma, with death occurring from cerebral haemorrhage.

Amphetamines are administered orally, intranasally, or by intravenous injection; methylamphetamine can also be smoked. Amphetamines may be taken to reduce fatigue and improve social performance. High doses may make the user feel that they have infinite power.

Intravenous amphetamine use causes rapid and intense effects, referred to as a 'rush' or 'flash'. Cravings for the amphetamine 'rush' or 'flash' may lead to repeated administration to sustain the effects, commonly referred to as a 'speed run'. Intravenous administration may continue for up to a week until supplies are exhausted or adverse effects of amphetamines develop (e.g. excessive fatigue and paranoia) and end the 'speed run'. Following the 'speed run', users may sleep for 24 to 48 hours and, on waking, extreme hunger is experienced. This may be followed by severe depression, leading to further amphetamine use. Intravenous amphetamines are often used in combination with other drugs of misuse. The combination of amphetamine with heroin is sometimes referred to as a 'speedball' or 'snowball'.

Amphetamines may also be used by intranasal administration ('snorting' or 'sniffing') in a similar fashion to cocaine (see Cocaine below). Intranasal administration induces a similar amphetamine 'rush' or 'flash' to intravenous administration. Crystalline methylamphetamine is the preferred form for intranasal administration.

Misuse in pregnancy

Amphetamine misuse in pregnancy is associated with the development of congenital abnormalities, including heart defects, biliary atresia, and oral cleft defects. Microcephaly in association with mental retardation and motor dysfunction has also been reported with methylamphetamine use during pregnancy. Babies born to mothers who use amphetamines may be premature and have a lower than average birth-weight.

Amphetamine misuse in pregnancy may result in the development of intoxication in the newborn or withdrawal signs depending on the time of use. Manifestations of intoxication in the newborn include profuse sweating, restlessness, and miotic pupils. These signs usually resolve within a few days. Neonates may become lethargic, which may necessitate tube feeding.

Dependence, tolerance, and withdrawal symptoms

Prolonged use of amphetamines may cause psychological dependence, characterised by the compulsion to seek further supplies of the drug. However, amphetamine use can be occasional and may not always lead to dependence.

Tolerance to the euphoric, anorexic, and hyper-thermic effects of amphetamines can occur; cross-tolerance between amphetamines and related stimulants, including cocaine, is also exhibited. In contrast, an increased sensitivity to some of the CNS effects of amphetamines may also develop. However, tolerance does not develop to the psychotoxic effects of amphetamines, and a toxic psychosis may occur after weeks or months of continued use.

Withdrawal symptoms following amphetamine use include lassitude, apathy, anxiety, and depression. Withdrawal symptoms, which may continue for some weeks, may be severe in the early stages and require careful observation of the patient; suicidal tendencies may develop as a result of severe depression. Other symptoms include craving, excessive hunger and eating, and prolonged sleep.

Management of withdrawal

For those patients who have become dependent on prescribed amphetamines or appetite suppressants, an agreed dosage reduction regimen may be instigated. Supportive therapy, counselling, and psychotherapy may also be beneficial. For those individuals who use intravenous amphetamines, or large doses of stimulants, and who are actually or incipiently psychotic, in-patient care may be necessary to provide a safe environment.

Antimuscarinic drugs

Antimuscarinic drugs are widely used in the treatment of parkinsonism and to reduce the extrapyramidal side-effects of antipsychotic drugs. In addition, antimuscarinic drugs, taken by mouth, may produce mild euphoria or toxic psychosis characterised by hallucinations and disorientation. It is known that some other drugs of misuse (e.g. cannabis and opioids) act in part by decreasing cholinergic activity, which supports the concept of antimuscarinic drugs as potential drugs of misuse.

The extent of antimuscarinic drug misuse is not known, although it appears to be most common in patients being treated with antipsychotic drugs.

Actions and methods of administration

Antimuscarinic drugs commonly produce euphoria, and in some instances, hallucinations and disorientation.

Other effects described by users include relaxation, a sense of well-being, and increased sociability. The stimulant properties of antimuscarinic drugs may result in individuals feeling more energetic. Blurred vision, flushing, tachycardia, memory impairment (especially affecting recent memory and learning capacity) may occur following antimuscarinic drug misuse.

The use of high doses of antimuscarinic drugs may result in the development of a toxic psychosis. It is characterised by profound visual hallucinations, illusions, distortion of the sense of time, dehydration, excessive thirst, feelings of persecution, blurred vision, and tachycardia.

Benzhexol is the most commonly misused anti-muscarinic drug. However, it is also the most frequently prescribed drug of its class for the treatment of extrapyramidal side-effects of antipsychotic drugs. Other antimuscarinic drugs (e.g. biperiden, benztropine, orphenadrine, and procyclidine) are also misused.

Misuse of antimuscarinic drugs may be more common among schizophrenic patients and individuals who misuse a range of drugs. Patients on antipsychotic therapy may fake extrapyramidal symptoms, or their intensity, in order to obtain antimuscarinic drugs; requests for prescriptions or supplies to replace 'lost drugs' or 'drugs running out quickly' may also be an indication of misuse. Patients may also be reluctant to stop antimuscarinic drug treatment or have their dose reduced. In some cases, patients may stop taking their antipsychotic medication and increase the dose of antimuscarinic drug, in order to achieve a feeling of euphoria and well-being.

Dependence, tolerance, and withdrawal symptoms

Physical and psychological dependence can occur with antimuscarinic drugs. Tolerance develops, with the need to increase doses to achieve a similar degree of mood elevation. Withdrawal symptoms associated with antimuscarinic drugs include myalgia, profuse sweating, gastro-intestinal disturbances, anxiety, hallucinations, nightmares, headache, insomnia, dysphoria, and paraesthesia; rebound extrapyramidal effects may occur in patients receiving antipsychotic drugs, or motor function deterioration in patients with parkinsonism.

Management of withdrawal

Withdrawal from the use of antimuscarinic drugs should be gradual, although the rate of withdrawal is dependent on individual circumstances and medical opinion. Supportive therapy, counselling, and psychotherapy may be beneficial.

Barbiturates

The barbiturates were widely prescribed until the 1960s when their dependence potential and consequences of overdosage were fully realised. Barbiturates have a narrow therapeutic margin beyond which life-threatening toxicity may occur and they have been involved in many overdose fatalities and suicide attempts.

The introduction of the benzodiazepines provided a safer alternative, and thereafter the number of prescriptions for barbiturates steadily declined. Barbiturates became common drugs of misuse during the 1970s, especially by young people, and this led to the establishment of stricter controls on supply. Although misuse of barbiturates has declined since then, it is still frequently encountered.

Barbiturates can be divided into the following categories:

- Short-acting

  Short-acting barbiturates include methohexitone and thiopentone; they are used in anaesthesia.

- Intermediate-acting

  Intermediate-acting barbiturates include amylobarbitone, butobarbitone, and quinalbarbitone; they are used in the treatment of severe intractable insomnia in people already taking barbiturates.

- Long-acting

  Long-acting barbiturates include methylphenobarbitone and phenobarbitone; they are used in the treatment of epilepsy.

Actions and methods of administration

Barbiturates have anxiolytic and sedative properties; memory and thought impairment may also occur. At higher doses, intoxication occurs with slurred speech, unsteady gait, and progressive muscle incoordination. Other effects that may occur include dizziness, ataxia, nystagmus, and headache; paradoxical excitement and confusion may also arise. Toxic doses result in CNS and respiratory depression. Hypothermia may also occur, with fever on recovery. Cardiorespiratory collapse is the commonest cause of death following overdosage.

A hangover effect can occur with long-acting barbiturates, and is similar to that following alcohol use; signs include feelings of discontent, headache, and impaired concentration. The hangover effect discourages the misuse of long-acting barbiturates. Short-acting barbiturates are also rarely misused; intermediate-acting barbiturates are the agents most commonly encountered. Common street names for barbiturates, which sometimes relate to specific proprietary preparations, include 'barbs', 'downers', 'sleepers', 'blue heaven', 'red devils', and 'rainbows'.

Barbiturates are commonly taken orally, especially by people dependent on them as a result of long-term use. However, use by injection is also encountered, especially in those who inject other drugs as well. The contents of a capsule are dissolved, usually in tap water, and injected intravenously; the femoral vein may be used when veins in the arms have been destroyed by repeated injection.

Injection of barbiturate solutions pose particular problems as a result of their alkalinity, and barbiturates are highly irritant to tissues. If injected outside a vein, ulcers and gangrene can develop (commonly referred to as a 'barb burn'). If injected inadvertently into an artery, intense vasospasm can occur and result in ischaemia and gangrene of the tissue supplied by that artery.

Misuse in pregnancy

Barbiturates cross the placenta, and foetal concentrations are higher than maternal concentrations as a result of poor barbiturate metabolism by the foetus. Therapeutic doses of barbiturates in pregnancy have been associated with a marginal increase in the risk of congenital abnormalities but larger doses can cause more severe defects (e.g. dysmorphic facial features, digital hypoplasia, and growth retardation). Chronic barbiturate use has also been associated with folate deficiency in the neonate. Neonatal hypoprothrombinaemia can occur if barbiturates are used during pregnancy and, in addition, there may be thrombocytopenia with an increased risk of haemorrhage.

The use of barbiturates during the six-hour period before delivery can result in adverse effects in the neonate, including diminished responsiveness, poor sucking, and inadequate weight gain. A neonatal withdrawal syndrome can occur in babies born to barbiturate-dependent mothers and symptoms include restlessness, irritability, tremor, hyperreflexia, sleep disturbances, hyperphagia, and vomiting; convulsions may also occur.

Dependence, tolerance, and withdrawal symptoms

Barbiturates can induce both physical and psychological dependence. Tolerance develops rapidly because barbiturates induce liver microsomal enzymes, which increase barbiturate metabolism. Tolerance is further increased by CNS adaptation to the effects of barbiturates. However, tolerance to the sedative effects tends to develop more rapidly compared to depressant actions on vital centres, and therefore increases the possibility of serious toxicity of increasing barbiturate doses. Cross-tolerance between the barbiturates, benzodiazepines (*see below*), alcohol, and other hypnotics and anxiolytics is also exhibited.

Withdrawal symptoms associated with abrupt cessation of barbiturate use are similar to those experienced with benzodiazepine use (*see below*), although the symptoms and course of events may be more severe and intense. Withdrawal symptoms may include anxiety, restlessness, pyrexia, and insomnia; hallucinations, disorientation, tremulousness, and seizures can also occur. Barbiturate withdrawal symptoms commonly start within 24 hours of stopping use and reach a peak in 48 hours. Death can occur from cardiovascular collapse or inhalation of vomit during convulsions.

Management of withdrawal
Ideally, withdrawal from barbiturates should be managed under medical supervision, although this may not always be possible. A long-acting barbiturate, commonly phenobarbitone, is substituted for the misused drug and a reducing regimen instigated. The patient should be told that their sleep will deteriorate for a while, but will eventually return to normal. Occasionally, shorter-acting barbiturates may be used in withdrawal regimens that are managed entirely in specialist units. Supportive therapy, counselling, and psychotherapy may be beneficial.

Benzodiazepines

The benzodiazepines are used therapeutically for their anxiolytic, hypnotic, anticonvulsant, and muscle relaxant properties. They are the most commonly prescribed anxiolytics and hypnotics; barbiturates are no longer recommended because benzodiazepines have fewer side-effects and are much less dangerous in overdosage. However, dependence and tolerance to benzodiazepines does occur, which has led to concern among the medical professions and the general public.

In general, drug misuse is associated with the administration of excessive and increasing doses of psychoactive substances that have not been prescribed. However, benzodiazepine misuse is primarily associated with inappropriate and long-term prescribing of benzodiazepines. Nevertheless, there is also a recognised black market for these drugs and high doses of benzodiazepines are often used in combination with other psychoactive drugs.

Benzodiazepines were introduced approximately 30 years ago; they were regarded as safer alternatives to the barbiturates, and during the 1960s and 1970s prescribing of barbiturates fell and that of benzodiazepines increased. Benzodiazepine prescribing peaked in 1979, and thereafter has been slowly declining.

The Committee on the Safety of Medicines (CSM) has issued the following advice on the prescribing of benzodiazepines:

- Benzodiazepines are indicated for the short-term relief (2 to 4 weeks only) of anxiety that is severe, disabling, or subjecting the individual to unacceptable distress, occurring alone or in association with insomnia or short-term psychosomatic, organic, or psychotic illness.
- The use of benzodiazepines to treat short-term 'mild' anxiety is inappropriate and unsuitable.
- Benzodiazepines should be used to treat insomnia only when it is severe, disabling, or subjecting the individual to extreme distress.

The Council of the Royal Pharmaceutical Society of Great Britain recommends that pharmacists should take every opportunity to discuss any problems they encounter over the use of benzodiazepines with the medical practitioner concerned. Taking into account the CSM guidelines, pharmacists are advised to counsel patients who are receiving prescriptions for benzodiazepines where, on the evidence available, it is considered appropriate to do so. In advising patients, pharmacists should bear in mind the need not to impair the patient's confidence in their medical practitioner.

Benzodiazepines vary in their duration of action, and this is used in their classification. Generally, long-acting benzodiazepines (e.g. diazepam, clobazam, clorazepate) have a half-life greater than 24 hours and have active metabolites (e.g. desmethyldiazepam), which accumulate during repeated administration. Intermediate or short-acting benzodiazepines (e.g. nitrazepam, lorazepam, temazepam) have a half-life of between 5 and 25 hours and active metabolites are uncommon. Accumulation of these benzodiazepines may be a problem in the elderly. Ultra short-acting benzodiazepines (e.g. triazolam) have a half-life of less than five hours and are not associated with any degree of accumulation.

In addition to the benzodiazepines and barbiturates (*see above*), other hypnotics and anxiolytics that are misused include chlormethiazole, chloral hydrate, dichloralphenazone, glutethimide, and meprobamate. The problems associated with their misuse are generally similar to those described for the benzodiazepines and barbiturates.

Actions and methods of administration

Benzodiazepine misuse commonly occurs as a result of inappropriate prescribing. Patients are often on long-term therapy, but only rarely take escalating doses.

Benzodiazepine misuse may also be associated with concurrent use of other drugs such as alcohol, cyclizine, or buprenorphine. Benzodiazepines are sometimes used to reduce the effects of opioid and alcohol withdrawal and, in some cases, to relieve stress and emotional disturbances. Injection of oral dosage forms of benzodiazepines is thought to be a feature of illicit use; the dissolved contents of a capsule, or a crushed and dissolved tablet, may be used.

The effects of intravenous benzodiazepines are described by drug users as exhilarating, and include excitement and talkativeness; aggression, hostility, and anti-social behaviour may also occur. Benzodiazepines may cause paradoxical effects including increased anxiety and perceptual disorders. They also impair cognition and psychomotor function.

Side-effects of benzodiazepines include amnesia, drowsiness, lightheadedness, confusion, and ataxia. Other reported side-effects include headache, vertigo, hypotension, gastro-intestinal disturbances, rashes, visual disturbances, and urinary retention. High doses of benzodiazepines reduce libido. Intravenous injection of benzodiazepines is associated with pain and thrombophlebitis.

Long-term benzodiazepine administration may impair psychomotor function, which may be permanent and has been thought to be associated with intellectual impairment. Ataxia and confusion, especially in the elderly, may result in falls and accidents.

Endocrine disorders may also occur with long-term benzodiazepine use and produce increased secretion of cortisol, prolactin, and growth hormone; effects of these include menstrual irregularities, premenstrual syndrome, breast engorgement, gynaecomastia, and galactorrhoea.

Misuse in pregnancy

Benzodiazepine use in pregnancy is commonly associated with persistent plasma-benzodiazepine concentrations in the neonate (e.g. for 1 to 2 weeks) caused by inefficient foetal and neonatal benzodiazepine metabolism. A neonatal benzodiazepine withdrawal syndrome has been described and is characterised by convulsions, tremor, irritability, hyperactivity, hypertonicity, tachypnoea, and frantic sucking.

Although benzodiazepines are probably not teratogenic in humans, a woman planning a pregnancy should be encouraged to discontinue her benzodiazepine use before conception. Benzodiazepine use in the first trimester of pregnancy has been associated with oral cleft defects.

Dependence, tolerance, and withdrawal symptoms

Long-term use of benzodiazepines is associated with dependence and the development of severe withdrawal symptoms in about 30% of people. Long-term users are predominantly women and there may be associated physical illness, depression, or history of other psychoactive drug use. The elderly are also more susceptible to the side-effects and long-term consequences of benzodiazepine use.

Tolerance to the sedative and hypnotic effects of benzodiazepines occurs as a result of neuroadaptation. Cross-tolerance between the different benzodiazepines is exhibited; cross-tolerance between the benzodiazepines and the barbiturates, alcohol, and other hypnotics and anxiolytics may also occur, although it may be partial.

Withdrawal symptoms associated with discontinuation of benzodiazepine use may occur following 4 to 6 weeks treatment. Therefore, prescribing monthly repeat prescriptions is inappropriate and puts patients at risk of developing dependence. Dependence on benzodiazepines can consist of both psychological and physical dependence. It is also postulated that benzodiazepines are no longer effective for the treatment of anxiety after 1 to 4 months of continued use.

Withdrawal symptoms associated with abrupt discontinuation of benzodiazepines may include toxic psychosis, confusion, tremor, convulsions, and delirium. Other symptoms may include insomnia, muscle spasm, rebound anxiety, and sleep disturbances. The symptoms are of varying intensity and are more severe with short-acting and ultra short-acting benzodiazepines compared to long-acting benzodiazepines. This may be because of a more rapid reduction in plasma-drug concentrations with short-acting and ultra short-acting benzodiazepines.

Management of withdrawal

Substitution of a short-acting or ultra short-acting benzodiazepine with diazepam is the first step in the management of benzodiazepine withdrawal. A reducing regimen (commonly in steps of 2.0 or 2.5 mg at fortnightly intervals) is then agreed with the user, although the precise schedule depends on individual circumstances. The time required for withdrawal can vary from about four weeks to several months depending on the duration of benzodiazepine use; withdrawal symptoms may persist for a year or more. Supportive therapy, counselling, and psychotherapy are necessary requirements to assist benzodiazepine withdrawal. Drug treatment (e.g. phenobarbitone) may be necessary for the prevention or treatment of convulsions.

Cannabis

Cannabis (Indian hemp) is the dried flowering or fruiting tops of the pistillate plant *Cannabis sativa*. In the UK, cannabis can be described as any part of any plant of the genus *Cannabis*. The plant grows in hot, dry conditions; suitable climates exist mainly outside Europe and major supplies originate from the West Indies, India, Pakistan, Afghanistan, the Middle East, Far East, Africa, and parts of North and South America.

Cannabis consists of male and female plants, both of which contain active ingredients (cannabinoids). A series of cannabinoids (over 60) have been isolated from the plant, the most active being delta⁹-tetrahydro-cannabinol (THC), which is found in all parts of the plant except the seeds; the highest concentration of THC is found in the flowering shoots of the female plant. However, the THC content is variable and depends on the conditions, place of growth, and storage; cannabis plants grown in the UK have a low THC content as a result of unfavourable climate.

Although a range of cannabis preparations exist, there are three main forms of illicit cannabis commonly used:

- Marijuana (herbal cannabis)

  Dried leaves and flowering tops of uncultivated cannabis plants. Marijuana is smoked; when it is infused and drunk, the preparation is known as bhang. The concentration of THC may be between 5 and 10%.

- Cannabis resin (hashish)

  Resin extracted from the flowering tops and leaves of female plants. The concentration of THC may be up to 20%.

- Cannabis oil (hashish oil)

  Liquid extract of cannabis resin having a high THC content (up to 85%).

Marijuana is usually obtained as the dried plant, or it may be compressed into blocks. Compressed marijuana commonly includes the whole plant; female plants represent the better quality product. A characteristic appearance of compressed marijuana (e.g. shape and size) is associated with the country of origin; for example, compressed marijuana from Malawi comes in

the form of sticks, and that from Jamaica comes in the form of small blocks.

Cannabis resin varies in its appearance depending on the country of origin. The resin is commonly formed into blocks, sticks, or cakes, which may be soft and pliable, or hard and dry, crumbling into a powder. Cannabis resin from Pakistan and Afghanistan is characteristically dark brown or black in colour; resin from the Lebanon is usually a compressed golden powder; and resin from Morocco is usually a golden to greenish-brown coloured slab or powder. The many street names for cannabis preparations include 'bhang', 'dope', 'ganja', 'grass', 'hash', 'kif', and 'pot'.

The large scale use of cannabis has led to the campaign to legalise its use, with claims of its relative safety, and counter-claims of its potentially harmful effects. There is a continuing debate on the rights and wrongs of legalising cannabis use. Some of the arguments for legalisation of cannabis use, however ill-founded, are:

- moderate use is not harmful
- far more dangerous substances (e.g. alcohol and tobacco) are legal
- costs of not legalising cannabis use (e.g. police and court time) exceed those of legalising use
- legalising its use will not cause an increase in the number of users.

Some of the arguments against legalisation of cannabis use, however ill-founded, are:

- cannabis use is associated with anti-establishment and anti-society culture
- legalisation of cannabis will convey a negative message with respect to drug misuse generally
- cannabis use is likely to proceed to misuse of other drugs
- cannabis use may impair driving ability
- social and health problems associated with cannabis use (e.g. crime, promiscuity, and psychosis) precludes legalisation.

It is well recognised that drug misuse is often sequential. Cannabis use is often thought of as a first step towards use of other more harmful drugs, although this is controversial. It would appear that only a minority of cannabis users go on to use other drugs and the presence of particular personality traits is more likely to predispose users to sequential drug use.

Actions and methods of administration
The psychological effects of cannabis are dependent on the dose, personality, expectations, previous experience,

and the environment in which it is taken. In isolation, cannabis may cause euphoria, relaxation, and somnolence. In a group situation, it may result in increased social interaction, friendliness, and laughter. Sensory perceptions (e.g. touch, smell, sight, and hearing) tend to become enhanced and perception of time is altered causing time to appear to pass slowly. Vigilance, coordination, and reaction times are diminished, all of which impair task performance (e.g. driving). At higher doses, cannabis is associated with more intense effects, including tremulousness, altered self-identity, hallucinations, and paranoia, especially in inexperienced users.

High levels of use may cause a cannabis psychosis, which is characterised by confusion, delusions, hallucinations, and emotional disturbances; it may occur with small doses in susceptible individuals. Cannabis psychosis commonly lasts from a few hours to days and almost invariably resolves within a week of stopping cannabis use. In the presence of regular, heavy cannabis use, cannabis psychosis may occur in repeated episodes. In some cases, cannabis psychosis may be maintained for prolonged periods. However, it has not been established whether cannabis use can lead to the development of a chronic and persistent psychosis.

In the presence of chronic cannabis use, a group of features sometimes referred to as the amotivational syndrome may occur; signs include lack of drive, decreased concentration, apathy, chronic lethargy, and indifference to social values. However, it is uncertain whether the cause is cannabis use or the syndrome is related to personality or the way of life chosen by those people who use the drug.

Cannabis used in low doses may cause irritation of the bronchial mucous membrane, tachycardia, hypertension, dry mouth, thirst, increased appetite, constipation, decreased intra-ocular pressure, and ataxia; rarely, photophobia and nystagmus may also occur. Higher doses produce drowsiness, bradycardia, bronchodilation, hypotension, hypothermia, peripheral vasoconstriction, infection and irritation of the conjunctiva, and ptosis.

Chronic cannabis use may lead to impaired lung function, emphysema, and lung cancer. Cannabis contains a higher concentration of polyaromatic hydrocarbons than tobacco, which are thought to be responsible for its carcinogenic effect. Cannabis is also commonly mixed with tobacco and then smoked.

The effects of cannabis on sexual function are controversial. A reduction in the number and motility of spermatozoa has been reported.

A cannabis cigarette is usually prepared by mixing cannabis resin with tobacco and rolling it into a cigarette (called a 'joint' or 'reefer') although marijuana may be used on its own. Alternatively, cannabis oil may be spread onto the outside of a tobacco cigarette, impregnated into the cigarette paper, or used to soak the tobacco. 'Joints' are usually prepared using large-size cigarette papers, or alternatively, 3 or 4 small cigarette papers are stuck together. In order to prevent the hot cannabis smoke from burning the throat, a large filter or support made of thin cardboard ('roach') is included at one end.

Pipes in all shapes and sizes are also used to smoke cannabis. They often have a long stem, through which smoke is inhaled, to reduce the burning effect of the hot smoke by allowing it to cool. Pipes may be designed to allow the smoke to pass through water and cool before inhalation ('hubble-bubble' pipes).

The technique employed in smoking cannabis preparations is designed to ensure maximal absorption. The smoke is inhaled deeply and the breath held (usually for 20 to 30 seconds), which facilitates absorption of the highly fat-soluble cannabinoids; on average, 18% of the THC content is absorbed. The effects are rapid following inhalation and appear within minutes. In contrast, oral ingestion is associated with a lower bioavailability of the cannabinoids as a result of significant first-pass metabolism. The onset of action is much slower (between 30 and 120 minutes) but the duration of action is more prolonged.

Cannabis can be taken as a tea, which is made by boiling cannabis in water. It is also sometimes mixed in cakes and sweets; rarely, it may be administered by the intravenous route. Cannabinoids are fat-soluble and therefore rapidly distributed to adipose tissue. They are released slowly into the bloodstream, and metabolites can be detected in the urine for several days after only a single use of cannabis.

Misuse in pregnancy
Tetrahydrocannabinol crosses the placenta and the foetus may be exposed to cannabinoids for long periods. In addition, smoking cannabis results in elevated blood-carboxyhaemoglobin concentrations, which reduces the availability of oxygen to the foetus. The smoking of tobacco present in cannabis cigarettes (see above) may also contribute to the adverse effects on the foetus (see Chapter 5). Cannabis use causes increased blood pressure and tachycardia, both of which can lead to diminished placental blood flow. It may also impair foetal growth and result in reduced birth-weight, an increase in the incidence of small-for-gestational-age babies, and preterm delivery.

Dependence, tolerance, and withdrawal symptoms
Psychological dependence can develop with cannabis use, although physical dependence is thought not to

occur. However, dependence is not a major feature of cannabis use. Tolerance to the initial psychological effects and tachycardia may occur, especially with chronic use. Withdrawal symptoms can occur following discontinuation of cannabis use and may include restlessness, insomnia, loss of appetite, anorexia, mild nausea, and weight loss.

Management of withdrawal
Most individuals who use cannabis can stop without any untoward effects, and those claiming to be dependent will not usually have any symptoms other than anxiety. Drug treatment is not required and supportive therapy, counselling, and psychotherapy are more appropriate.

Cocaine

Cocaine is an alkaloid obtained from the leaves of the coca plant *Erythroxylum coca* and other species of *Erythroxylum*. The coca plant is indigenous to Bolivia and Peru, although it is now cultivated in other South American countries as a result of the rapid expansion in the illegal world trade of cocaine during the 1970s. Coca is also grown in other parts of the world, including Taiwan, Java, India, and some regions of Africa.

South American Indians chew coca leaves for the relief of fatigue and hunger, and as part of religious ceremonies. It is intended primarily to improve work performance and induce a feeling of well-being. The leaves usually contain less than 2% cocaine, which results in low plasma-cocaine concentrations. This form of use releases cocaine slowly and avoids rapid increases in plasma-cocaine concentrations. Problems associated with cocaine use in this form are not often seen in the native populations of South America.

Cocaine was initially used for the treatment of depressive disorders and morphine dependence until the dangers of cocaine use and dependence were realised. Cocaine was also marketed in various forms that included both medicinal and non-medicinal products. Coca-cola, for example, contained cocaine until the coca component was removed in 1903.

Cocaine was formerly linked to high-income groups and the 'elite society', because of its expense. It was portrayed as a 'recreational drug' used by the 'jet set', factors which glamorised cocaine use. However, cocaine use now appears to have spread to other sections of society. Common street names for cocaine hydrochloride include 'C', 'Charlie', 'snow', and 'white lady'.

The production of cocaine base ('crack') from the hydrochloride salt is called freebasing. The purity of the cocaine base is dependent on the quality of the cocaine hydrochloride used. Street names for cocaine base include 'rock' (because the crystals resemble small pieces of rock), 'crack' (because cocaine base makes a cracking sound when heated and smoked), and 'nuggets'.

Adulterants are often found in illicit cocaine and consist of a wide-range of substances. The role of adulterants in the medical consequences of drug misuse is discussed above, under Routes of administration and associated adverse effects.

Actions and methods of administration
The effects of cocaine occur in two phases: a euphoric phase followed by a dysphoric phase. Cocaine blocks neuronal re-uptake of catecholamines (especially dopamine and noradrenaline) in both the central and peripheral nervous systems. Increased availability of these neurotransmitters is thought to account for the euphoric phase, which is commonly described as the 'cocaine high'. Depletion of neurotransmitters, and consequently reduced availability, is thought to be responsible for the dysphoric phase, which is commonly described as the 'cocaine crash'. At present, however, it remains uncertain whether the dysphoric phase is actually a withdrawal feature as a consequence of the neuroadaptive reaction to the acute effects of cocaine. The euphoric effects of smoking cocaine base are more intense compared to intranasal administration or even intravenous use, although dysphoric symptoms are also more intense with smoking cocaine base.

The euphoric phase is characterised by CNS stimulation, which gives rise to intense euphoria and a sense of well-being, and increased physical and mental capacity. Other effects of the euphoric phase include appetite suppression, insomnia (with a decrease in REM sleep), hyperactivity, mydriasis, increased muscle activity, and sexual excitement, although at high doses, impotence and loss of libido may occur in men. Women may have difficulty achieving orgasm.

High doses may also cause psychotic states (*see below*), hallucinations, anxiety, panic attacks, restlessness, profound insomnia, agitation, and gastro-intestinal disturbances. Prolonged insomnia may lead to confusion and exhaustion. Formication (feelings of insects crawling on the skin) may also occur and is commonly described as 'cocaine bugs'. Stimulation of the peripheral nervous system results in tachycardia, hypertension, vasoconstriction, and pulmonary oedema, although CNS stimulation may also be a contributory factor. Fever may occur as a result of the disturbance of temperature regulating systems and increased muscle activity.

The dysphoric phase is characterised by depression and anxiety. Other effects of the dysphoric phase include somnolence, hunger, and an increase in REM sleep (which is associated with increased dreaming). Severe depression following use of cocaine base may also occur. When large doses have been used, or after a period of prolonged and continued use, dysphoria may develop into cocaine psychosis as a result of high plasma-cocaine concentrations. It may be characterised by the presence of hallucinations (auditory, olfactory, tactile, or visual), delusions, and paranoia, and is relieved when plasma-drug concentrations decline.

The effects of cocaine on the cardiovascular system (e.g. hypertension and tachycardia) are thought to be contributory factors in the development of cocaine-induced myocardial infarction or ischaemia. Cocaine may precipitate cardiac arrhythmias as a result of a direct toxic effect on cardiac muscle or its effect on catecholamine metabolism. Fever associated with cocaine use may also be a contributory factor. Arrhythmias related to cocaine use include sinus tachycardia, ventricular tachycardia, ventricular fibrillation, and ventricular asystole; they may be life-threatening and require treatment with anti-arrhythmic drugs.

Death as a result of respiratory failure, may occur in rare cases if vital medullary centres become depressed in the dysphoric phase. Death may also be caused by cerebral haemorrhage, convulsions, cardiac arrhythmias, or myocardial infarction.

Cocaine hydrochloride is predominantly administered by the intranasal route. Subcutaneous injection or rectal administration may also be employed, although these methods are infrequently encountered. Intravenous administration of cocaine hydrochloride is uncommon but it does occur.

The onset and duration of effect depends largely on the route of administration. Smoking cocaine base or the intravenous injection of cocaine hydrochloride results in a rapid onset of action, typically within 15 to 60 seconds, which lasts about 20 minutes. In contrast, intranasal administration is associated with a much slower onset of action, which lasts up to 1.5 hours.

The most common means of administration of cocaine hydrochloride is by the intranasal route, which usually involves placing a small quantity of cocaine hydrochloride powder on a small mirror. The powder is then formed into a thin line with a razor blade and snorted into a nostril through a thin glass tube, straw, or rolled-up paper (sometimes a bank note). Street terms for intranasal administration include a 'snort', 'hit', or 'line', each referring to a single dose. The repeated use of cocaine by this route may cause ulceration and perforation of the nasal septum as a result of vasoconstriction.

Cocaine base or 'crack' is obtained as small pellet-like crystals called 'bits'. Each 'bit' weighs approximately 250 mg and is commonly wrapped in aluminium foil or 'cling film'. It is ready for smoking and can be mixed with cigarette tobacco, or heated in a water pipe or on a piece of aluminium foil and the vapour inhaled. The vascular network of the lungs allows effective absorption after smoking cocaine base. Users often indulge in binges ('runs') in which consecutive doses are taken for prolonged periods until either the supply of cocaine or the money to buy it is exhausted.

Oral use of cocaine (e.g. chewing coca leaves) results in absorption from the mucous membranes within the mouth and from the gastro-intestinal tract following ingestion.

Cocaine hydrochloride is sometimes injected in combination with heroin or another opioid ('speedballing').

Misuse in pregnancy

Women sometimes use cocaine in the ill-founded belief that it will shorten labour and that they will derive more pleasure from the delivery. Cocaine misuse can cause premature detachment of the placenta (abruptio placentae) and spontaneous abortion. Cocaine use is also associated with preterm labour and delivery, and newborn babies may have growth retardation, lower birth-weight, smaller head circumference, decreased length, and decreased Apgar scores compared to babies of non-cocaine using mothers. Babies born to mothers who use cocaine may be irritable, have feeding problems, and be difficult to control.

Dependence, tolerance, and withdrawal symptoms

Psychological dependence has long been associated with cocaine use. The evidence to support the development of physical dependence is less convincing. Psychological dependence appears to be more intense and common in heavy users, and also in those who smoke cocaine base. In contrast, the chewing of coca leaves by the native population of South American countries does not appear to induce psychological dependence, and these people have little difficulty in discontinuing use.

The risks of developing psychological dependence to cocaine appear to be higher following intravenous use and smoking compared to intranasal use. Although the risk may be higher with the use of cocaine base, it does not occur as rapidly as often implied in the popular press.

Tolerance to the cardiovascular, respiratory, and convulsant effects of cocaine has been documented. Tolerance to the euphoric effects of cocaine base is characterised by an inability of misusers to derive pleasure and enjoyment from use of the drug (anhedonia). Cross-tolerance occurs between cocaine, amphetamines, and some other stimulants.

Withdrawal symptoms associated with cocaine use closely resemble those of the dysphoric phase described above. At present, it remains uncertain whether the dysphoric phase is actually a withdrawal feature consequent on a neuroadaptive reaction to the effects of cocaine. Some cocaine users may use other drugs (e.g. opioid analgesics) in an attempt to reduce the intensity of the dysphoric effects of cocaine use.

Craving for cocaine occurs as a result of memory of the euphoric effects ('cocaine high'); memory of the dysphoric effects ('cocaine crash') is apparently lost. Cocaine craving can return after months or years following the last cocaine use.

Management of withdrawal

The management of cocaine withdrawal is mainly directed towards controlling the intense dysphoria and craving. Drug treatment (e.g. tricyclic antidepressants and lithium) may be tried, although supportive therapy, counselling, and psychotherapy are more commonly used.

Designer drugs

Designer drugs are substances intended for recreational use, which are derivatives of existing drugs. Designer drugs are synthesised with the intent of avoiding legal restrictions. They may be drugs that were developed by legitimate pharmaceutical research, but have been acquired for misuse. Most, if not all, designer drugs originate in the US and are subsequently introduced into the UK. However, not all designer drugs that are established in the US gain popularity in the UK.

The designer drugs most commonly encountered are phenylethylamines (mescaline analogues), which include methylamphetamine, MDA (3,4-methylenedioxy-amphetamine), and MDMA 3,4-methylenedioxymeth-amphetamine).

MDA was synthesised and misused as a 'love drug'. It produces mild intoxication, euphoria, and empathy. However, large doses resulted in delirium, agitation, and hallucinations; death has also been reported. MDA can be used to synthesise other analogues including MDMA.

MDMA is commonly referred to as 'ecstasy' and has become increasingly popular in the UK. It is a hallucinogenic amphetamine derivative. Initially, MDMA use was confined to middle-class groups but younger people across all sections of the community are now involved as a result of decreasing price and increasing promotion. Street names of MDMA, in addition to 'ecstasy', include 'Adam', 'XTC', 'MDM', and 'M & M'.

MDMA has been reported by users to produce euphoria, empathy, and increased self-esteem. Other reported effects include enhanced perceptions of vision, sound, and touch. The onset of action of MDMA is within 20 to 60 minutes, and the duration of action is approximately two hours. MDMA use has been associated with anorexia, bruxism, hypertension, tachycardia, profuse sweating, and blurred vision. Nausea, anxiety, insomnia and, as a delayed effect, lethargy have also occurred. Chronic paranoid psychosis has also been reported following long-term MDMA use. Deaths have been associated with MDMA use, although underlying disease may have been a contributory factor. In some cases, MDMA has been reported to elicit a strong reaction characterised by sensory dislocation, which can recur many weeks after use (flashbacks).

MDMA is used in the form of capsules or tablets containing between 75 and 150 mg of MDMA. It has gained public awareness in the UK as a result of its association with music cultures, especially so-called 'acid house parties'. A 'binge' pattern of use may sometimes be encountered, in which MDMA is used continually until supplies are exhausted. Some users wait at least 2 to 3 weeks between doses of the drug, reporting that the effects of MDMA use diminish and the side-effects increase if the drug is taken too frequently.

Another phenylethylamine designer drug, called DOM (2,5-dimethoxy-4-methylamphetamine) became known as STP (referring to 'serenity, tranquillity, and peace'). At low doses, it produced mild sympathetic stimulation, euphoria, and perceptual distortions. However, it had a narrow margin of safety, and at slightly higher doses, produced hallucinations and significantly increased sympathetic stimulation. The use of DOM did not escalate.

Methylamphetamine (*see* Amphetamines and related stimulants above) is another example of a phenylethylamine designer drug.

Synthetic opioid derivatives of fentanyl and pethidine have been synthesised, and have resulted in numerous deaths from overdosage.

Another class of designer drugs are the arylhexylamines, which include phencyclidine (*see below*) and its analogues. The complex pharmacological properties of arylhexylamines produce a confusing array of symptoms in the intoxicated user. Overdosage may result in extreme agitation, psychosis, fever, and CNS and respiratory depression.

Hallucinogens

Hallucinogenic drugs produce hallucinations. In addition, they alter perception of sensations (illusions), induce false beliefs that are firm (delusions), and cause mood alterations.

Hallucinogenic mushrooms (also called 'magic mushrooms') contain the active ingredients, psilocybin and psilocin. The mushroom *Psilocybe mexicana* grows in Mexico, but related species containing the active ingredients are also found in Europe. In the UK, the most common variety is the Liberty Cap (*Psilocybe semilanceata*), which is harvested between September and November. Hallucinogenic mushrooms may be eaten raw, cooked, or made into a drink; they may also be dried to preserve them for later use. In the UK, it is not an offence to possess and eat these mushrooms in their raw state, although it is an offence to make preparations from them.

The effects of hallucinogenic mushrooms range from excitement and euphoria with small doses to hallucinations and perceptual disorders at larger doses. A sensation of body parts swelling may also occur. The consumption of about 30 mushrooms produces an effect similar to a mild dose of lysergide. The hallucinations are commonly visual, although may also be auditory or tactile. Other effects of hallucinogenic mushrooms may include mydriasis, dysphoria, hyperreflexia, tachycardia, and drowsiness; nausea, and abdominal pain may also occur.

One important aspect of hallucinogenic mushroom misuse is the accidental ingestion of poisonous mushrooms picked in error. 'Bad trips' and flashbacks (*see* Lysergide, below), and rarely, transient psychosis may also occur.

Mild to moderate psychological dependence may occur with hallucinogenic mushroom use; physical dependence and withdrawal symptoms have not been reported. Tolerance to the effects of hallucinogenic mushrooms develops rapidly; cross-tolerance is exhibited between hallucinogenic mushrooms and other hallucinogens (e.g. lysergide).

Mescaline is a hallucinogenic alkaloid contained in the cactus *Lophophora williamsii* found in Mexico and some parts of the USA; slices or buttons (called 'peyote' or 'peyotl') are chewed by the native populations. Mescaline produces hallucinations and sympathomimetic effects similar to those of lysergide (*see below*), but it is less potent.

Myristicin is a hallucinogen contained in mace and nutmeg. Mace is the arillus (extra seed covering) of the seed of *Myristica fragrans* and nutmeg is the dried kernels of the seeds of the same plant. Mace and nutmeg are both used as food flavouring agents, but at high doses produce excitement, hallucinations, dry mouth, tachycardia, and dilated pupils.

Other drugs that produce hallucinations include lysergide and phencyclidine, and are discussed below in detail.

Khat

Khat (catha) is the leaves of the shrub, *Catha edulis*, which contains the stimulant alkaloids, cathinone and cathine; other constituents include celastrin, choline, tannins, and inorganic salts. Khat is cultivated in the Yemen and nearby regions of Africa, and the native populations chew the leaves for their stimulant effects. Khat use in other countries is rare, although immigrant communities may continue khat use in their country of settlement.

Khat leaves are transported moistened and wrapped in banana leaves to keep them fresh; drying results in loss of active constituents, and the leaves are therefore stored in domestic deep freezers to reduce deterioration.

Actions and methods of administration

Khat leaves are chewed into a large mass (quid), which is held inside the cheek. Generally, chewing lasts for only a few hours, but, in some cases, may continue for days.

The active constituents of khat resemble amphetamine in their actions. The stimulant actions of khat are mediated by increased noradrenaline release and inhibition of its uptake. Initially, feelings of well-being, talkativeness, and excitement are the predominant effects. Dry mouth commonly occurs, necessitating the consumption of large quantities of water. Further chewing results in diminished appetite, dilated pupils, tachycardia, tachypnoea, and constipation. Prolonged chewing of khat may cause mania, insomnia, hypertension, and hyperactivity. Khat psychosis may occur with prolonged use.

Dependence, tolerance, and withdrawal symptoms

Tolerance to the effects of khat may develop as a result of depletion of noradrenaline stores, and reduced sensitivity and number of noradrenaline receptors. Withdrawal symptoms include lethargy and nightmares.

Lysergide

Lysergide (lysergic acid diethylamide) is a synthetic compound derived from the alkaloids found in ergot (*Claviceps purpurea*). Lysergide was first synthesised in 1938 by Albert Hoffman in his search to find stimulant drugs related to lysergic acid. Lysergide was the twenty-fifth such derivative and was called LSD 25. Lysergide was subsequently marketed and became widely used by psychiatrists in the 1950s and early 1960s, particularly for the treatment of drug and alcohol dependence.

Lysergide was used in the belief that it could release repressed thoughts from the subconscious. Other uses included personality disorders, sexual disorders, autism, and terminal illness. However, well-controlled studies failed to demonstrate any therapeutic benefit.

The misuse of lysergide achieved increasing popularity, which peaked in the 1960s and early 1970s. Lysergide was withdrawn from the market in 1966 following increasing concern about its misuse. The incidence of misuse declined dramatically in the late 1970s, following a police operation to break a manufacturing and distribution network.

Lysergide is illicitly synthesised in home laboratories and is distributed in a range of forms. In solution, it can be absorbed onto any suitable material (e.g. sugar cubes, blotting paper, or small flakes of gelatin). Small pieces of absorbent paper, the size of postage stamps, are impregnated with one dose of lysergide; they are commonly decorated with a motif such as a cartoon character and may, therefore, easily be mistaken for transfers commonly used by children. A variety of tablets and capsules may also be produced. Pinhead-sized tablets called 'microdots' containing a single dose of lysergide are sometimes distributed on a strip of sticky tape. Common street names for lysergide preparations include 'acid drops', 'blotter acid', 'tab', 'paper mushrooms', and 'window panes'.

Actions and methods of administration

The lysergide molecule resembles serotonin and the catecholamines, adrenaline and noradrenaline. It is the activation of serotonin pathways that are thought to be responsible for the psychological effects of lysergide. Sympathomimetic effects of lysergide include dilated pupils, slight increase in blood pressure, and tachycardia; tremor, pilo-erection, muscle weakness, nausea, and hyperthermia may also occur.

The psychological effects of lysergide (commonly described as a 'trip') are not predictable and depend on numerous factors including the users attitude, emotional state, expectation, personality, and previous experiences. There is a disturbance of perception relating to body image, time, and space; body parts (or the whole body) may appear to enlarge or contract. Almost all sensory faculties are heightened, and mood changes are intense, variable, and unstable. Euphoria, ecstasy, and excitement may also occur. Thought control is disturbed, producing loss of short-term memory and emergence of the memory of events in the distant past. Synaesthesia, which is the distortion of sensory perception characterised by one sensory stimulus evoking a response in another (e.g. sounds are visual and colours heard), may also occur.

As a result of the effects of lysergide, especially disturbance of thought control, users believe they are having a mystical experience. They may relate it to death and reincarnation; strange, imaginative thoughts and ideas may also be manifested.

Lysergide can induce 'unwanted' experiences (commonly described as a 'bad trip'), although it is not known why they occur. Characteristic features include dysphoria, paranoia, acute panic reactions, delusions, and distressing hallucinations; confusion and loss of contact with reality are also prominent. The effects of 'bad trips' appear to diminish with time. 'Bad trips' are more common with higher doses, although the dose is not thought to be the sole cause as some individuals appear to have an increased susceptibility. 'Bad trips' may occur in persons who have previously enjoyed using lysergide and are experienced with it. 'Bad trips' may also lead to accidental fatalities, although suicide is rare. Impulsive and irrational behaviour, which can be sudden and dangerous, may occur in a few cases. Violence and aggression, which may be directed towards others or towards themselves, may also occur.

Flashbacks are described by some users as recurrences of the psychological effects of previous lysergide use in the absence of drug intake. Flashbacks can occur months or years later. The cause is not known, although there may be precipitating factors (e.g. cannabis use or stress). Flashbacks tend to occur more commonly following the use of large doses of lysergide.

Severe depressive disorders associated with anxiety and panic may occur following lysergide use. Psychosis resembling schizophrenia in its manifestations may also occur, and can be a brief or prolonged episode. The condition usually resolves completely in time.

Lysergide is almost invariably taken by mouth, although it can be injected or administered by the intranasal route. Minute quantities of lysergide are able to elicit an effect; a dose of 10 μg will produce a noticeable effect. Lysergide is commonly used on an intermittent basis; users rarely resort to lengthy 'binges'.

Lysergide is well absorbed following oral administration. Peak effects are seen between 30 to 90 minutes following lysergide ingestion. The duration of effect is in the order of 8 to 12 hours, although these diminish after 4 to 6 hours.

Misuse in pregnancy

Lysergide use in pregnancy has been associated with congenital abnormalities, although the evidence is conflicting.

Dependence, tolerance, and withdrawal symptoms

Physical dependence is thought not to occur with lysergide use, although there have been some reports of psychological dependence. However, in such cases, there may be an underlying personality disorder. Tolerance to the effects of lysergide occurs within 3 to 4 days and larger doses of up to 800 μg may be required to elicit the same response; the development of rapid tolerance may be the reason for the intermittent pattern of lysergide use. Tolerance is lost after 4 to 6 days. Cross-tolerance is exhibited between lysergide and other hallucinogens (e.g. hallucinogenic mushrooms). There are no withdrawal symptoms associated with discontinuation of lysergide use.

Management of withdrawal

No treatment is necessary, except for any underlying disorder that may be present. Supportive therapy, counselling, and psychotherapy may be beneficial.

Non-prescription medicines

The misuse potential of a large number of non-prescription medicines is clearly recognised, and some of the common constituents of non-prescription medicines are discussed here.

The misuse of non-prescription medicines is thought to be widespread, although the true extent is not known; this is primarily because of lack of reporting. Some non-prescription medicines are commonly misused in conjunction with alcohol and other drugs in order to potentiate their individual effects.

The Council of the Royal Pharmaceutical Society of Great Britain has issued a statement on the misuse of non-prescription medicines (Fig. 7.1).

Non-prescription medicines that are liable to misuse usually contain one or more of the following constituents:

- antihistamines
- emetics
- laxatives
- opioids
- stimulants.

Antihistamines (e.g. cyclizine and diphenhydramine) are often misused on their own or in combination with other drugs of misuse. They commonly cause sedation, dizziness, and incoordination. In some cases, especially in children, CNS stimulation can occur causing insomnia, nervousness, tachycardia, tremor, and convulsions.

The use of antihistamines in combination with other depressant drugs may lead to coma, cardiorespiratory collapse, and even death.

There has been much concern in recent years over the misuse of cyclizine-containing products, which when used in large doses, may cause euphoria; some users may inject solutions of crushed tablets. Cyclizine potentiates the euphoric effects of opioids and has also been used

---

Some over-the-counter medicines and non-medicinal products are liable to be abused, which in this respect usually means

(a) consumption over a lengthy period, and/or,

(b) consumption of doses substantially higher than recommended.

Such products should be sold personally by the pharmacist and sales should be refused if it is apparent that the purchase is not for a genuine medicinal purpose or if the frequency of purchase suggests overuse. A pharmacist should not attempt on his own to control an abuser's habit, but should liaise with bodies such as drug dependency clinics in any local initiative to assist abusers.

An up-to-date list of products known to be abused nationally appears in the 'Medicines, Ethics and Practice' guide. The products which are abused are subject to change and pharmacists should keep abreast of local and national tends.

Fig. 7.1
Council statement on abuse of over-the-counter medicines.

with benzodiazepines, alcohol, and stimulants such as ephedrine. There have been several case reports suggesting that psychotic reactions may develop following misuse of cyclizine and that dependence may occur. The Council of the Royal Pharmaceutical Society of Great Britain recommends that medicines containing cyclizine should be sold personally by the pharmacist.

Ipecacuanha may be misused as an emetic by patients suffering from eating disorders (e.g. anorexia nervosa and bulimia nervosa). Young women in their early teens to mid-twenties are most commonly affected. Ipecacuanha is taken following a binge meal in an attempt to induce vomiting and, therefore, avoid the absorption of food. **Laxatives** are also commonly misused by patients suffering from eating disorders. Laxatives may reduce gastro-intestinal transit time and impair the absorption of food. Misuse of laxatives produces weight loss, dehydration, and disturbance of electrolyte balance. Hypokalaemia can occur and symptoms include fatigue, muscle weakness or cramps, headache, palpitations, and abdominal pain; adynamic paralytic ileus may also occur.

Opioids (e.g. codeine, dextromethorphan, and morphine) are included in many non-prescription medicines for their analgesic, cough suppressant, and antidiarrhoeal properties. The pattern of misuse of opioids in non-prescription medicines is the same as that described under Opioids (*see below*).

Stimulants (e.g. ephedrine, pseudoephedrine, and phenylpropanolamine) are included in a range of non-prescription products, particularly cold and 'flu' remedies. These products are commonly misused when amphetamines or similar stimulants are not available.

Non-prescription stimulants may be marketed as 'look alike' amphetamines (sometimes called 'pseudo speed'). Misuse of stimulants may cause paranoid psychosis with delusions and hallucinations (auditory, visual, or tactile); consciousness commonly remains unaffected. Cardiac arrhythmias may also occur. Severe hypertensive episodes have occurred following phenylpropanolamine ingestion.

In children, therapeutic doses of stimulants contained in cough mixtures have been shown to cause agitation, insomnia, and visual hallucinations.

The misuse of stimulants such as ephedrine and pseudoephedrine has been associated with the development of tolerance and dependence. The management of withdrawal from stimulants is similar to that described under Amphetamines and related stimulants (*see above*).

Opioids

Opioids are compounds that possess morphine-like activity; the term opiates was previously used to describe naturally occurring alkaloids from the opium plant *Papaver somniferum*. Opioids are used primarily for their analgesic, cough suppressant, and antidiarrhoeal properties. Opioids may also be found in non-prescription medicines and these are also subject to misuse (*see above*).

Opium is now rarely seen in the UK but it does continue to be used in other countries. The opium poppy grows in many countries (e.g. Afghanistan, Pakistan, Thailand, China, and Indonesia) and is used to prepare raw opium, which may be smoked, eaten, or drunk as an infusion. Opium is rarely used therapeutically.

Morphine is the principal alkaloid present in opium and is the standard opioid to which the activity of other opioids is related. Morphine was isolated from raw opium in 1803 and became established as an analgesic. In 1874, diamorphine, then called diacetylmorphine, was synthesised from morphine. Throughout this chapter, the name heroin has been used to describe the misused product, and diamorphine has been reserved to denote the therapeutically used product.

Heroin dominates as the opioid obtained on the black market from illicit, imported sources, reflected by the large increase in heroin seizures, although a black market also exists for diverted medical supplies of opioids including diamorphine and morphine. Illicit heroin comes in a variety of forms; it can be in powder form and off-white to dark brown in colour or a black, tar-like substance. Common street names for heroin include 'Big Harry', 'Chinese white', 'dragon', 'scag', 'smack', and 'white stuff'.

There are many other opioids that are synthesised from sources other than opium; buprenorphine, methadone, and pethidine are examples.

Actions and methods of administration

Different opioids may vary in their onset and duration of action, rate of absorption, distribution, metabolism, and excretion. These properties are generally conferred by the fat solubility and basicity of each compound.

Opioids exert their effects on the CNS, which accounts for their misuse potential. Heroin crosses the blood-brain barrier rapidly compared to other opioids and consequently has a shorter onset of action. It is hydrolysed to morphine in brain tissue, and it is probably morphine that accounts for its actions. Heroin is approximately 2.5 times more potent than morphine but has a shorter duration of action.

The euphoria following injection or smoking of opioids is intense (commonly described as a 'rush' or 'buzz'), providing relief from anxiety or stress, and producing intense pleasure; feelings are often described by users to be similar to sexual orgasm. Euphoria is followed by somnolence and lassitude, commonly described as being 'on the nod'. Other effects of opioids at normal therapeutic doses include nausea and vomiting, constipation, drowsiness, confusion, dry mouth, sweating, facial flushing, vertigo, bradycardia, palpitations, orthostatic hypotension, palpitations, hypothermia, restlessness, mood changes, and miosis. Difficulty in micturition and biliary or ureteric spasm may also occur. At higher doses, respiratory depression and hypotension with circulatory failure may occur.

Sexual dysfunction associated with opioid misuse includes loss of libido and is commonly associated with prolonged dependence. Females may experience amenorrhoea.

After heroin, methadone is the most commonly misused opioid. It is extensively bound to plasma proteins and has a longer duration of action than morphine. Buprenorphine is also highly bound to plasma proteins. It is a partial opioid agonist, which can produce withdrawal symptoms in persons severely dependent on other opioids. Pethidine has a shorter duration of action than morphine but may cause more excitatory effects, including hallucinations, muscle twitches, agitation, and convulsions. The intense euphoria experienced with pethidine compared to other opioids is commonly described as 'edgy', 'jangly', or 'rough'.

Overdosage is the main consequence of opioid misuse and is commonly inadvertent. It may be caused by lack of awareness of the degree of purity of the drug. Street samples of heroin differ in their purity and overdosage can result from using a product with a high concentration of heroin. Loss of tolerance following withdrawal can also result in overdosage if the user returns to the same dose used before withdrawal. Initial use of a dose similar to that used by a friend who has developed substantial tolerance can also result in overdosage. Symptoms of overdosage include stupor, respiratory depression, coma, pulmonary oedema, and respiratory arrest.

The opioids are administered orally, intranasally, by injection, or smoked; the preferred route depends on the particular opioid and the prevailing 'craze' or fashion. Liquid preparations or solutions of crushed tablets may be injected. When the desired opioid is not available, users will commonly resort to other opioids. Street heroin is commonly bought in small amounts (called 'wraps', 'ching bags', or 'street deals').

Heroin is commonly administered by intravenous injection (referred to as 'mainlining'); it may also be injected just below the skin surface ('skin popping'). Heroin tablets, powder, or ampoule contents are mixed with a small quantity of tap water and heated, commonly in a teaspoon using a match. A syringe is used to inject the solution, which is likely to contain impurities and undissolved material; a piece of cotton wool is sometimes inserted into the bottom of the syringe as a filter. If a syringe is not available, glass droppers from ear or eye drop bottles may be used with a syringe needle attached to the end. Heroin base is relatively insoluble, and citric acid or lemon juice are occasionally added by misusers to increase its solubility.

Heroin can be mixed with cigarette tobacco and smoked or, more commonly, it can be heated on a piece of aluminium foil and the vapour inhaled. This latter method is referred to as 'chasing the dragon' because the vapour released on heating the heroin forms curling wisps that supposedly resemble the tail of a dragon. Heroin may also be administered by the intranasal route ('snorting'). Misuse of buprenorphine by the intranasal route appears to be gaining in popularity. These methods may appear relatively harmless to some individuals in comparison to injection and can therefore lead to experimentation.

Heroin or other opioids may be mixed with other drugs of misuse; a 'speedball' is a mixture of an opioid with a stimulant (e.g. cocaine). Such mixtures may enhance the psychoactive effects and prevent the severe depression that often follows stimulant use. Antihistamines such as cyclizine are sometimes used to enhance the effects of opioids.

Misuse in pregnancy

Opioids are thought not to be teratogenic and the incidence of congenital abnormalities is the same in opioid-dependent mothers as that in the general population. However, in the third trimester, there is evidence that heroin causes placental insufficiency leading to episodic intra-uterine foetal distress and sometimes stillbirth. Many opioid users experience episodes of amenorrhoea, which may make dating the pregnancy difficult.

Abrupt withdrawal of opioids in dependent pregnant women may precipitate uterine irritability and premature labour, and a programme of controlled withdrawal on an in-patient basis is essential; out-patient programmes are only applicable if the user has good support at home. It is correct practice for any doctor confirming pregnancy in an opioid user to prescribe a temporary maintenance dose of methadone linctus immediately, without waiting for the results of urine analysis to confirm drug misuse. Oral methadone should be substituted for all opioids in a dose sufficient to prevent the occurrence of withdrawal symptoms. Methadone has a long duration of action, making it less likely that the mother and foetus will experience intermittent withdrawal symptoms. Reduction of opioid use should ideally be undertaken in the second trimester. Pregnant women should be advised about the risk of premature labour should they withdraw from the opioid too quickly.

The development of neonatal withdrawal symptoms depends on the dose of opioid taken by the mother, the duration of dependence, and the timing of the last dose in relation to parturition. Opioid dependence in pregnancy represents a high risk of obstetric complications and adverse effects on the foetus. The degree of complications and adverse effects is related to the opioid used and its route of administration; other contributory factors include poor nutritional status, poor health, and inadequate antenatal care.

Neonatal opioid withdrawal symptoms commonly occur in babies born to mothers dependent on opioids. The onset of withdrawal symptoms is variable depending on the opioid and can develop within minutes of delivery to 1 or 2 weeks later, although the onset is commonly within 24 to 72 hours; the onset is later in babies born to mothers maintained on methadone.

Effects of the mother's opioid misuse on the foetus include low birth-weight, short length, and small head circumference as a result of intra-uterine growth retardation; however, long-term development appears to be unaffected. In the third trimester, heroin misuse may cause placental insufficiency and foetal distress, and sometimes stillbirth. Transmission of diseases acquired as a result of drug misuse (e.g. HIV infection) may also occur.

Neonatal withdrawal symptoms include irritability,

restlessness, tremor, persistent high-pitched crying, constant sucking of the fingers, diarrhoea, fever, respiratory distress, muscular hypertonia (with occasional hypotonia), hyperreflexia, yawning, sneezing, nasal congestion, vomiting, and sweating. Sleep and feeding difficulties are also commonly present. Convulsions can occur in severe withdrawal and can be life-threatening.

Dependence, tolerance, and withdrawal symptoms

The euphoric effects of opioids lead to the need to repeat the experiences and therefore to dependence and tolerance. Psychological and physical dependence develop gradually; users are often unaware of their manifestation and believe that they are in control. The use of smokable forms of heroin carries an increased risk of dependence because users commonly relate dependence to injection and the dangers are, therefore, not realised.

Tolerance develops to almost all the effects of opioids; it can develop to a substantial degree where dependent users will be taking doses that would be fatal to those that have not developed tolerance. The euphoric and pleasurable effects, which diminish in duration and intensity as tolerance develops, become non-existent or brief. Tolerance is lost to a large extent following withdrawal from the opioid.

Generally, there is substantial cross-dependence and cross-tolerance between different opioids that act at the same opioid receptors; the extent is variable as a result of opioid selectivity and affinity profiles for the different opioid receptors. There may be little, if any, cross-tolerance and cross-dependence between some opioids that act primarily at different opioid receptors.

Withdrawal symptoms associated with abrupt withdrawal of opioids in dependent users are variable in intensity, duration, and onset, and also depend on the opioid used; other factors include total daily dose, interval between doses, duration of use, health status, and personality characteristics. Generally, withdrawal symptoms in morphine-dependent subjects begin within a few hours, reach a peak within 36 to 72 hours, and then gradually subside; withdrawal symptoms associated with methadone dependence develop more slowly and may be less intense, but they may also be more prolonged.

Common withdrawal symptoms include anxiety, craving, depression, restlessness, disturbed sleep or insomnia, and lassitude; other features include yawning, mydriasis, lachrymation, rhinorrhoea, sneezing, muscle tremor, sweating, irritability, anorexia, nausea, vomiting, weight loss, dehydration, diarrhoea, leucocytosis, bone pain, muscle cramps, abdominal pain, tachycardia, increased respiratory rate, hypertension, and an increase in body temperature. Alternate feelings of hot and cold in combination with pilo-erection (gooseflesh) may occur. Some physiological values may not return to normal for some months following withdrawal. Craving for opioids may last for several months, and sleep disturbances often take longer than other withdrawal symptoms to resolve.

The symptoms described above are referred to as 'nonpurposive behaviour', and are not directed towards obtaining the opioid. In addition, other behavioural features directed towards obtaining the opioid and relieving withdrawal symptoms may be apparent. This is referred to as 'purposive behaviour' and includes pleas, demands, faking of withdrawal symptoms, and manipulation; they are dependent on the observer and the environment.

Dependence on opioids is also associated with general self-neglect and loss of appetite, which can result in nutritional deficiency.

Management of withdrawal

The management of opioid withdrawal depends on the degree of dependence. Young heroin users with a short history of use (from six months to one year), and who have used relatively small amounts daily, can stop using heroin abruptly. The intensity of withdrawal symptoms may be similar to an episode of influenza, and general supportive care may be all that is required. This form of opioid withdrawal is commonly referred to as 'cold turkey'.

Symptomatic treatment may be necessary. Short-term administration of benzodiazepines may be necessary for insomnia. Non-opioid analgesics (e.g. paracetamol and ibuprofen) may be administered for pain relief and antispasmodics (e.g. dicyclomine) for colicky abdominal pain.

Cross-tolerance between the opioids enables the administration of opioids other than the one to which dependence is present, and thereafter gradually reducing the dose of the substituted opioid. Codeine and dihydrocodeine have been used, although they themselves are also subject to misuse and dependence. Generally, the use of dihydrocodeine or codeine for the treatment of withdrawal is to be deprecated.

Methadone substitution is the commonest therapy used for opioid withdrawal and dependence. Methadone has a long half-life, which allows supervised once daily administration; it also has effects similar to other opioids that are misused (e.g. heroin). Doses that suppress withdrawal signs are administered in place of the opioid that the individual is dependent upon; a reducing regimen is agreed with the user and strictly adhered to, although in exceptional circumstances, the reducing schedule may be altered. The rate of reduction depends on the opioid used, length of use, and whether the treatment is on an in-patient or out-patient basis.

In some cases, methadone maintenance in which there is no aim of reducing the dose or treating dependence may be appropriate, and is a long-term measure to stabilise and improve the life-style of the user. Users suitable for methadone maintenance include those with a long history of opioid dependence, and who have had several attempts at treatment for dependence. Methadone maintenance may also be used in pregnancy (*see above*).

Clonidine is an alpha$_2$-adrenergic receptor agonist that has been used for the symptomatic treatment of opioid withdrawal. Hypotension is a troublesome side-effect for some patients, so clonidine is only useful in a setting where the blood pressure can be monitored. Clonidine inhibits the release of rebound noradrenaline that is thought to be responsible for causing many of the withdrawal symptoms. Clonidine treatment may shorten the withdrawal period to about seven days in heroin dependence, and 10 to 14 days in methadone dependence.

The opioid antagonist naltrexone may be used for the maintenance of detoxified, formerly opioid-dependent patients. It blocks the euphoric actions of opioids and is given to former users to prevent further dependence. Treatment should be initiated in a drug addiction or specialist centre. Naltrexone should not be given to patients currently dependent on opioids since an acute withdrawal reaction will be precipitated. Naltrexone has also been tried in combination with clonidine.

In all cases, supportive therapy, counselling, and psychotherapy are beneficial in addition to the withdrawal regimen. Acupuncture or related treatments have been used to treat opioid withdrawal, although evidence for their effectiveness is not clear. These forms of therapy may be suitable adjunctive measures.

Phencyclidine

Phencyclidine was marketed as an anaesthetic agent during the 1960s but had to be withdrawn as a result of adverse postoperative effects (e.g. delirium and hallucinations). However, the widespread misuse of phencyclidine in the USA during the 1970s did not manifest in the UK and, although still a part of the 'drug scene' in USA and Canada, misuse in the UK is relatively rare.

Solutions of phencyclidine are sometimes sprayed onto other drugs (e.g. cannabis) or plant leaves (e.g. oregano), or the powder may be manufactured into pills or tablets. The powder may be mixed with, or disguised as, other drugs of misuse (e.g. lysergide or cocaine). Many analogues of phencyclidine have been synthesised and misused.

Actions and methods of administration
The effects of phencyclidine are often described by users as a pleasurable experience, characterised by sensory isolation, detachment, weightlessness, and altered perceptions; euphoria and a sense of enhanced strength are also reported. Users are often observed to have a blank stare, nystagmus, and an exaggerated gait; hypertension and tachycardia may also occur.

The effects of phencyclidine are dose-dependent. At high doses, or in overdosage, vomiting, disorientation, hallucinations, synaesthesia, convulsions, and respiratory depression may occur.

Violence is often associated with phencyclidine use and may be directed towards others or to themselves. Auditory hallucinations and distortion of images may result in paranoia and violence; feelings of impending doom may also occur. The feeling of enhanced strength and resistance to pain may contribute to violent behaviour.

Phencyclidine use may result in the development of psychosis. It is characterised by thought disorder, disorientation, hallucinations, paranoia, and depersonalisation, and may last for a few hours or up to a few weeks. Depressive disorders may occur following phencyclidine psychosis.

Phencyclidine can be administered orally, intra-nasally, by injection, or by smoking. It is sometimes mixed with cannabis and smoked, as it is thought that cannabis potentiates the action of phencyclidine. Phencyclidine is also commonly used in combination with other drugs (e.g. lysergide and cocaine).

Common street names for phencyclidine include 'angel dust', 'elephant tranquilliser', and 'rocket fuel'.

Misuse in pregnancy
Phencyclidine use in pregnancy may result in agitation in the newborn; consciousness may also be affected.

Dependence, tolerance, and withdrawal symptoms
Psychological dependence and tolerance are features of phencyclidine use. In chronic misuse, withdrawal symptoms similar to those of the amphetamines (*see* Amphetamines and related stimulants above) may occur.

Volatile substance misuse

Volatile substance misuse refers to the intentional inhalation of volatile substances to achieve a state of altered mood, perception, and behaviour. Many other terms are used to describe volatile solvent misuse, including solvent misuse, solvent abuse, 'glue sniffing', inhalant misuse, and volatile solvent misuse. However, the term volatile substance misuse is perhaps the most appropriate as it encompasses glues, solvents, and other volatile substances (e.g. aerosol propellants).

In the UK, volatile substance misuse became widespread in the 1970s and began to cause great public concern in the early 1980s. At that time there was no legislation aimed directly at preventing volatile substance misuse because the need was not recognised. In the UK, volatile substance misuse was associated with 848 deaths between 1971 and 1988; the annual figure rose steadily from 31 deaths in 1980 to a peak of 134 deaths in 1988. This alarming increase has led to calls for urgent consideration of methods to prevent volatile substance misuse.

Volatile substance misuse is almost invariably associated with young people between 11 and 15 years of age, although adult cases have been reported. In the UK, an estimated 3.5 to 10% of young people have experimented with volatile solvent misuse and 0.5 to 1% are regular users. Volatile solvent misuse occurs across all sections of the community, although contributory factors (e.g. family problems and antisocial behaviour) may play a part.

Volatile substance misusers can be divided into two broad groups:

• Experimental users

Young people may become involved in volatile substance misuse through curiosity, excitement, experiment, or as a result of peer pressure. Those involved are generally male in their early teenage years. These subjects usually practise volatile substance misuse in group situations and generally stop after a short period of time.

• Regular users

The second type of person involved with volatile substance misuse often has underlying problems (e.g. behavioural or family difficulties), and volatile solvent misuse may provide an escape from reality. These subjects are generally male and tend to be older than the people in the first group; they are also more likely to resort to volatile substance misuse in isolation, and on a frequent and more hazardous basis.

In England, Wales, and Northern Ireland, the Intoxicating Substances Act (1985) makes it illegal for a person to supply, or offer to supply, a substance to a person under 18 years of age if such a person knows or has reasonable grounds for believing that those substances are likely to be used for volatile substance misuse. This legislation controls the supply of potential products involved in volatile substance misuse. It is not an offence to indulge in volatile substance misuse, but other legislation may be involved in the event of crimes arising as a result of volatile solvent misuse. In Scotland, volatile substance misuse legislation is under Scottish common law and the Solvent Abuse (Scotland) Act 1983, which permits prosecutions where supply to children is involved, although volatile substance misuse itself is not an offence.

The Council of the Royal Pharmaceutical Society of Great Britain has issued a statement on solvent misuse (Fig. 7.2).

Considerable attention has been given to the current problem of solvent misuse, known as glue sniffing. Pharmacists are reminded that many products containing organic solvents are capable of being misused, and are advised that particular attention should be paid to sales.

The products involved include adhesive plaster remover, colloidions, dry cleaning fluids, organic solvents, certain glues and shoe cleaning fluids, and aerosols (which are misused because of their propellant content).

Pharmacists are advised to prohibit the sale of such products by self-selection, to question regular purchasers, and to investigate demands for large quantities, and to be particularly vigilant if the demand is from teenagers.

Fig. 7.2
Council statement on solvent misuse.

Nitrite inhalants (amyl and butyl nitrite) are not used therapeutically, although amyl nitrite was formerly used as a vasodilator in angina pectoris, as a smooth-muscle relaxant in biliary and renal colic, and in the emergency treatment of cyanide poisoning. Nitrite inhalants are used by male homosexuals in the belief that they improve sexual performance and enjoyment.

Actions and methods of administration
All of the volatile substances listed in Table 7.1 are subject to misuse. Many of the products are readily available, cheap, and easily concealed.

The range and magnitude of the effects of volatile substance misuse are dependent on the circumstances of use. Important factors include the state of mind of the individual, the environment, the absence or presence of other people, and the relationship with other misusers in a group situation.

TABLE 7.1
Preparations that are subject to misuse and their common volatile constituent(s)

Preparation	Volatile constituent(s)
Acrylic paints	Toluene
Adhesives	Acetone
	Ethyl acetate
	n-Hexane
	Methyl ethyl ketone
	Methylene chloride
	Toluene
	1,1,1-Trichloroethane
	Xylene
Aerosol propellants	Chlorodifluoromethane (Halon 22)
	Dichlorodifluoromethane (Halon 12)
	Dichlorotetrafluoroethane (Halon 114)
	Trichlorofluoromethane (Halon 11)
Anaesthetics	Enflurane
	Halothane
	Isoflurane
	Nitrous oxide
Anti-freeze products	Isopropanol
Bottled fuel gases	n-Butane
	Isobutane
	Propane
Car paints and thinners	n-Hexane
	Toluene
	Xylene
Chewing-gum remover	Trichloroethylene
De-greasing fluids	Tetrachloroethylene
	1,1,1-Trichloroethane
	Trichloroethylene
De-icing products	Isopropanol
Dry-cleaning fluids	Tetrachloroethylene
	1,1,1-Trichloroethane
	Trichloroethylene
Fire extinguisher	Bromochlorodifluoromethane (BCF) propellants
Lacquers	Methylene chloride
	Toluene
	1,1,1-Trichloroethane
Nail polish remover	Acetone
Paint strippers	Dichloromethane
	Toluene
Petrol	Aliphatic hydrocarbons
Refrigerants	Dichlorodifluoromethane (Halon 12)
	Trichlorofluoromethane (Halon 11)
Shoe dyes	n-Hexane
	Methylene chloride
	Toluene
	1,1,1-Trichloroethane
Solvents	Acetone
	Carbon tetrachloride
	Chloroform
	Diethyl ether
	n-Hexane
	Methyl ethyl ketone
	Methyl isobutyl ketone
Spot removers	Carbon tetrachloride
	Tetrachloroethylene
Woodwork adhesives	Xylene
Typewriter correcting fluid and thinners	1,1,1-Trichloroethane
White spirit	Aliphatic hydrocarbons

The characteristic feature of volatile substance misuse is the rapid onset of action (the 'high') followed by an equally quick recovery; the high can be maintained by repeated use for several hours. The initial effects following inhalation (the excitatory phase) include euphoria, a sense of well-being, disinhibition, blurred vision, and a feeling of invulnerability; visual or auditory hallucinations may also occur. Other effects in the excitatory phase may include nausea and vomiting, dizziness, flushing, cough, sneezing, and excessive salivation.

The excitatory phase is followed by CNS depression, which is rarely severe, although the user may fall asleep for several hours. Muscular incoordination, ataxia, slurred speech, nystagmus, and epileptiform seizures may also occur.

The local effects of volatile solvent misuse are commonly chronic, and include recurrent epistaxis, rhinitis, conjunctivitis, halitosis, nasal and mouth ulceration, and perioral eczema ('glue sniffers rash'). Systemic effects may include anorexia, weight loss, loss of concentration, depression, irritability, paranoia, and fatigue.

Volatile substance misuse carries a risk of sudden death, especially with high doses. The possible causes include vagal inhibition, respiratory depression, and cardiac arrhythmias, all of which are caused by the direct effects of volatile substances. Indirect causes of sudden death associated with volatile substance misuse include anoxia, trauma, asphyxiation, and inhalation of vomit. The volatile substances and products predominantly involved in causing deaths are bottled fuel gases (especially butane), toluene, 1,1,1-trichloroethane, and aerosol propellants (especially Halon 11 and Halon 12).

The method used to inhale volatile substances depends on the product. Adhesives, cleaning fluids, and petrol may be poured onto a piece of cloth (e.g. a handkerchief or coat sleeve) and the vapour inhaled. More viscous substances may be poured into a plastic bag or an empty potato-crisp packet, and the vapour inhaled by placing the bag over the mouth and squeezing the bag gently to force the vapour into the mouth, or nose, or both. This method may also be used for other non-viscous volatile substances to maximise inhalation.

Aerosol propellants and bottled fuel gases are misused in a variety of ways including spraying the contents into a large plastic bag and inhaling the contents. A particularly dangerous method of inhaling bottled fuel gas, aerosol propellants, and fire extinguisher contents is to spray the contents directly into the mouth or nostril. Large body bags may also be used; these enable the body and volatile substance to be totally enclosed within the bag.

Physical damage associated with toluene misuse includes reduced lung function as a result of damage to the alveoli and the vascular network of the lungs. Aplastic anaemia has been reported to occur following toluene use and, rarely, liver and kidney failure. Neurological consequences of toluene misuse include the development of a cerebellar syndrome with ataxia affecting the gait and arms; nystagmus may also be present. These symptoms may persist in some cases, especially following severe and prolonged use. Toluene can also cause mild peripheral neuropathy, although it is rare and only thought to occur with very prolonged use. Cognitive impairment may occur with chronic, long-term toluene use, although its severity is not related to the duration of use. Psychomotor function may also be impaired.

In addition to sensitisation of the heart muscle, the misuse of n-hexane can result in the development of peripheral neuropathy involving both motor and sensory systems.

Tetrachloroethylene is irritant to the eyes, nose, and throat and may cause persistent nausea and vomiting. It has also been associated with the development of liver and kidney dysfunction; pulmonary oedema may also occur. Trichloroethylene sensitises the heart muscle and at high doses can cause renal and hepatic toxicity resulting in hepatic necrosis and nephropathy. Chronic misuse of trichloroethylene has been associated with the development of optic neuropathy, cranial nerve palsy, and cognitive impairment.

Some products may contain substances that are more harmful than the volatile substance itself; the additional substances include copper, lead, vinyl chloride, and zinc.

Nitrite inhalants are rapidly absorbed following inhalation; effects include smooth-muscle relaxation, vasodilatation, headches, flushing, hypotension, and reflex tachycardia; euphoria may also occur and is described by users as a 'rush'. The nitrite inhalants are used to produce altered consciousness and for their stimulant action. However, their use as a 'sex aid' is predominant, especially by male homosexuals, and includes use to heighten libido, prolong erection, relax rectal smooth muscle, and reduce the anal sphincter tone; all of these effects are unsubstantiated.

Nitrite inhalants have been reported to cause syncope, acute psychosis, raised intra-ocular pressure, transient hemiparesis, methaemoglobinaemia, and coma; rarely, sudden death can occur. The use of nitrite inhalants has been implicated in the development of opportunistic infections and Kaposi's sarcoma in homosexual men with HIV infection. Nitrites are thought to diminish immune response and may facilitate the replication of HIV.

Amyl nitrite is a yellow, clear, volatile liquid and is available in glass capsules (vitrellae). Butyl nitrite is primarily an imported product from the USA, where it is marketed as a 'room deodoriser' to avoid legal restrictions. Street names for amyl nitrite include 'poppers' or 'snappers' as a result of the need to break the glass capsules to inhale the product.

Misuse in pregnancy
All volatile substances cross the placenta and there is a risk of congenital abnormalities as a result of misuse. Toluene misuse during pregnancy has been reported to cause effects similar to the foetal alcohol syndrome (see Section 6.3).

Dependence, tolerance, and withdrawal symptoms
Psychological dependence may occur with volatile substance misuse, especially in individuals who are regular users. Tolerance develops to the effects of volatile substances with the need to use increasing doses. Withdrawal symptoms may rarely occur, and include craving and a general feeling of dysphoria.

Nitrite inhalants are associated primarily with recreational use, and dependence, tolerance, and withdrawal symptoms have not been reported.

Management of withdrawal
No treatment for withdrawal symptoms that may be associated with volatile substance misuse is necessary. Supportive therapy, counselling, and psychotherapy may be beneficial.

7.5 THE ROLE OF THE PHARMACIST

The pharmacist is in a position to sell or supply equipment for injection, provide information leaflets on drug misuse and prevention of HIV infection and hepatitis B, and offer advice to anyone concerned about drug misuse.

The Advisory Council on the Misuse of Drugs has identified the need for pharmacists to be involved in regional and district plans for the reduction of harm from problem drug use, especially in the reduction in the spread of HIV infection. The Advisory Council points out that training will be necessary, and bodies responsible for training (e.g. the Royal Pharmaceutical Society of Great Britain) should review the training in drug misuse received by pharmacists at undergraduate and postgraduate level.

The role of the pharmacist in preventing drug misuse and problems associated with drug misuse includes the provision of information on all aspects of drug misuse to other professionals, drug users, and anyone else interested (e.g. parents or friends of a user). Pharmacists are ideally placed to be at the centre of effective prevention programmes and initiatives (e.g. needle exchange schemes) designed to prevent the harm caused by drug misuse.

A sensitive and sympathetic attitude towards drug users is needed by pharmacists; there is still a view that drug users are undesirable customers who are unpleasant, dishonest, and a nuisance. The needs of drug users, and their relatives and friends, are essential considerations for pharmacists who are involved with drug misuse. Pharmacists should be aware of the services that are available, including NHS management and rehabilitation, and self-help and community groups. One or more of these services will be appropriate for users, but the choice depends on the extent and pattern of drug use; for example, a user who has taken drugs only a few times and is anxious that the use will develop may benefit from advice, information, and counselling, whereas a user with established dependence may benefit from advice, information, and counselling, and, in addition, NHS management and rehabilitation. It should be noted at this stage that private, fee-paying organisations exist for the management of drug users and may be able to assist users.

Self-help and community groups play a vital role in the management of drug misuse, and should be recommended at an early stage to all users; see appropriate national organisations in Section 7.6. These organisations may be able to provide information on local groups, or other appropriate organisations if they are unable to help.

Parents of drug misusers often feel helpless and frightened following the discovery of drug use by their child; self-help and community groups will be able to provide advice, information, and counselling to cope with the stress invariably associated with the discovery and management of drug use by their child.

Information on the local trends and extent of drug misuse can be obtained from drug treatment centres, community drug teams, and general practitioners. Liaison and cooperation with local authority services, community based drug agencies, and other health-care professionals is essential in the management of drug misuse. The dissemination of information between community pharmacists, on local trends of drug misuse, is also of great importance.

Needle exchange schemes

The role of the pharmacist in the prevention of complications associated with drug misuse is clearly highlighted by the need to discourage the sharing of injection equipment. It has been suggested that approximately 75% of pharmacies in England and Wales are prepared to sell injection equipment to users in line with the guidance from the Royal Pharmaceutical Society of Great Britain. The guidance states that pharmacists can, at their discretion, sell injection equipment to drug misusers, although it is also important to collect used equipment and dispose of it safely; a sharps container is suitable for the collection of used equipment brought in by users.

The sharing of injection equipment cannot be attributed solely to ignorance of the associated risks of infection, especially HIV infection. The most common reason for sharing is the difficulty in obtaining new equipment. Other reasons include the need to use drugs to avoid withdrawal symptoms and sharing may be the only means of obtaining the drug. There also appears to be a social acceptance of sharing injection equipment among friends and sexual partners; users feel that friends may be insulted if they refuse to share, and some users are convinced by friends claiming their needles to be 'clean'.

Financial constraints may also contribute to the sharing of injection equipment; there may be a choice between buying new equipment or more drugs. This emphasises the need for the supply of free injection equipment to users in needle exchange schemes. Some users may also believe that their previous injection habits have already increased their risks of infection and may continue sharing as a result. However, many users claim they are more careful about sharing, and share only with people they know, or only in an 'emergency' when they do not have their own equipment.

Some community pharmacies are already participating in free 'new for old' syringe and needle exchange schemes in order to reduce the sharing of contaminated injection equipment. Such schemes are usually operated in collaboration with the health authority or local authority services.

Pharmacists who decide to become involved in needle exchange schemes should follow guidance from the Council of the Royal Pharmaceutical Society of Great Britain (Fig. 7.3).

Participation in syringe and needle exchange schemes is generally considered to be an important role for community pharmacists in the prevention of the spread of HIV infection, hepatitis, and other infections. In the short term, at least, measures aimed to control the spread of HIV infection should take precedence over the reduction of drug misuse. The main criterion for providing needle exchange schemes is the fact that users who inject drugs will do so under any circumstances. Providing free equipment may, therefore, reduce

1. Normally schemes will be promoted by health authorities and local pharmaceutical committees. In other cases the existing facilities should be researched and the pharmacist should liaise with the Local Pharmaceutical Committee (Area Pharmaceutical Committee), the Local Medical Committee (Area Medical Committee), and any local drug abuse teams and clinics in order to establish how many pharmacists need to take part based on how many drug users are actually injecting.

2. The supply of syringes and needles, and the receipt of used equipment should always be dealt with by the pharmacist, and supplies should always be accompanied by advice and encouragement to make use of any local drug advisory services. Any leaflets from health education agencies, local drug dependency clinics, or 'walk-in centres' should be available.

3. All persons requesting syringes and needles should be encouraged to surrender used equipment.

4. If a pharmacist decides to accept used syringes and needles for disposal then only a properly designed 'sharps' disposal container should be used and pharmacists should not participate in any scheme where such containers are not available.

5. Drug misusers should be encouraged to sheath or otherwise enclose needles before returning them to the pharmacy. The waste should not be handled by anyone other than the person wishing to dispose of it, and that person should be told to place it in the 'sharps' disposal container which should be located well away from customers and in a place known to staff but where they will not have inadvertent contact. It should not be located in the dispensary.

6. If at all possible, used contaminated material should be brought to the pharmacy by drug misusers in a personal, sealed 'sharps' container.

7. Staff should be carefully instructed about the risk of infection and advised to refer all inquires to the pharmacist. It is important that pharmacists consider having themselves and their staff vaccinated against hepatitis.

8. Pharmacists should comply with any other guidance issued in respect of the particular scheme they are participating in.

Fig. 7.3
Guidelines for pharmacists involved in schemes to supply clean syringes and needles to drug users.

sharing and use of contaminated equipment. An argument against needle exchange schemes is that the incidence of misusers choosing to inject drugs may rise as a result of increased availability; this may be true in some cases because some users may be refraining from inject- ing because of the risks associated with using shared injecting equipment.

Needle exchange schemes should not be instituted in a form that is threatening to misusers; in this respect pharmacies are ideally placed to provide easy access, and are not associated with authority (e.g. compared with hospital-based needle exchange schemes). Pharmacies are seen by users as being free of the stigma associated with specialist services and, in addition, allow for anonymity. Pharmacists are commonly approached for the purchase of injection equipment, and it follows that pharmacy needle exchange schemes will be effectively utilised. In schemes that are not pharmacy related, the users attracted tend to be those with a lower risk of complications associated with injecting drug use; it is thought that pharmacy needle exchange schemes will attract, and therefore reach, those users with higher risks.

Pharmacists have expressed some concerns about their involvement with needle exchange schemes and these include the need for:

- Education and training, which many pharmacists feel is necessary to alleviate the apprehension associated with dealing with users.
- Liaison with specialist services to provide support for pharmacists and a place to which pharmacists could refer users for further advice.
- Pharmacy involvement in any given area to be wide, with a reasonable number of pharmacies taking part.
- Ensuring adequate arrangements for the supply of sharps containers, and their collection and disposal.
- Remuneration issues to be resolved with respect to needle exchange schemes.

These issues must be resolved in order to obtain the fullest support from all pharmacists. The most important aspect of the involvement of pharmacists in the prevention of complications associated with drug misuse by injection is their ability to reach those misusers in the high risk groups. In addition, by providing advice and information, pharmacists are able to influence the misuser's practice of injection, and those who do not inject may be influenced never to attempt it.

Dispensing for drug misusers

The Misuse of Drugs (Notification and Supply to Addicts) Regulations 1973 also provide that only medical practitioners who hold a special licence issued by the Home Secretary may prescribe diamorphine, dipipanone (Diconal™), or cocaine for addicts; other practitioners must refer any addict who requires these drugs to a treatment centre. General practitioners and other doctors may still prescribe diamorphine, dipipanone, and cocaine for patients (including those dependent on these drugs) for relief of pain due to organic disease or injury without a special licence. Whenever possible the drug misuser will be introduced by a member of staff from the treatment centre to the pharmacist whose agreement has been obtained and whose pharmacy is conveniently sited for the patient. Prescriptions for weekly supplies will be sent to the pharmacy by post and will be dispensed on a daily basis as indicated by the doctor. If any alteration of the arrangements are requested by the drug misuser, the portion of the prescription affected must be represcribed and not merely altered.

A special form, FP10(HP)(ad), in Scotland HBP(A), is available to doctors in the NHS drug treatment centres for prescribing cocaine, dextromoramide, diamorphine, dipipanone, methadone, morphine, or pethidine by installments for addicts. In Scotland, general practitioners can prescribe by installments on form GP10. In England and Wales forms FP10 and FP10 (HP) are not suitable for this purpose but form FP10(MDA) is available.

Forged prescriptions

The pharmacist should be aware of the lengths to which drug misusers may go to obtain supplies. It can be extremely difficult to detect a forged prescription, but every pharmacist should be alert to the possibility that any prescription calling for a misused product could be a forgery.

The forger may make a fundamental error in writing the prescription or the pharmacist may get an instinctive feeling that the prescription is not genuine because of the way the patient behaves.

If the prescriber's signature is known, but the patient has not previously visited the pharmacy, or is not known to be suffering from a condition that requires the medicinal product prescribed, the signature should be scrutinised and, if possible, checked against an example on another prescription known to be genuine. Large doses or quantities should be checked with the prescriber in order to detect alterations to previously valid prescriptions.

If the prescriber's signature is not known, the prescriber must be contacted and asked to confirm that the prescription is genuine. The prescriber's telephone number must be obtained from the telephone directory, or from directory enquiries, not from the headed notepaper, as a forger may use false letter headings.

The dispensing of a forged prescription for a controlled drug or prescription-only medicine can constitute a criminal offence.

7.6 USEFUL ADDRESSES

DAWN (Drugs, Alcohol, Women, Now)
Omnibus Workspace
39–41 North Road
London N7 9DP
Tel: 071-700 4653

INSTITUTE FOR THE STUDY OF DRUG DEPENDENCE (ISDD)
1 Hatton Place
Hatton Garden
London EC1 8ND
Tel: 071-430 1991

MIND (NATIONAL ASSOCIATION FOR MENTAL HEALTH)
22 Harley Street
London W1N 2ED
Tel: 071-637 0741

NARCOTICS ANONYMOUS
P.O. Box 417
London SW10 0RP
Tel: 071-351 6794/6066

NAYPCAS (National Association of Young People's Counselling and Advisory Services)
17–23 Albion Street
Leicester LE1 6GD
Tel: (0533) 558763

PARENTLINE-OPUS (Organisations for Parents Under Stress)
Rayfa House
57 Hart Road
Thundersley
Essex SS7 3PD
Tel: (0268) 757077
A telephone helpline for parents experiencing any kind of a problem with a child.

RELEASE
169 Commercial Street
London E1 6BW
Tel: 071–377 5905

RE-SOLV
St. Mary's Chambers
19 Station Road
Stone
Staffordshire
ST15 8JP
Tel: (0785) 46097
The society for the prevention of solvent and volatile substance abuse.

SCODA and STANDING CONFERENCE ON DRUG ABUSE
1–4 Hatton Place
Hatton Garden
London
EC1N 8ND
Tel: 071-430 2431

TACADE
1 Hulme Place
The Crescent
Salford M5 4QA
Tel: 061-745 8925
The advisory council on alcohol and drug education.

TERENCE HIGGINS TRUST
52—54 Grays Inn Road
London WC1X 8JU
Tel: 071-242 1010
To provide support and help for people living with AIDS and
HIV infection.

TRANXCALL
P.O. Box 440
Harrow
Middlesex
Tel: 081-861 2164
To advise and support those dependent on medically prescribed
minor tranquillisers.

TURNING POINT
CAP House
4th Floor
9—12 Long Lane
London EC1A 9HA
Tel: 071-606 3947

7.7   FURTHER READING

Arif A, ed. *Adverse health consequences of cocaine abuse.*
Geneva: WHO, 1987.
Banks A, Waller TAN. *Drug misuse: a practical handbook for
GPs.* Oxford: Blackwell Scientific Publications, 1988.
Cox BM. Drug tolerance and physical dependence. In: Pratt
WB, Taylor P, eds. *Principles of drug action. The basis of
pharmacology.* 3rd ed. New York: Churchill Livingstone,
1990: 639—90.
DHSS. *AIDS and drug misuse Part 1. Report by the Advisory
Council on the Misuse of Drugs.* London: HMSO, 1988.
DoH. *AIDS and drug misuse. Part 2. Report by the Advisory
Council on the Misuse of Drugs.* London: HMSO, 1989.

Ghodse H, Maxwell D, eds. *Substance abuse and dependence.
An introduction for the caring professions.* Basingstoke:
Macmillan Press, 1990.
Gossop M, Grant M, eds. *Preventing and controlling drug
abuse.* Geneva: WHO, 1990.
Gudex C. Adverse effects of benzodiazepines. *Discussion paper
65.* York: Centre for Health Economics, University of York,
1990.
Hindmarch I, *et al.,* eds. *Benzodiazepines: current concepts.
Biological, clinical and social perspectives.* Chichester: John
Wiley & Sons, 1990.
Home Office. *Prevention. Report of the Advisory Council on
the Misuse of Drugs.* London: HMSO, 1984.
Home Office. *Problem drug use: a review of training. Report
by the Advisory Council on the Misuse of Drugs.* London:
HMSO, 1990.
Home Office. *Tackling drug misuse: a summary of the
government's strategy.* 2nd ed. London: Home Office, 1986.
Hopkinson N. Fighting the drug problem. *Conference report
based on Wilton Park Conference 331: 23—27 January 1989.*
London: HMSO, 1990.
Jaffe JH. Drug addiction and drug abuse. In: Gilman AG *et al.,*
eds. *Goodman and Gilman's The pharmacological basis of
therapeutics.* 8th ed. New York: Pergamon Press, 1990:
522—573.
Koren G, ed. *Maternal-fetal toxicology. A clinicians' guide.*
New York: Marcel Dekker, 1990.
Lee J, *et al. Perspectives - three views on drug education.*
Salford: TACADE, 1989.
Maddock DH. *Drug abuse. A guide for pharmacists.* London:
The Pharmaceutical Press, 1987.
Peroutka SJ, ed. *Ecstasy: the clinical, pharmacological and
neurotoxicological effects of the drug MDMA.* Boston:
Kluwer Academic Publishers, 1990.
Reynolds JEF ed. *Martindale. The extra pharmacopoeia.* 29th
ed. London: The Pharmaceutical Press, 1989.
Rice W. *Dealing with solvent misuse - the role of education in
a prevention strategy.* Stone and Salford: Re-Solv and
TACADE, 1990.
The Royal College of Psychiatrists. *Drug scenes. A report on
drugs and drug dependence by the Royal College of
Psychiatrists.* London: Royal College of Psychiatrists, 1987.
Stockley D. *Drug warning. An illustrated guide for parents and
teachers.* London: Macdonald, 1986.
UK Health Departments, HEA. *HIV and AIDS. An assessment
of current and future spread in the UK.* London: HMSO,
1990.

Chapter 8

SPORT AND EXERCISE

8.1 PROMOTION OF SPORT AND EXERCISE FOR HEALTH

It is well recognised that regular physical activity induces a variety of physiological changes (*see* Section 8.2) that promote good health whereas lack of activity has a deleterious effect. Various authorities have recognised the need to promote an improvement in the level of physical activity in the population as part of the strategy to improve the overall health of the nation. During the 1960s the Council of Europe put forward a charter, 'Sport for All', which was followed in the UK by the creation of a Minister for Sport (a junior minister in the Department of Environment) and the Sports Council. The 'Sport for All' campaign in the UK was officially launched in 1972. The Sports Council works together with health authorities and local authorities to undertake projects and campaigns to promote health through an increase in physical activity. In addition, the government seeks to promote physical activity as a means of improving public health through the Health Education Authority (HEA), which also deals with other health aspects (*see* Chapter 1). However, the ultimate aim of

'Sport for All' is still a long way off. Despite the improvements made in the facilities available (e.g. a steady increase in the number of indoor sports centres, swimming pools, and golf courses since 1970), it has been estimated that only about a quarter of the population in the UK undertakes some form of physical activity.

In some instances, physical activity may be a regular part of a person's normal working life (e.g. dancing, building, or mining) or home life (e.g. gardening). However, increasing automation and the use of labour-saving devices significantly reduces the amount of activity required in some occupations, and many involve no physical work at all. It is therefore essential that anyone involved in sedentary occupations should reserve some of their leisure time for recreational physical activity. Sport and exercise are considered as two subcategories of physical activity, and are ideal for those who are otherwise unable to achieve the desired levels of activity in their working life. Department of Employment surveys have shown that the average annual holiday entitlement for most full-time manual employees has doubled over the last 25 years from 2 to 4 or more weeks, and the average number of hours in a basic working week has dropped from 42.8 to 38.9 hours. There is therefore more leisure time available for a greater number of people than ever before, but more campaigns are required to bring to the attention of individuals the need to devote some of this time to regular physical activity.

It is not necessary to exercise at the level of elite athletes to attain health benefits, and fitness may be improved at any age. Many people are not prepared to make time or do not have the inclination to take up a sport; they should be encouraged to seek alternative methods of exercise (*see* Section 8.5), either in the privacy of their own homes, or just by walking briskly at every available opportunity. In fact, the annual General Household Surveys in Great Britain have shown that the most popular sporting activity in the years for which figures are available was walking two or more miles. However, learning a sport and participating in organised events may provide additional benefits for the mental state as a result of the efforts made to meet challenges; self-esteem and self-confidence may also improve. Belonging to a sports club may also improve social skills as a result of interaction with other people.

Pharmacists can play a valuable part in promoting an increase in physical activity by being readily available to answer questions and offer advice to members of the public who wish to take up sport or exercise. Those suffering with chronic conditions or disabilities that preclude intensive exercise but who nevertheless wish to partake in some form of physical activity will, in particular, require careful counselling. Advice may also be sought about the management of minor sports injuries or about drugs and dressings needed to stock sports club medical bags.

8.2 THE PHYSIOLOGY OF EXCERCISE

In order to understand the reasons for the benefits of sport and exercise (*see* Section 8.3) it is necessary to understand the physiology of exercise. Sports and exercise are not without their own health-risks (*see* Section 8.4), and a knowledge of physiology will also enable an assessment to be made of an individual's capacity for activity, and whether or not medical referral is essential before taking part.

Energy is necessary to enable all functions of the body to be carried out, and is derived from the oxidation of glucose. Glucose is obtained from the metabolism of carbohydrates, fats, and proteins and undergoes oxidation in all cells of the body (cellular respiration) to produce carbon dioxide, water, and energy. The energy

is used to convert adenosine diphosphate (ADP) to adenosine triphosphate (ATP); the phosphate bonds of ATP store energy, which is yielded when required by hydrolysis of the terminal bond, forming ADP in the process. Complete oxidation of glucose proceeds through three stages (Fig. 8.1): glycolysis to produce pyruvic acid, the Krebs' cycle, and the electron transport chain. Oxygen is required for the latter two stages, and this process is therefore termed aerobic respiration. Oxygen is taken into the body during respiration at the same time that carbon dioxide is expelled. The heart pumps oxygenated blood received from the pulmonary circulation to the rest of the body, and deoxygenated blood to the lungs for oxygenation. Oxygen binds with haemoglobin in erythrocytes for transportation in the systemic circulation to the tissues. It therefore follows that during exercise, which increases the overall energy demand, all these processes must increase in efficiency to provide the extra oxygen required.

Anaerobic respiration occurs during sustained muscle activity when there is insufficient oxygen to meet the requirements of aerobic respiration. The pyruvic acid produced by the oxidation of glucose cannot be completely oxidised, and is converted to lactic acid (*see* Fig. 8.1). Approximately 80% of the lactic acid is transported to the liver for conversion to glucose or glycogen, and the remainder accumulates in the muscles.

Most forms of exercise utilise both aerobic and anaerobic respiration.

Aerobic exercise   Exercise involving aerobic respiration requires that the oxygen demands of the active muscle must be fully met once the initial period of adjustment is over. To achieve this, there must be increases in respiration rate and depth, cardiac output, and blood-flow to the muscles. Regular aerobic exercise induces adaptive changes so that future exercising becomes comparatively easier. However, this is not a long-term effect, and previous levels of unfitness will return if exercise sessions are discontinued. Aerobic fitness is measured by the maximal oxygen uptake (VO_2 max), which is defined as the maximum rate of utilisation of atmospheric oxygen during continuous activity. Inactivity decreases VO_2 max whereas aerobic training for a few weeks can improve it substantially. VO_2 max improves as the maximum cardiac output increases (*see below*). VO_2 max starts to decline after 20 years of age, but the rate of decline can be decreased by regular exercise.

Anaerobic exercise   Exercise involving anaerobic respiration does not rely on a supply of oxygen to the muscles from the circulation, but can only be sustained

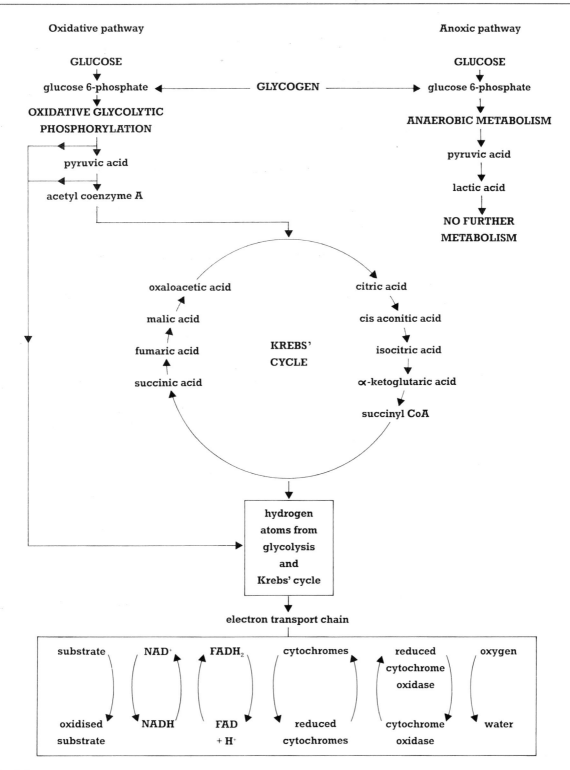

Fig. 8.1
Outline pathways of glucose metabolism.

for 1 to 2 minutes, as opposed to aerobic exercise, which in a fit subject can be sustained for hours. Anaerobic respiration occurs during short bursts of extremely strenuous activity (e.g. 100 metres sprint), when the supply of oxygen is insufficient to keep up with the exercising muscles (*see also* Muscles below).

Isotonic exercise   Isotonic (endurance or dynamic) exercise involves muscle work during movement (e.g. cycling, running, or swimming) and is of value in improving stamina and endurance. Isotonic exercise is dependent mainly on aerobic respiration.

Isometric exercise   Isometric (power or static) exercise (e.g. handgrip or weight lifting) involves a sustained increase in contraction of antagonistic muscles without movement. It is primarily employed to increase muscle strength. As a result, those that train regularly using isometric exercises are likely to be heavier than endurance athletes. They also tend to have more deposits of body fat. Isometric exercise is dependent mainly on anaerobic respiration.

Most forms of exercise employ both isometric and isotonic techniques.

Respiratory system

The total lung capacity (TLC) in adult males is approximately six litres but at rest only 10% of this is used. The tidal volume is the amount of air that moves into and out of the lungs with each breath, and at rest is 500 mL. Of this, 150 mL occupies the dead space (i.e. those parts of the airway not involved in gaseous exchange), which means that only 350 mL reaches the alveoli. The tidal volume increases during exercise, and at maximal breathing, when the largest proportion of the TLC is used, it is referred to as the vital capacity (VC). This may be between 3 and 5 litres in adult males, which still leaves a residual volume of 1 to 1.5 litres. The VC of males is 50% greater than that of females. The effort required for respiration is minimal at rest, but obviously increases as activity increases, and additional muscles are employed.

The average respiration rate at rest is 12 respirations/minute. Since the TV is 500 mL, the average volume of air inspired every minute is six litres. The maximum breathing capacity (maximum ventilation volume) in adult males in a normal atmosphere is 125 litres/minute. The volume of air taken in during a deep inspiration may be as much as 3.6 litres. Exercise increases the rate of respiration and the volume of air inspired per minute.

Respiration rate is controlled primarily by the concentration of carbon dioxide in the blood. Thus, if the concentration falls, respiration rate decreases until the blood-carbon dioxide concentration rises to normal levels. Oxygen only acts as a stimulus if there is a severe reduction in blood-oxygen concentration because haemoglobin remains at least 85% saturated until quite low oxygen concentrations are approached. However, with further reductions in oxygen concentrations to extremely low levels, anoxia of the inspiratory area in the medulla results in a diminished response to impulses received from chemoreceptors, and breathing may stop altogether.

Overbreathing immediately before an event is thought by some athletes to improve performance because a few vital seconds may be gained by temporarily removing the desire to breathe. Carbon dioxide is flushed out from the lungs, reducing the blood concentration to such an extent that respiration temporarily stops. The oxygen remaining in the lungs diffuses slowly into the blood but eventually, a very low blood-oxygen concentration stimulates breathing. At about the same time, or shortly afterwards, the blood-carbon dioxide concentration rises sufficiently to act as a further stimulus. The interaction of both stimuli are required to maintain respiration. It is possible to hold one's breath for up to a minute after a deep inspiration, and this too may be used to gain time, especially in swimming. Eventually, respiration is stimulated by rising blood-carbon dioxide concentrations. Athletes may combine breath-holding with overbreathing in an effort to further increase the time of non-breathing. However, this practice should not be encouraged as it may produce anoxia severe enough to cause syncope, which is particularly dangerous for swimmers.

Alveolar diffusion capacity, which is a measure of the gaseous exchange efficiency of the alveoli, varies even among healthy subjects, and training cannot increase this function above an individual's inherent maximum. Thus, the oxygen saturation of blood will be different among highly trained athletes. However, through intensive training, the muscles can adapt to a certain amount of oxygen lack (*see below*).

Cardiovascular system

The cardiac output (CO) is the volume of blood pumped into the aorta from the left ventricle of the heart every minute. It is equal to the pulse rate (PR) multiplied by the stroke volume (SV), which is the volume of blood ejected by the ventricles at each heartbeat.

$$CO = PR \times SV$$

In a normal adult heart, the resting pulse rate is about 70 beats/minute, and the stroke volume about 70 mL. The cardiac output at rest is therefore about

5.25 litres/minute. To increase oxygen perfusion of the tissues to cope with the increased demand created by exercise, the cardiac output must be increased by raising the stroke volume or the pulse rate, or both.

The pulse rate is controlled in part by the autonomic nervous system: the sympathetic division increases the rate; and the parasympathetic division lowers it. In people who have not been used to regular vigorous exercise, the cardiac output is mainly raised by an increase in the pulse rate. Physical training, however, increases the parasympathetic tone of the vagus nerve, and there is a much smaller rise in pulse rate for a given work-load. Trained subjects therefore feel more comfortable than untrained individuals. In order to achieve the desired increase in cardiac output, trained individuals show a greater rise in stroke volume, which is produced by an increased ventricular capacity of up to 30%. This causes the heart to enlarge, but must be distinguished from enlargement caused by cardiac disease in which the increased size is a result of muscular hypertrophy. The increase in size of the ventricular chamber reduces the pressure developed during systole. The resting pulse rate of highly trained individuals also falls, and may be as low as 40 beats/minute in elite athletes.

The cardiac reserve is the maximum that the cardiac output can be increased above normal during vigorous activity, and is expressed as a percentage. In the average adult, this reserve may be 400%, but trained athletes may achieve a 600% cardiac reserve. The actual cardiac output in trained athletes may reach 30 litres/minute or more during exercise. These cardiac changes reduce the work that the heart has to perform for a given work-load and makes exercising progressively easier. These effects occur as a result of long-term isotonic exercise and may be apparent after a few weeks. In isometric exercise, the arterial pressure rises, which increases the tension on the wall of the left ventricle. The cardiac output changes little and isometric exercise does not greatly improve stamina.

Athletes may show abnormal ECG (electro-cardiogram) patterns as a result of altered physiology (as well as some temporarily deranged biochemical results), and this must be borne in mind if evacuation to hospital and testing subsequent to an event is necessary as a result of either collapse or injury.

The heart, brain, and skeletal muscles have increased oxygen demands during exercise, and blood must be redirected to these organs away from other parts of the body (e.g. gastro-intestinal tract). In vigorous activity, the blood supply to the heart tissue is increased by up to four or five times. The need for diversion of the systemic blood-flow decreases with training because the oxygen-extracting ability of the muscles improves (*see below*). The result is that the individual feels more comfortable during exercise as a result of fewer gastro-intestinal symptoms.

Regular exercising increases the network of blood capillaries supplying the muscles and improves the overall efficiency of the circulation. This has the added effect of lowering the peripheral resistance, which has a beneficial effect on blood pressure.

The principal function of haemoglobin, which is contained in erythrocytes, is to transport oxygen in the blood. The normal blood-haemoglobin concentration is 14 to 18 g/100 mL of blood for males, and 12 to 16 g/100 mL of blood for females. A constant enhanced demand for oxygen by the tissues (e.g. as a result of physical training) increases the number of erythrocytes, and consequently the amount of haemoglobin, present. Plasma volume may also rise with the result that the haemoglobin concentration remains constant or may even drop, suggesting anaemia ('sports anaemia'). However, the actual oxygen-carrying capacity is higher because the total amount of haemoglobin present is greater. These rises in highly trained individuals may approach 40% above average values. Carbon monoxide, present in tobacco smoke and exhaust fumes from motor vehicles, binds with haemoglobin much more strongly than oxygen and therefore substantially reduces the oxygen-carrying capacity of the blood. Exercise can aid the removal of carbon monoxide from haemoglobin.

The core temperature, which is the deep body temperature measured by the oral or rectal method, may rise up to 41°C (105.8°F) during intensive exercise. In order for this heat to be lost by conduction, convection, and radiation from the skin, the volume of blood perfusing the skin increases during strenuous activity. Heat is also lost by evaporation of sweat. If any of these mechanisms are blocked, or the individual is unfit, heat stroke (*see* Section 8.4) or even sudden death may occur.

Muscles

With regular training, local adaptive changes enable the muscles to increase the quantity of oxygen extracted from blood, and improve its utilisation. There is an increase in the number of muscle capillaries, and the number and size of muscle mitochondria. In the average person at rest, about 15% of the cardiac output is used by the muscles. This percentage increases with exercise, and in trained athletes at maximal exercise may approach 90%. Muscles are also able to adapt to use greater amounts of lipids as an energy source. Training increases the bulk, strength, and stamina of muscles, which are able to function longer aerobically (*see above*) as a result of improved oxygenation. The increase in muscle size is more likely to be a result of an increase in fibre size rather than number of fibres. Training also improves the strength of tendons and ligaments.

The lactic acid that accumulates as a result of anaerobic metabolism (*see* Fig. 8.1) during sustained muscle activity must eventually be catabolised, and the extra oxygen required for this process is termed the 'oxygen debt'. The additional oxygen is 'repaid' at the end of the activity by a continued increase in the depth and rate of respiration. Muscle fatigue and pain is caused by a combination of factors including the build up of lactic acid and carbon dioxide in the tissues, and a reduced supply of oxygen. The response of the muscle filaments becomes progressively weaker in the face of sustained contraction, and activity must either cease or switch to the slower aerobic pace. Proponents of the 'burn' as the goal to be attained in 'aerobics' (aerobic exercises) are, in fact, promoting an anaerobic activity.

Sprinting is a particular athletic event in which a short distance (e.g. 60 to 100 metres) is run at high speed. However, sprinting may also be employed in everyday life, (e.g. in running for a bus or, at its most extreme, to escape from danger). Sprinting requires anaerobic metabolism in the muscles, and for unfit individuals, any increase in activity above their normal level may be comparable to a 'sprint' in terms of muscle metabolism and fatigue. If oxygen were provided at a sufficient rate to keep pace with oxidative processes to produce enough energy for a sprint, the blood supply to the muscles would have to increase to such an extent that there would be no room in the muscles for sufficient myofibrils to sustain the contraction, or enough mitochondria to cope with the oxidative processes. Anaerobic metabolism, therefore, is a means of allowing short periods of sustained muscle contraction. Longer periods require aerobic metabolism and the activity must therefore continue at a slower pace (e.g. marathon running). Regular aerobic training will, however, increase the capacity for sprinting by increasing the number of capillaries in the muscles.

There are two types of fibre present in skeletal muscles: fast fibres, which contract quickly and with great strength, and are suitable for anaerobic exercise; and slow fibres, which are more suitable for aerobic exercise. The proportion of each type of fibre present in the muscles of an individual is genetically determined, and a born sprinter is unlikely to become an elite marathon runner or vice versa. However, training does improve performance above baseline in both types.

8.3   THE BENEFITS OF SPORT AND EXERCISE

Exercise and the prevention of ill-health

Physical activity does not necessarily increase the life expectancy of an individual, but it does offer some measure of protection against developing disease and therefore improves the quality of life. The functioning of muscles and the respiratory and cardiovascular systems is improved by regular exercise (*see* Section 8.2), and many studies have shown that this is a major contributory factor to the reduction in risk for ischaemic heart disease. Generally, the forms of exercise of most benefit to the heart are those that involve the movement of large muscles and an increase in blood-flow to the tissues (i.e. aerobic exercises). Exercise is also of value in maintaining ideal body-weight, which is itself of benefit in reducing the risk for ischaemic heart disease. Exercise cannot replace cardiac tissue that is already damaged but may aid in the improvement of residual performance (*see* Exercise in the management of disease below). Other studies have shown reduced risks for cancer, hypertension, and stroke, and improved glucose tolerance.

Exercise increases the plasma-HDL concentration, which has a beneficial effect on cholesterol levels, and reduces the concentration of the more harmful LDLs (*see* Section 2.2.2). It also increases fibrinolysis and therefore aids in the dissolution of blood clots. These properties may help to explain the epidemiological evidence linking sustained regular exercise with the prevention or slowing of atherosclerosis.

Inactivity is associated with loss of bone mass whereas exercise has been shown to increase bone mass and may aid in the prevention of osteoporosis. This effect may occur at any age, and in the elderly, the increase in bone mass is greater than the amount of bone lost. Similarly, exercise can prevent the muscle atrophy that occurs with inactivity as well as reducing the stiffness associated with arthritis or other conditions that limit joint movement. However, exercise is contra-indicated during the acute stages of inflammation in osteoarthritis or rheumatoid arthritis.

Exercise has psychological benefits, which are particularly marked in depressed or anxious patients. Some workers have claimed that this is caused by the release in the brain of endorphins, although the evidence is still inconclusive. Others have postulated that exercise may promote feelings of increased self-confidence or reverse the feelings of apathy commonly experienced by depressed individuals. Whatever the mechanism, it is generally agreed that regular exercise is of benefit in the prevention and management of depressive disorders.

Some studies have shown that exercise is of value in stress management and prevention, although the evidence is inconclusive and the mechanism unclear. There may be an action through the same pathways that improve anxiety and depression, or it may simply be that exercise represents an active form of relaxation (i.e. by concentrating on something different for a short while an individual is able to clear the day's problems from his or her mind). It may also be a positive way of relieving frustrations. However, it is important that the chosen form of exercise does not represent additional stress, and it is suggested that for those with stressful life-styles, aggressive competitive sports should be avoided unless the subject finds them particularly enjoyable and rewarding.

Exercise during pregnancy is of benefit to delivery, and has been associated with a reduced incidence of abortion and prematurity; it does not appear to adversely affect the well-being of the newborn. However, careful consideration of the type of activity undertaken is necessary, and anaerobic exercises, contact sports, horse riding, skiing, water skiing, SCUBA diving, or any activity involving extreme environmental changes are not recommended. Any other form of physical activity that may have been carried out before pregnancy may be continued in moderation, avoiding vigorous exercise, particularly during the third trimester. The intensity and duration of exercise should be reduced as pregnancy proceeds. For those who previously did not undertake regular exercise but wish to start a programme during pregnancy, walking and swimming are the best options. It has been suggested that three sessions a week lasting no more than 30 minutes each is adequate and should not be exceeded. The risks of exercise during pregnancy are discussed in Section 8.4.

Exercises can be tailored to meet the capacity and abilities of most subjects, and the disabled will benefit as much from physical activity as able-bodied people. It is a misconception that people with disabilities are fragile creatures not able to do anything for themselves. This attitude is likely to lead to a worsening of the disability with a concomitant degradation in the level of the individual's independence. In fact, for such individuals, exercise may have an even greater impact in improving the quality of life by increasing stamina, strength, dexterity, and coordination, thereby maximising residual capacities. The effort required to carry out everyday tasks may be reduced, resulting in increased independence and self-confidence. It may also help prevent the emergence of a secondary disability. Where possible, aerobic exercises involving the movement of large muscles to improve cardiopulmonary performance

and exercises to work the joints should be carried out. Exercises in water are particularly advantageous as they are non-weight-bearing. However, there will be those with some types of disability that make many exercises impractical or difficult, and exercises of sufficient intensity to significantly improve cardiovascular fitness are just not possible. This should not, however, preclude them from engaging in physical activities of low intensity, increasing the programme gradually to remain within their capabilities and comfort at each stage. It is now not uncommon for physically disabled people to learn a sport, and there are many organisations and clubs that can help. The added advantage of sports participation is that it brings people with disabilities together, and they can learn and benefit from each others experiences in coping with the tasks of everyday life.

People with mental handicaps suffer impairment of learning processes, and there may also be associated physical disabilities (e.g. impaired coordination). However, once again, there is no reason why they should not participate in sports or exercise, which in addition to improving physical fitness, may well have beneficial effects in improving learning ability, mood, and self-confidence. They may also simply find it enjoyable, and for the energetic young, it may prove a valuable means of 'releasing energy' and relieving frustrations that they are unable to channel in other directions. Skilled help is necessary for both physically and mentally handicapped people to participate in sports and exercise safely and effectively, particularly when first starting. A medical assessment should be undertaken initially to assess the most suitable form and appropriate intensity of sport or exercise to ensure that the individual is not put at risk of further injury.

Physical activity naturally falls with advancing age, and with it there is a decline in fitness, stamina, strength, suppleness, and coordination. Eventually the deterioration may be such that everyday tasks cannot be carried out (e.g. carrying shopping or doing housework) and the individual loses independence. It has been estimated that 20% of the decline is as a result of inactivity. This degenerative process may be retarded by maintaining a reasonable level of activity to suit the ability of the individual. Movement of each joint through its full range each day maintains joint mobility; swimming or stair-climbing increases strength; and activities such as digging, swimming, walking, or housework carried out at least three times a week improves stamina. Elderly people who regularly undertake some form of exercise often show improved concentration and mood compared to more sedentary individuals, and may also be afforded some degree of protection against hypothermia during the winter because of the effect that physical activity has in raising body temperature. Additional social benefits may be gained through attending local exercise classes for the elderly.

Elderly people are not precluded from participating in many sporting activities, and are likely to gain additional benefits from the excitement and challenge of competition, and joining in any social events organised by their particular club. It is recommended that anyone contemplating a programme of vigorous exercise should first seek medical advice to ensure that there is no underlying condition that first requires treatment, or which may contra-indicate intensive physical activity. Enquiry must also be made about any medication as the effects of some drugs (e.g. antihypertensive drugs, beta blockers, calcium-channel blockers, diuretics, some psychotropic drugs, and insulin and oral antidiabetic drugs) may compromise the safety of exercise. Warming-up and cooling-down exercises are recommended for anyone exercising, but their importance must be particularly stressed for the elderly. It is also important to emphasise that elderly people should not exercise in extremes of environmental temperature, which may precipitate hypothermia or hyperthermia because the homoeostatic control mechanisms may not function as efficiently as in younger adults.

Exercise only produces long-term benefits if it is carried out regularly. Protection against disease stops when regular activity ceases; cardiovascular disease is not prevented in old age because of a high level of fitness when young unless fitness is maintained during the intervening years.

Exercise in the management of disease

Exercise is not necessarily contra-indicated in the presence of established disease, although a temporary curtailment of physical activity may be required until certain conditions are brought under control (*see* Section 8.4). Controlled exercise may even be beneficial in the management of some conditions (e.g. diabetes mellitus, depressive disorders, and obesity).

Exercise may be of benefit after myocardial infarction in reducing the oxygen requirements of the residual heart muscle for a given work-load. Patients are therefore more able to cope comfortably with everyday activities, and meet the demands imposed by occasional increased effort. It is not recommended that cardiac patients undertake isometric exercise (*see* Section 8.2) because the increase in blood pressure during exercise may place too great a strain on the heart. Patients should not attempt to design their own exercise programmes, but should be trained under medical supervision.

Regular exercise has a beneficial effect in hypertension as it eventually brings about a reduction in blood pressure. The decrease is of the order of 13/12 mmHg, although the fall is not so substantial in normotensive subjects. Regular exercise also reduces the blood pressure response to a given work-load. Hypertensive patients should avoid severe, prolonged isometric exercises (*see* Section 8.2) because of the association with a rapid increase in blood pressure. Moderate isotonic exercises (*see* Section 8.2) are permissible once blood pressure is under control with antihypertensive drugs. However, the response of patients must first be determined.

Obesity has been linked with adverse effects on health (*see* Section 2.1), and is generally associated with lack of exercise. However, inactivity cannot really be considered a sole aetiological factor of obesity, but rather a consequence, as once obesity is established the level of exercise tends to fall. Regular exercise is of benefit in the management of obesity if combined with a suitable weight-reducing diet (*see* Section 2.3). This is particularly important for those individuals whose rate of weight-reduction appears to be slowing despite a drastic reduction in dietary energy intake. As the fat-free mass (FFM) decreases with reducing weight, so too does the basal metabolic rate (BMR), which means that slimmers have to further reduce their energy intake to continue losing weight (*see* Section 2.3). This may be offset to some extent by increasing the level of physical activity, which increases the overall energy expenditure. Exercise does not, however, increase the BMR and the increase in energy expenditure as a result of physical activity is not sufficient to be used as a means of reducing weight alone; it is only of benefit as an adjunct to dietary measures.

Studies have shown that regular exercise improves glucose tolerance and insulin sensitivity, which may be of value in both Type I (juvenile-onset) and Type II (maturity-onset) diabetes mellitus. However, Type I diabetics must be particularly aware that hypoglycaemia may result from strenuous activity and preventive measures must be taken (*see* Section 8.4). Short periods of activity or intermittent sporting events are more suitable than prolonged endurance-type activity for diabetics.

A supervised and controlled programme of exercises has been shown to be beneficial in those with obstructive airways diseases (e.g. asthma or chronic bronchitis) in reducing dyspnoea and improving exercise tolerance. The most suitable exercises are those that can be performed at home (e.g. stair-climbing) with regular assessments at out-patient clinics.

8.4   THE RISKS OF SPORT AND EXERCISE

The most drastic adverse effect that may occur during exercise is sudden death, which is usually the result of heart failure. However, this is not a common event; the risk of sudden cardiac death during strenuous activity is greatest in those who do not regularly exercise (e.g. less than 20 minutes/week). The risk may be reduced by building up a programme of exercise of gradually increasing intensity.

Other adverse effects that may arise are generally as a result of attempting to do too much exercise while still unfit, poor preparation for a sports event, failure to take into account prevailing environmental conditions, or over-exercising when suffering from certain diseases. In some instances, particularly in elite athletes, there may be adverse biochemical or hormonal changes as a result of altered physiology.

General adverse effects

Some individuals experience abdominal cramps, and nausea and vomiting with hard exercise. These effects may be caused by the diversion of blood away from the gastro-intestinal tract to the heart, lungs, and muscles, although the exact mechanism is unclear. It may be an indicator of poor fitness, although some people are more susceptible than others. Gastro-intestinal disturbances are more often associated with running than cycling or swimming. 'Runner's diarrhoea' is also not uncommon, and is related to the severity of the exercise. There are also reports of gastro-intestinal bleeding (melaena or haematemesis) in marathon runners and other endurance sports (e.g. long-distance cycling). The mechanism is unclear, and it is essential to exclude serious pathology (e.g. peptic ulceration or colorectal cancer) before attributing this symptom to the stresses of the exercise. For those who appear to be susceptible, training programmes should be rescheduled to be less intense, increasing gradually to the required level. Non-steroidal anti-inflammatory drugs should be avoided, particularly during the few days before a race.

Haemoptysis occasionally occurs during strenuous exercise, and may simply be caused by irritation of the airways. This is especially likely to occur on repeated inspiration of cold, dry air in the winter. However, medical investigation is necessary to exclude a serious disorder (e.g. bronchiectasis or tuberculosis).

Chest pain may occur for a variety of reasons (e.g. angina pectoris, indigestion, musculoskeletal injury within the chest, oesophagitis, or referred spinal pain), and should always be investigated before continuing further exercise. Exercise is not contra-indicated in controlled angina pectoris provided that the exertion is not too vigorous. Regular attacks of palpitations should always be referred for investigation, although they are not uncommon in athletes, either during recovery from intensive exercise or at rest, and do not necessarily represent any serious pathology.

Syncope may occur at the end of a period of intense physical exercise (e.g. marathon run), and is usually the result of a dramatic fall in blood pressure caused by the abrupt cessation of activity. The pumping action of the muscles on the blood circulation is suddenly stopped and a large volume of blood pools in the dilated vessels of the lower legs. Falling from the vertical to the horizontal position will restore the blood-flow, and there is no cause for alarm provided that no injury is sustained in the fall. Occasionally, collapse may be caused by cardiac arrest, which should always be excluded. Syncope during physical activity should always be thoroughly investigated and all forms of exercise discontinued until the cause has been elicited.

Anaemia may often be diagnosed in athletes on the basis of a reduced blood-haemoglobin concentration (see Section 8.2). Medical investigation of anaemia is necessary, particularly in men, to exclude serious pathology (e.g. peptic ulceration). In women, anaemia may be a true diagnosis if pregnant or experiencing regular heavy menstrual losses, and requires treatment with iron supplements. Diets deficient in iron may also be a contributory factor. Haematuria is associated with long-distance running, although the underlying reason is not clear. All patients with haematuria should be referred for medical investigation but reassured that 'exercise haematuria' is not necessarily serious. Haemoglobinuria, which also produces a reddish-coloured urine, may occur in long-distance runners or karate players. It is caused by repeated severe jarring resulting in local haemolysis, and is more common in men than women. The oxygen-carrying capacity of the blood does not fall below normal and treatment is not required. Prevention may be effected by the use of some means of protection (e.g. springy insoles in running shoes or changing from road running to cross-country running).

Amenorrhoea and oligomenorrhoea may occur in women who regularly undertake intensive endurance exercising (e.g. long-distance running), and may be caused by impairment of cyclical secretion of luteinising hormone, although there are insufficient data to conclusively support this. Women with low body-weight and low body fat are particularly prone; emotional disturbances caused by intensive training schedules and competition may also be a contributory factor. Amenorrhoeic athletes should be referred for medical investigation, although menses generally resume on reduction of exercise, and fertility is not usually impaired.

Exercising in conditions of high air temperature and relative humidity can be dangerous, especially for the unfit, and may result in heat stroke (sunstroke). The core temperature rises and relies on various mechanisms to lower it (see Section 8.2). Anything that acts to block these mechanisms (e.g. heavy clothing, a still or humid atmosphere, or dehydration) causes the core temperature to rise further, and eventually brain cells may be destroyed. Severe cases may result in some degree of permanent brain damage on recovery. Some drugs (e.g. antimuscarinics, barbiturates, and phenothiazines) or diseases (e.g. diabetes mellitus) may also impair the heat regulatory mechanisms. Heat stroke is characterised by a core temperature around 41°C (105.8°F) or more, confusion, headache, irritability, and a hot dry skin. Blood pressure is usually normal to start with but eventually falls during the final stages. Immediate treatment is necessary, and the patient should be sponged with tepid water and fanned with cool air to lower the core temperature to about 38°C (100.4°C). Further decreases by these means should be avoided to prevent the risk of precipitating hypothermia. It is preferable not to use cold water for sponging or cold air for fanning because the resultant cutaneous vasoconstriction may impair the mechanism of heat transfer from the centre of the body to the surface. Administration of fluids and electrolytes may also be necessary.

Vigorous activity in hot conditions causes profuse perspiration and results in excessive loss of salt and water from the body. The average loss of sweat during light work is 2 to 3 litres/day but during heavy physical activity in hot weather the maximum rate of production may reach 2 to 4 litres/hour. The rate does, however, fall off as perspiration continues and may be as little as 0.5 litres/hour after 24 hours of sustained sweating. Sweat contains salt, and large salt losses may occur at maximal sweating rates. If these losses of salt and water are not replaced heat exhaustion results, which can be classified as salt-depletion heat exhaustion and water-depletion heat exhaustion; both may occur together.

Salt-depletion heat exhaustion occurs if there are excessive salt losses during intense activity, and is characterised by painful contractions in exercised muscles during the post-exercise phase (heat cramps). Additionally, there may be fatigue, headache, nausea and vomiting, postural hypotension, and weakness. Treatment involves the oral or parenteral administration of sodium chloride.

Water-depletion heat exhaustion is characterised by dehydration and thirst. The face and eyes may have a sunken appearance, and the skin feels cool and clammy; the condition may be complicated by heat stroke. The concentration of electrolytes in the body fluids rises and death occurs when the amount of fluid lost approaches 15 to 25% of the initial body-weight. Treatment requires rehydration by the oral administration of water or, in more severe cases, the administration of glucose 5% intravenous infusion. Losses of body fluid during a marathon run may approach 3 to 4 litres (or more in hot weather), and hypovolaemic shock may occur if inadequate fluid is taken during a race. Runners should ensure that they have taken plenty of fluid before the start of a race, and take advantage of all drinks available during the event. Shock may not become apparent until as long as 20 minutes after completion of the race.

Heat exhaustion may be prevented by drinking plenty of fluids before, during, and after prolonged sessions of intensive physical activity, particularly if undertaken in hot conditions. Salt supplementation may also be necessary in some individuals although, for many, the daily intake of dietary sodium is far in excess of requirements. Salt cannot be absorbed from the gastro-intestinal tract during exercise and should be taken before or after an event. Replacement salt solutions must be hypotonic, and a sodium choride 0.5% solution is generally considered adequate. Sodium Chloride Tablets (B.P.) are available and should be dissolved in water before administration. It is essential that plenty of fluid should be taken with salt supplements, and if this is not available, salt supplementation is not recommended. Salt solutions may cause nausea and vomiting, and sustained-release formulations are available to minimise the gastro-intestinal side-effects. There is no advantage to be gained by excessive salt supplementation, which in the short-term causes fluid retention, and in the long-term has been linked with the development of hypertension (see Section 2.2.5). Regular training or acclimatisation in a hot climate causes an increase in overall sweat production and a decrease in sodium concentration of sweat. Highly trained athletes may not, therefore, require as great a salt supplementation as might be expected.

Hypothermia may develop during a marathon race in the presence of cool weather, wind, or rain, particularly if the athlete is ill-clad or running slowly. The runner should avoid early fatigue caused by starting the race at too fast a pace because fatigue lowers the rate of heat production. If necessary, a lightweight garment that is both waterproof and windproof should be carried. Hillwalkers, climbers, and skiers may also be at risk of hypothermia if inadequately dressed or injured in ambient temperatures close to 0°C (32°F). As the air temperature drops below freezing point, there is the additional hazard of frost-bite.

Mild hypothermia occurs with a core temperature below 35°C (95°F), and is characterised by shivering and an intense feeling of cold. However, the subject is usually still alert and, unless injured, should be self-motivated to take action to keep warm. A core temperature of below 32°C (89.6°F) results in severe hypothermia, which causes apathy, impaired judgement, coma, and eventually fatal ventricular fibrillations. Treatment is required when the core temperature falls below 34°C (93.2°C); recovery is unlikely if the core temperature falls below 26°C (78.8°F). The patient should be thoroughly dried and reclothed in warm dry clothing, and then wrapped in a foil blanket if available. Rapid rewarming (e.g. by immersion in hot water) can be dangerous in some situations and should be avoided. Warm drinks, preferably containing sugar, should also be given once the core temperature has risen above 31°C (87.8°F).

Alcohol should never be given to hypothermic patients or ingested following exercise in cold conditions because this can accentuate or precipitate hypothermia. After a period of vigorous exercise the subject will almost certainly have used up most of the carbohydrate reserves and be reliant on the formation of glucose from amino acids (gluconeogenesis) as an energy source. This reaction involves pyruvic acid as an intermediate product. However, alcohol metabolism also utilises pyruvic acid, which is then unavailable for conversion to glucose. There is consequently insufficient pyruvate to replace the glucose used during the period of exercise. The result is hypoglycaemia, which adversely affects the homoeostatic mechanisms controlling core temperature, and hypothermia may develop. Hypoglycaemia also contributes to the patient's mental confusion.

Frost-bite is marked by areas of hard white skin, usually on the extremities, although severe cases may extensively involve the limbs. Small areas may be treated by immersion in hand-hot water to induce thawing, but more severe frostbite requires evacuation of the patient to an intensive care unit in hospital and should not be treated by rapid rewarming.

The risks in specific medical conditions

Anyone suffering with anaemia, chronic disorders of the cardiovascular, renal, or respiratory systems, metabolic disorders, or thyroid disorders must consult their doctor and have a full medical examination before undertaking any exercise programme. It is generally considered that exercise is contra-indicated in such disorders until the condition has been brought under control. Medical assessment is also advised for patients recovering from acute conditions, and in those with hypertension or musculoskeletal disorders.

Exercising is contra-indicated during infections, particularly viral infections because there is often an associated risk of myocarditis. The extra work-load placed on the inflamed heart results in reduced exercise tolerance characterised by breathlessness and fatigue, and can be responsible for sudden death during exercise. Exercise may also prolong convalescence and increase the incidence of postviral depression (e.g. following influenza or Epstein-Barr virus infection). Patients should not, therefore, resume exercising until fully recovered.

Sport and exercise may uncover underlying cardiac defects or disease (e.g. when a person collapses while running or playing sports). Cardiac disorders (e.g. ischaemic heart disease, myocardial disease, and valvular heart disease) reduce the cardiac reserve of the heart. Faulty valves (either as a result of incompetence or stenosis) increase the work-load of the heart muscle under normal conditions, and exercising causes further increases. A person with valvular heart disease is therefore unable to cope with the same level of physical activity as someone with a normal heart. Chronic myocarditis may lead to cardiomyopathy and possibly cause sudden death during exercise. However, a controlled and supervised exercise programme may be of benefit in preventing further cardiac damage following myocardial infarction (see Section 8.3).

Exercise tolerance is reduced in those with obstructive airways disease because more work is required to force air through constricted passages. Also, any disorder that increases the dead space of the lungs reduces the efficiency of respiration. Fluid accumulates in the air spaces of the lungs in pulmonary infections, reducing the efficiency of gaseous exchange. Emphysema results in reduced elasticity of the alveoli, which lowers the amount of air expelled. Some diseases (e.g. asthma, bronchitis, and emphysema) influence the distribution of blood to different parts of the lungs, which reduces exercise tolerance because alveolar gaseous exchange is dependent on adequate perfusion. Similarly, exchange can only take place across healthy alveolar walls, and any disease that affects the lining (e.g. emphysema, pulmonary fibrosis, or viral infections) reduces the efficiency of respiration. Carbon dioxide diffuses into the alveoli faster than oxygen diffuses into the blood, so the primary effect of impaired gaseous exchange is reduced oxygenation of the blood rather than an increase in the blood-carbon dioxide concentration. Exercises may, however, be beneficial in the management of obstructive airways disease but full medical supervision is necessary (*see* Section 8.3).

Exercise may cause attacks of asthma in susceptible individuals, and for some asthmatics this is the only provocative factor. Breathlessness and wheezing characteristically occur after exercise, or may arise after a few minutes into continuous exercise. Exercise-induced asthma (EIA) usually peaks about 5 to 10 minutes after exercise and abates after 30 to 60 minutes. The severity of the attack is related to the intensity of exercise, but further exercise 2 to 4 hours later (the refractory period) fails to elicit the same intensity of response. This property is made use of by some asthmatic athletes who induce asthma some time before an event. EIA does not necessarily occur every time a susceptible individual exercises, but may be precipitated by specific factors. Cold, dry conditions are more likely to induce an attack than a warm, moist atmosphere, and it is noteworthy that swimming is less likely to induce asthma than running. EIA may also be related to stress or the presence of certain allergens (e.g. pollens) in the air. Known precipitating factors should be avoided, and prophylactic therapy administered (but *see* Table 8.2 for a list of drugs banned in sports competitions).

Exercise may precipitate hypoglycaemia in Type I diabetes mellitus, and it can occur up to several hours after physical activity unless preventive measures are taken. A patient should be medically assessed before undertaking a programme of sport or exercise. It may be necessary to reduce the insulin dose before anticipated exercise and to inject at a site not being exercised (to minimise the increase in absorption that occurs from exercising muscles, presumably as a result of increased blood-flow). Doses should not be administered less than one hour before exercise. Some diabetics, especially the lean, may need to ingest carbohydrate before exercising and during prolonged sessions, and a meal should always be taken within three hours of completing the activity. It may be helpful for those who wish to regularly undertake vigorous exercise to monitor their blood-glucose concentrations before, during, and after exercise, in order to assess their personal response to physical activity and to allow reasonably accurate predictions of future requirements to be made. Type II diabetics on diet therapy alone do not generally experience problems related to altered blood-glucose concentrations, and need only observe the same precautions related to taking up exercise as the general population. However, those on oral antidiabetic agents may experience hypoglycaemia during prolonged physical activity, and should first seek medical advice. Exercise has, however, been shown to be beneficial in both types of diabetes mellitus (*see* Section 8.3) and should be encouraged.

Vertigo during exercise may simply be related to stress or it may be indicative of a serious disorder (e.g. iron-deficiency anaemia or cardiac disease), particularly if it occurs on changes in posture. Exercise is contra-indicated until medical investigations have been carried out.

Exercise during pregnancy may pose some risks for the mother or foetus, although if carried out sensibly and in moderation, has been shown to be of benefit (*see* Section 8.3). A pregnant woman should seek medical advice to assess whether or not it is safe for her to exercise. Absolute contra-indications include any factors that predispose to prematurity (e.g. incompetent cervix, more than one foetus, or a history of premature labour), or any factors that cause decreased oxygenation of the uterus or placenta (e.g. pregnancy-induced hypertension or smoking). Relative contra-indications should be assessed on an individual basis taking into account all other factors present, and include anaemia, arrhythmias, diabetes mellitus, essential hypertension, thyroid disorders, or extremes of weight. Vigorous exercise by pregnant women has been seen to produce foetal bradycardia and should therefore be avoided. Hyperthermia may have an adverse effect on the foetus and pregnant women should avoid exercising to such a level or in conditions that significantly raise the core temperature. For the same reason, post-exercise saunas or hot baths are not recommended.

It may be necessary to consider the effects of any medication on performance or ability to partake in sports or strenuous exercise programmes. Some drugs (e.g. morphine) depress the rate of respiration, which ultimately slows down the rate of gaseous exchange between the alveoli and the blood. Alterations in fluid and electrolyte balance affect the plasma concentrations of some drugs (e.g. lithium), and toxic effects may arise if the patient becomes dehydrated during intense exercise. Studies have shown increased absorption of medication from transdermal delivery systems (e.g. glyceryl trinitrate patches) during hard physical activity, which may be related to an increase in cutaneous blood-flow and increased skin temperature. For the performance-enhancing effects of drugs in sport *see* Section 8.5.

Sports injuries

The types of injury that occur during sports and exercise may also occur during the course of everyday activity, and pharmacists can apply the principles of treatment or referral discussed in this Section to any such injury. Injuries are more likely to occur in the unfit, and the risks may be significantly reduced by improving strength, stamina, suppleness, and playing skill. The different reasons for injuries arising during sports or exercise are:

- trauma
- overuse
- environmental factors.

The type of injury occurring during sports and exercise generally varies with the type of activity being undertaken. Trauma is more likely to occur during combat or contact sports (e.g. boxing, judo, or rugby), whereas overuse injuries are more commonly a feature of sports involving repetitive movements (e.g. golf or tennis). Traumatic and overuse injuries mainly involve bone and soft tissue, with soft-tissue injuries accounting for over 80% of all sports injuries. There are more injuries involving the limbs than head and trunk, and the incidence in the lower limbs is greater than in the upper. Overuse injuries occur most commonly in the tendons of the ankle, hip, knee, shoulders, and wrist. Environmental injuries occur during activities that expose the subject to adverse conditions for a prolonged period of time (e.g. heat stroke in marathon runners, hypothermia in hillwalkers and long-distance swimmers, or altitude sickness and frost-bite in mountain climbers). Environmental injuries generally affect the homoeostatic mechanisms of the body and, if severe, may endanger life (see General adverse effects above).

The principles of treatment

Injury to soft tissues causes the release of prostaglandins (especially prostaglandin E_2) and other inflammatory mediators (e.g. bradykinin, histamine, and serotonin), which cause swelling, pain, and bruising.

The principal aim in the treatment of soft-tissue injuries is to reduce the risk of infection where the skin has been broken, minimise initial swelling and pain, and promote rapid healing. It is also important to reduce the risks of secondary damage. The injured area should be examined periodically for signs of inflammation, which is characterised by erythema, swelling, and tenderness. There may be decreased mobility and pain. More ominous findings that warrant referral include fever, infection, severe pain on movement, persistent pain at rest, direct injury to a joint, or sounds on movement of the joint.

The four essential elements in the early management of soft-tissue injuries can be remembered by the mnemonic **RICE.**

- Rest
- Ice
- Compression
- Elevation

The **RICE** regimen may then be followed by other measures (e.g. heat treatment and drug treatment) and rehabilitation.

Rest   Immobilisation is recommended for the first 24 hours to avoid aggravating the lesion, prevent further bleeding, and minimise inflammation and swelling. It may be necessary to avoid bearing weight on an affected limb. If longer-term immobilisation of an area is indicated, it is essential to ensure that this does not prevent movement in unaffected joints, as this will promote atrophy of tissues and loss of coordination. Soft-tissue injuries should not be massaged or manipulated at this stage, which could aggravate the lesion. Prolonged rest for muscle injuries is usually discouraged because the collagen scar tissue formed is unable to contract, and repair is associated with some loss of flexibility.

Ice   Cooling the injured area (cryotherapy) reduces the local blood-flow and decreases the metabolic rate in peripheral cells, thus limiting the extent of inflammation and degree of pain. Commercial ice-packs or home-made packs containing crushed ice may be used, or if nothing else is to hand, cold water will help. Cooling sachets are available, and contain two separated chemicals that undergo an endothermic reaction when brought into contact with each other. However, these are not as efficient in cooling the body and do not last long enough to be effective. Cold treatment should be administered for up to 30 minutes and repeated every two hours over the first 24 hours. For large lesions it may be necessary to continue the applications for 48 hours. Ice and ice-packs should always be wrapped in damp cloths to prevent skin burns, and should not be left on for longer than the recommended time. Cooling aerosol sprays are also available, but their effect is likely to last for less time than ice-packs. Injuries should not be cooled if the patient suffers with atherosclerosis or a peripheral vascular disease (e.g. Raynaud's syndrome).

Compression   Compression involves the application of pressure over the injured area, and is employed to decrease bleeding and the flow of inflammatory exudate, and therefore reduce swelling. A compression bandage should be applied after the ice has been removed. It is necessary to extend the bandage 20 centimetres above and below the injured area, but it is vital that the bandage is not applied so tightly that blood-flow is totally impeded. Compression should be applied for at least 24 hours, although large lesions may require compression for longer.

Elevation   The injured area should be raised above the level of the heart to aid drainage of fluid and reduce swelling.

Other measures   Heat treatment (thermotherapy) is the application of heat for 20 to 30 minutes by means of an infra-red lamp, hot-water bottle, or heat-pad. Heat causes vasodilatation, which increases the flow of blood to the injured area, and is of benefit to relieve the pain produced by muscle spasm. Heat is of value in promoting relaxation of muscles before exercising, and therefore reduces the risk of further injury. If applied to joints, heat improves mobility by reducing the viscosity of synovial fluid. However, heat should not be used during the first 48 hours following a soft-tissue injury because of the risk of rebleeding. Heat treatment should not be used for open wounds or in patients with reduced skin sensation who would be unable to detect a burn. Alcohol is a vasodilator and should be avoided for up to 72 hours following an injury in order to minimise bleeding into the damaged area. Ideally, it should also be avoided before or during exercise. Hot baths should also be avoided initially in favour of showers or tepid baths to avoid the risk of rebleeding.

Ultrasound treatment and laser therapy increase blood-flow and reduce inflammation. Non-steroidal anti-inflammatory drugs may be of benefit, but to be effective should be administered for up to 3 to 5 days starting as soon as possible after the injury. Prolonged administration in most cases is unnecessary. Topical counter-irritant products, which produce a sensation of warmth, are widely available but are of limited value and should never be used under a dressing or on open wounds.

Rehabilitation   Prolonged rest leads to loss of suppleness, strength, and stamina. Gentle exercise, dictated by the extent of pain, should commence after 24 hours (or longer where indicated, *see below*) to restore the full range of movement of a part and minimise the permanent loss of strength associated with the formation of scar tissue. Controlled isometric exercises (*see* Section 8.2) of increasing intensity are beneficial in aligning the randomly orientated collagen fibres of new scar tissue. Injured areas may require support (which does not involve compression) during rehabilitation by means of suitable bandages.

Prevention   Sports injuries may be prevented by warming-up properly before exercising to increase the blood-flow to the tissues and by gentle cooling-down exercises afterwards. Warming-up has the effect of raising the temperature of the tissues making them more elastic and therefore less susceptible to tearing. Suitable warm-up exercises include muscle stretches, running on-the-spot, and loosely shaking all joints. Protective equipment is essential for those activities where direct contact with playing equipment or other players is associated with a high risk of injury. Correct footwear is also important, including the use of cushioned insoles to act as shock-absorbers and reduce the stress on joints. Different sports require different designs of footwear, and sports shoes should not be used interchangeably. The Amateur Athletic Association has ruled that children should not participate in running events longer than 5 kilometres on the basis that severe injury to rapidly growing tissue may result in permanent deformity.

Table 8.1 lists suggestions of items that may be included in a sports medical bag to cover the basic requirements of first-aid in the event of sports injury. However, there may be more specific requirements for a particular sport, and some governing bodies actually lay down rules dictating the contents of sports club medical bags.

Management of specific injuries

Strains   A strain is tearing apart of muscle fibres, and is characterised by pain and swelling. Muscle strains may be graded according to severity: grades 1 and 2 involve damage to the fibres only and the muscle sheath remains intact; grade 3 is partial rupture of the fibres and sheath; and grade 4 is complete rupture. Treatment of muscle strains involves the **RICE** regimen and an early encouragement back to activity. Grades 3 and 4 may require surgical repair.

Haematomas   As muscle fibres rupture, blood pools into the interstitial spaces to form haematomas, which cause pain and loss of function. Haematomas should be treated by the **RICE** regimen. Large haematomas may require immobilisation of the injured area for 24 to 48 hours. They are eventually resorbed although, in some cases, this may not happen and surgical aspiration may be necessary.

A haematoma may be invaded by osteoblasts (possibly derived from the periosteum), which initiate ossification in the soft tissue. This condition is termed myositis

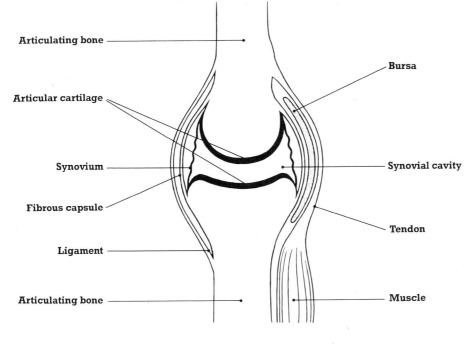

Articulating bone

Bursa

Articular cartilage

Synovium

Synovial cavity

Fibrous capsule

Ligament

Tendon

Articulating bone

Muscle

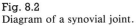

Fig. 8.2
Diagram of a synovial joint.

ossificans and is characterised by pain, stiffness, and reduction in movement. Massaging thigh injuries may predispose to this condition and should therefore be avoided. Ossification may be further encouraged by exercise, and treatment of myositis ossificans includes immobilisation. Gentle exercising may commence when ossification appears to have stopped or is receding. Surgery is only indicated in the later stages to remove an old lesion.

Sprains A sprain is an injury caused by overstretching or twisting a ligament, and may vary from damage of a few fibres to complete rupture. Symptoms include pain, swelling, and tenderness. A complete rupture (which may be relatively painless) usually produces abnormal or excessive movements. Initial treatment of sprains comprises the **RICE** regimen and administration of non-steroidal anti-inflammatory drugs, followed by gentle exercise of gradually increasing intensity. Immobilisation may be necessary for severely damaged ligaments, and a complete rupture must be repaired surgically.

Overuse injuries As the name implies an overuse injury is the result of doing the same activity for too long or too often. It may also be the result, in those

unaccustomed to a particular activity, of doing too much too quickly. Muscle pain and stiffness following exercise, bursitis, capsulitis, tendinitis and tenosynovitis, and blisters and friction burns are all examples of overuse injuries. In general, initial treatment comprises the **RICE** regimen and the administration of non-steroidal anti-inflammatory drugs. A programme of exercise of gradually increasing intensity should be implemented, except for those conditions where complete rest is indicated (*see below*). Some modifications in action may be necessary to prevent further injuries; these may include changes in playing technique, exercise schedule, or equipment (e.g. changing to padded running shoes), or modifications to the activity itself (e.g. cross-country running instead of road running).

Muscle pain and stiffness are not uncommon in muscles that have been subjected to unaccustomed intense physical activity, and characteristically appear 24 to 48 hours after the exercise. The mechanisms responsible are unknown, although it has been established that there is damage to the muscle fibres and membranes. Greater damage is caused by exercises that involve an increase in muscle length than those that rely on muscle shortening. Exposure of the muscle to similar exercise at a later date does not produce pain. There is

Table 8.1

Suggestions of items to include in a medical sports bag to administer basic first-aid in the event of sports injury

Item	Purpose	Examples	Comments
Wound cleansing			
Disinfectants and cleansers	to cleanse and disinfect skin and wounds	Cetrimide Chlorhexidine Povidone-iodine Sodium chloride 0.9% (sterile solutions may also be used for eye irrigation)	Chlorinated solutions (e.g. dilute sodium hypochlorite solution) are no longer recommended for wound cleansing as they are considered too irritant.
Swabs	to apply the disinfectants and cleansers	Gauze Swab BP Absorbent Cotton BP Absorbent Cotton Gauze BP	Absorbent cotton hospital quality should not be used for wound cleansing.
Wound dressing			
Absorbents	to absorb wound exudate and provide protection	Absorbent Cotton BP Absorbent Lint BPC Calcium Alginate Dressings (Drug Tariff) Gauze and Cotton Tissue BP Perforated Film Absorbent Dressing BP	
Haemostatic dressings	to stop bleeding	Calcium Alginate Dressings (Drug Tariff)	
Tulle dressings	to apply to abrasions, burns, and other skin injuries, usually beneath an absorbent dressing	Paraffin Gauze Dressing BP Chlorhexidine Gauze Dressing BP	
Retention bandages	to hold dressings in place and to aid in the application of pressure to stop bleeding	Cotton Conforming Bandage BP Elastic Net Surgical Tubular Stockinette (Drug Tariff) Elasticated Tubular Bandage BP Open-wove Bandage BP Triangular Calico Bandage BP	May also be used as a sling.

Table 8.1 *continued*

Item	Purpose	Examples	Comments
Standard dressings	comprises an absorbent pad and retention bandage in one complete sterile dressing, used for wounds that are bleeding severely		A selection of sizes is recommended, including an eye pad.
Adhesive dressings ('plasters')	an absorbent pad (which may be medicated) surrounded partly or completely by a piece of extension plaster, used to cover minor wounds	Elastic Adhesive Dressing BP Semipermeable Waterproof Plastic Wound Dressing BP	
Surgical adhesive tape	to secure dressings	Elastic Surgical Adhesive Tape BP Permeable Non-woven Surgical Synthetic Adhesive Tape BP Zinc Oxide Surgical Adhesive Tape BP	May also be used as a skin closure for small incision wounds. May also be used to immobilise small areas.
Management of soft-tissue injuries			
Cooling aids	to reduce the blood-flow in soft-tissue injuries, and minimise further damage and swelling	Ice Ice-packs Cooling sachets	
Compression bandages	to provide pressure to reduce the flow of blood and inflammatory exudate	Cotton Crepe Bandage BP Crepe Bandage BP Elastic Adhesive Bandage BP	
Support bandages	to provide support for an injured area during active movement	Cotton Crepe Bandage BP Crepe Bandage BP Elasticated Tubular Bandage BP Open-wove Bandage BP	Provides light support only.
Miscellaneous			
Wide-necked thermos flask or insulated bag	to carry ice or ice-packs		
Bucket, sponge, and towel	for general cleaning purposes		
Scissors, safety pins, and forceps	to cut up dressings and for general surgical use		

some risk of further injury if already damaged muscles are exercised vigorously, and the pain and discomfort experienced as a result may impair performance. It is therefore advisable to prevent delayed-onset muscle pain by gradually working up to a particular intensity of exercise.

Bursitis is inflammation of a bursa (a sac-like fluid-filled cavity surrounding soft tissues and protecting them from friction). It may be caused by trauma or overuse. Treatment comprises the administration of non-steroidal anti-inflammatory drugs or local corticosteroid injections. Surgical aspiration may be necessary in chronic cases.

Capsulitis is inflammation of a joint capsule and may be caused by trauma or overuse. General methods of treatment may be sufficient (i.e. rest and the application of heat or cold) together with the administration of non-steroidal anti-inflammatory drugs or local corticosteroid injections. Gentle exercises should be started once the pain and inflammation have subsided. Severe cases may require manipulation under anaesthetic.

Injuries to tendons may involve complete or partial rupture, which produces pain and, if rupture is complete, loss of function. Partial ruptures may allow limited, albeit painful movement. Tendon ruptures require immobilisation for 1 to 2 weeks or longer. Inflammation of the tendon itself produces tendinitis, and of its outer covering, tenosynovitis. There is pain on movement and swelling may be visible. Treatment comprises rest, either cold or heat treatment, and the administration of non-steroidal anti-inflammatory drugs or local corticosteroid injections into the tendon sheath to control the inflammation; this should be followed by regular exercise of gradually increasing intensity. Chronic cases may require immobilisation or surgical decompression.

Stress fractures may result from the repeated application of stress to a bone without any evidence of direct trauma. Pain appears after exercise initially, but may progress to more severe and continuous pain. There is local tenderness and in some cases a lump. X-rays may appear clear, although eventually callus formation may be evident indicating a healed stress fracture. It is essential to rest the affected bone for 4 to 6 weeks to prevent progression to complete fracture but isometric exercises (*see* Section 8.2) are recommended to prevent muscle atrophy.

A blister is the common name for a vesicle or, if large, a bulla. It is a fluid-filled sac on the surface of the skin, and may be formed during sports and exercise as a result of repeated friction between the skin and a hard object (e.g. ill-fitting shoes). Intact blisters are best left untreated, and further damage prevented, if necessary, by a non-adherent protective covering. If aspiration is undertaken, all equipment used should be sterile and the covering flap of skin left in order to further reduce the risk of infection. Friction burns may be treated by cooling the affected area and the oral administration of an analgesic. Broken skin may require cleansing and covering with a non-adherent dressing to prevent infection. If extensive areas are involved, hospital treatment may be required.

Specialist help for sports injuries is available from sports injury clinics (both in the NHS and on a private, fee-paying basis), and a list of addresses may be obtained from the Sports Council (*see* Section 8.6).

8.5   PARTICIPATION IN SPORTS AND EXERCISE

The effects of training are to increase the maximum capacity for work so that less effort is required for the same work-load, and the maximum intensity and duration of work increases. Changes only occur in those muscles that are exercised, including heart and respiratory muscles, and to be of benefit to health, physical activity must therefore be intense enough to significantly increase the heart rate and respiration rate. Regular physical activity can improve stamina, suppleness, and strength.

In healthy subjects, the maximum heart rate at peak exercise is about 200 beats/minute at 20 years of age, and decreases with age. The minimum amount of physical activity required to induce a training effect is three sessions of 20 minutes each week of aerobic exercise, during which time the heart rate should be increased to between 60 and 70% of the maximum. There is marked individual variation in maximum heart rate, and those over 35 years of age, the obese, or anyone with a pre-existing medical condition, may require a medical examination (including an ECG) before commencing (*see below*).

Exercising vigorously every day is neither necessary nor is it recommended because the risk of injury is increased. A refractory period of 24 to 48 hours is essential to allow the worked muscles to recover. Overtraining is also likely to cause fatigue and a loss of interest. Some individuals, however, prefer not to rest on the days between exercise sessions but alternate periods of light and hard exercise, or alternate sports that use different muscles. Those who are not used to vigorous activity should start exercising gently at first and increase the intensity in small stages at intervals of 8 to 10 weeks. Although the aim is to work the muscles and cardio-vascular and respiratory systems, the individual should not feel unduly distressed.

Injuries during sport and exercise may be prevented by warming-up before and cooling-down afterwards. Participants should be realistic in their choice of activity and choose within their capabilities. Progress in a new venture or in returning to an old one after a period of inactivity should be gradual, aiming for appropriate goals on the way. It is important to remember that many vigorous activities require a certain level of fitness for safe participation, and although such activities are of enormous benefit in improving and maintaining fitness, they may not be suitable for getting fit. Thus, it may be necessary to first undertake a graded programme of suitable training exercises.

Training is a long-term commitment, and individuals who stop it completely will soon return to being unfit, and possibly become obese if dietary adjustments are not made to meet the reduced level of physical activity.

Fitness tests

An initial routine medical examination to assess the safety of sport or exercise for an individual may include screening for, or testing of, the following:

- degree of obesity
- blood pressure
- heart and lung sounds
- ECG*
- tendon reflexes
- enlargement of lymph nodes
- herniation in groin.

Additional tests may be required if routine medical examination reveals abnormalities. Sport-specific tests (e.g. chest X-ray for SCUBA diving) may also be necessary.

Fitness tests are tests carried out under controlled conditions to assess an individual's fitness and, consequently, their capacity for exercise. Fitness may be assessed by measurement of various parameters including cardiovascular fitness, muscular endurance and strength, flexibility, and body composition (i.e. proportion of body fat).

The basis of all the different tests is to increase the work-load on the subject by a known amount and measure the response either during the test or at the end of it. The easiest parameter to measure is the final pulse rate. There is some risk of cardiac arrest attached to the tests, but when compared to the risk in the general population, these tests are considered to be relatively safe provided that they are supervised by trained personnel and adequate means of resuscitation are available.

The simplest test is the step test, which involves stepping on and off a step of predetermined height for a given time, followed by measurement of pulse rate. The results are read against standard tables to give the fitness index. There are many variations of step height, length of test, and intervals of final pulse measurement, but the most important point is that whatever parameters are chosen, they must remain constant to enable comparisons to be made.

Bicycle ergometry involves the use of a modified bicycle with a variable-resistance drive wheel that can be adjusted to different work-loads. The subject pedals against the resistance for a given time, after which the pulse rate is measured and compared against standard

tables. More sophisticated tests may involve the measurement of gases inhaled and exhaled to determine VO_2 max (*see* Section 8.2).

Many different types of treadmill are available to suit medical purposes or for training athletes. They may be horizontal or raised through successive gradients to increase the work-load. Pulse rate is usually measured before and after the test or, alternatively, experienced personnel can measure pulse rate and blood pressure during the test.

Diet and sport

Basic nutrition is as important in preparing athletes for events as physical training itself, and peak performance cannot be reached if there are any nutritional deficiencies. Women may be at a disadvantage if suffering from iron-deficiency anaemia as a result of heavy menstrual losses.

The dietary energy requirements of an athlete are much greater than those of a sedentary individual, particularly for those participating in endurance events. Adverse conditions (e.g. hot or humid weather) must also be taken into account and salt and fluid intake adjusted accordingly (*see* Section 8.4). The daily dietary energy requirements (*see* Section 2.1) of a young male athlete may be between 12.7 and 17.5 MJ (3024 and 4167 kcals) compared to about 10.6 MJ (2550 kcals) for a sedentary young man. The energy required for physical activity is provided by the oxidation of carbohydrates and fats. Excess dietary carbohydrate is stored as glycogen in muscles (about 350 g) and liver (about 100 g). Liver glycogen is broken down into glucose to maintain the optimum plasma-glucose concentration necessary for brain and nervous system function, and for use by muscles during exercise. Glycogen in muscles is converted when required to glucose-6-phosphate, which is metabolised to provide ATP. However, there is insufficient stored glycogen to last for more than about 90 to 120 minutes in trained individuals, and stores are only mobilised in those muscles actually in use. Fat stored in adipose tissue provides an additional source of energy for many hours of work, although it cannot be relied upon as the sole source because the oxidation of fat is only able to supply 50% of the energy required at any time.

Many special diets have been put forward as being essential for peak athletic performance, some of which may be extremely faddist. The nutrient requirements of an athlete are exactly the same as those of any other individual and there is nothing to be gained by taking megadoses of vitamins and minerals (*see* Section 2.2.6), or consumption of vast quantities of proteins. Excess

---

* This test is important to assess any cardiac malfunction, but it can be misleading unless interpreted by experienced personnel because some extremely fit athletes have abnormal ECG patterns.

protein is not laid down in muscle tissue but is used as an energy source or stored as glycogen òr fat. Carbohydrates are metabolised to glucose, which is used as a source of energy or stored as glycogen or fat. Fats are a highly concentrated source of energy able to supply twice as much energy weight for weight as carbohydrates and proteins, but are not metabolised fast enough to be of use in the shorter athletic events. The recommendations for intake of dietary fats are the same in athletes as for any other individual (*see* Section 2.2.2), and should not be exceeded. There is no advantage to be gained by laying down deposits of fat in the body in anticipation of endurance events. This is harmful to health in the long-term since obesity has been linked with many diseases (*see* Section 2.1), and merely increases the energy required by the athlete to move the extra body-weight.

It has been suggested that an increase in the intake of some vitamins is essential if physical activity is increased. This is only true for thiamine and niacin (nicotinic acid and nicotinamide), and the Reference Nutrient Intakes (RNIs) are related to dietary energy intake. The RNI for thiamine is 400 μg/4.2 MJ (1000 kcals) and for niacin is 6.6 mg/4.2 MJ (1000 kcals). The RNIs for other vitamins and minerals remain the same for all levels of activity (*see* Table 2.1). Carnitine is a dietary supplement that has been claimed to increase endurance and thereby improve athletic performance. These claims have not been adequately proven, although carnitine does have a role in long-chain fatty acid metabolism.

The average diet contains salt far in excess of the daily requirement and, in most cases, will be sufficient to meet the additional demands created by profuse sweating during exercise. If evaporation of sweat is inhibited (e.g. by heavy clothing), sweating will be excessive and sodium losses even greater. Salt supplementation (*see* Section 8.4) may be required in such instances, but is generally more efficient if taken prophylactically, rather than during exercise.

Anyone anticipating training sessions or exercise should not eat anything later than 2.5 to 3 hours beforehand, as this may cause gastro-intestinal discomfort during the event. Foods eaten at this stage should be rich in carbohydrates and low in fats and proteins, which take longer to digest. Carbohydrates ingested 0.5 to 1 hour before an event have the effect of stimulating a sudden increase in plasma-insulin concentration, which prevents mobilisation of fatty acids, and thus allows premature depletion of the glycogen reserves. However, glucose in solid form or solution may be taken immediately before exercise without adverse effect. Fluid replacement (*see* Section 8.4) is necessary during long events (e.g. marathon runs). Minerals are not absorbed during exercise because of gastro-intestinal stasis and should be taken with fluid before the event rather than during it. Marathon runners are only able to cope with small, but frequent, quantities of a dilute glucose solution (e.g. no more than 5 g/100 mL) during a race, and must rely on using body stores of glycogen and fat as a source of energy.

Carbohydrate loading diets have been devised for endurance events to double or treble the glycogen stores in the muscle. About seven days before an event, the athlete totally depletes his muscles of glycogen by intensive activity. The diet over the next 2 to 3 days is rich in proteins and fats but low in carbohydrates, which is followed by 3 to 4 days of a diet rich in carbohydrates and low in proteins. Training should be reduced during this phase, particularly when little carbohydrate is being ingested. Response to such a technique is varied, and individuals should assess their personal response well in advance of an event. However, it is unlikely to work more than twice in a 12-month period. Some authorities feel that the low-carbohydrate phase is unnecessary. Elite marathon runners undergoing intensive training sessions will regularly deplete their stores of muscle glycogen, and all that may be required before the event is to reduce activity and adopt a high- carbohydrate low-protein diet for 2 to 4 days.

Events that require short sessions of activity do allow for carbohydrate replacement between periods of activity (e.g. between heats in athletic events or at half-time in sports matches); glucose is generally used in the form of high-energy drinks. Those involved in activities involving a high degree of skill require regular glucose supplementation in order to avoid hypoglycaemia because the nervous system can only use blood-glucose as a source of fuel, and is unable to utilise the body's fat stores.

Isotonic drinks are used to replace fluid and electrolyte losses, and are generally low in carbohydrate. They are only of value in intermittent activity, when gastro-intestinal inhibition may be sufficiently reversed to allow absorption of the minerals. Cool drinks increase the chances of absorption by promoting peristalsis.

Drugs in sport

In high-level sports competitions, athletes are under enormous pressure to succeed, both for honour and financial rewards. To win and break records is the all-consuming goal and, in order to attain this, some athletes resort to the use of artificial means to increase performance without considering the ethical values or the risk-benefit ratio to themselves. Training for sports competition is not always synonymous with training for health. There is also a growing trend towards the use of ergogenic agents (*see below*) in non-competitive sports, and sources of anabolic steroids are frequently sought by body builders. Misuse of drugs causes unwanted side-effects, and in some cases even death; some adverse effects may not become apparent until years later. Sports authorities have introduced control measures to stop what is effectively cheating and also to protect the athletes themselves from irreparable damage to their health.

Difficulty in obtaining some agents through legitimate channels may drive athletes to black-market sources of dubious origin, further increasing the risk to their health. Health education for athletes is necessary to first explain that in many cases the evidence supporting the claims of enhanced performance is lacking or contradictory, and second that performance enhancement cannot be justified if, as a result, health is compromised.

There are several categories of drugs that an athlete may choose to use:

- Therapeutic drugs

  It may be necessary from time to time for athletes to take some form of medication to relieve the symptoms of minor illnesses or to treat more serious acute disorders or injuries. Some athletes may have a chronic condition (e.g. asthma) that requires the long-term administration of drugs. The side-effects of some drugs (e.g. nausea, drowsiness, or fatigue) may impair athletic performance or may have adverse effects during physical activity (*see* Section 8.4), and the benefits of exercise must be weighed against the potential risks. Where possible, alternative means of treatment should be sought, or if none are available, a programme of physical activity should be designed to minimise the associated risks. Prescribers also have the additional problem of making sure that they do not prescribe a substance that is included in a banned list for those participating in a registered sporting event.

- Illicit drugs

  The use of illicit drugs (e.g. amphetamines, heroin, cocaine, and cannabis) is a problem in society as a whole rather than one specifically confined to athletes, and has been discussed in Chapter 7.

- Ergogenic agents

  Some drugs may enhance performance (ergogenic agents) or improve mood, and have been misused for this purpose (often referred to as 'doping'). This confers an unfair advantage over those who choose not to resort to artificial means of improving performance, and also imposes serious health risks for those who do.

- Masking agents and techniques

  Substances or methods may be used to mask the detection of banned drugs during testing.

The governing bodies of sporting events have drawn up lists of banned classes of drugs. There are absolutely no exceptions to the rules, and doctors cannot prescribe any of the drugs covered by the list; they must seek alternatives for patients wishing to participate in sports competitions. Banned substances may be inadvertently taken, which is particularly likely to happen if non-prescription medicines are purchased or athletes do not tell prescribers that they intend to compete.

Subjecting athletes to tests to detect the presence of banned substances, and subsequent disciplinary action for those with positive results may act as a deterrent to some, but there are others whose determination is such that they devise ways and means of 'cheating' the test itself. Testing is usually carried out on a sample of urine because it is a non-invasive technique and therefore considered the most convenient and least obtrusive means of analysis. Urine also has the advantage that any drugs present are more concentrated than in blood, and there is less interference with the test from the normal constituents of urine than those of blood.

Laboratories undertaking drug-testing must be accredited by the International Olympic Committee (IOC), which guarantees that samples are analysed in accordance with recognised procedures and to the highest standards. The level of doping control in individual countries is variable, and the concern of many athletes is that urine analysis during the competition itself will not necessarily detect drugs that have been used during training (e.g. anabolic steroids). Many of those who misuse these substances have become knowledgeable about drug kinetics and can plan their dosage schedules ahead to minimise the risk of detection, or use masking agents when they know a test is likely to take place. As a result, some nations (including the UK) have introduced random drug testing during training for major competitions.

The Medical Commission of the IOC has drawn up a list of banned substances, classifying them into six categories:

- Class A - Stimulants
- Class B - Narcotic analgesics
- Class C - Anabolic steroids
- Class D - Beta blockers
- Class E - Diuretics
- Class F - Peptide hormones and analogues.

Stimulants   Stimulants have been shown to improve athletic performance in some studies, although others have shown conflicting results. They increase alertness and mood, and mask fatigue but do not prevent exhaustion. Judgement is impaired and eventually performance deteriorates. The effects of stimulants are not perceived by the subject who continues the activity with a significantly increased risk of injury.

Caffeine enhances performance in endurance events by releasing free fatty acids and thus exerting a glycogen-sparing effect. It also reduces fatigue. Its presence in urine is permitted up to a maximum concentration of $12 \mu g/mL$, and it is considered that normal social drinks of caffeine-containing beverages would not contain sufficient to exceed this limit.

Sympathomimetics in high doses improve blood-flow and act as mental stimulants. However, adverse effects include anxiety, increased blood pressure, headache, palpitations, and tremor. These compounds are often present in non-prescription medicines for coughs, colds, and influenza.

Narcotic analgesics   Narcotic or opioid analgesics may be used to mask pain and permit activity in the face of injury, which is not to be recommended. However, they are more likely to be misused for their euphoric effects. These agents also produce respiratory depression, which is a serious adverse effect for anyone contemplating intensive physical activity. The major risk of these drugs is their dependence potential (*see* Chapter 7).

Anabolic steroids   Anabolic steroids are synthetic derivatives of testosterone used to increase strength and lean body mass, and to decrease recovery time from exercise. These agents are used during training rather than the event itself, and are one of the most widely misused drugs in sport. The evidence for increase in muscle mass is conflicting, and additional factors of diet and sustained intensive exercise must also be taken into account. There are numerous adverse reactions associated with the use of anabolic steroids, some of which are irreversible, and others that may be fatal. Adverse effects include acne, aggressiveness, depression, enlargement of the clitoris, fatigue, foetal damage, gallstones, gynaecomastia, hypertension, increased plasma-LDL concentrations and decreased plasma-HDL concentrations, infertility,

jaundice, liver disorders, menstrual irregularities, oedema, premature closure of the epiphyses in adolescents, priapism, prostate enlargement, and testicular atrophy. Ischaemic heart disease, stroke, and liver cancer are adverse effects that may not appear until some years later. Irreversible masculinising effects in women include hirsutism, male-pattern baldness, and deepening of the voice. Anabolic steroids enhance the development of muscles but not tendons, which increases the risk for injuries.

Testosterone is also used as an ergogenic agent in the hope that as it is naturally present in the body its use will not be detected. The IOC has included it in the list of banned substances under anabolic steroids by requiring that the ratio in the urine of testosterone:epitestosterone should not exceed 6:1.

Beta blockers   Beta-adrenoceptor blocking drugs reduce heart rate, anxiety, and tremor, and are consequently used in precision sports (e.g. archery and snooker). They are included in the banned list with the provision that authorities may request testing in certain sports that do not involve a high level of physical activity. These are unlikely to include endurance events in which beta blockers would severely decrease performance capacity.

Diuretics   Diuretics may be used for one of two reasons. Firstly, they produce a rapid loss in weight as a result of fluid loss and therefore may be taken immediately before a weigh-in (e.g. in boxing). Secondly, they may also be used as masking agents to produce a dilute urine.

Peptide hormones and analogues   Chorionic gonadotrophin (HCG or human chorionic gonadotrophin) administered to males causes an increase in the concentrations of endogenous androgenic steroids, and its use in sport is therefore banned. Corticotrophin (ACTH) increases the concentrations of endogenous corticosteroids (which have a stimulant action), and its use in sport has consequently been banned.

Human growth hormone is used to increase size and strength, although the evidence for this effect in normal, healthy adults is lacking. Unlike anabolic steroids, the enlargement produced by growth hormone is non-specific and many organs may be involved. This is probably less likely to be a problem in adults, in whom most of the growth receptors will be inactive, than in children and adolescents. It is predicted that the long-term use of growth hormone could produce acromegaly, cardiomyopathy, diabetes mellitus, hypertension, and hyperhidrosis although, to date, there are only anecdotal reports available to confirm this. In some cases, other drugs (e.g. clonidine, propranolol, and vasopressin) may be used to stimulate increased release of endogenous growth hormone from the pituitary gland.

Other ergogenic aids   Blood doping is a technique to improve blood-haemoglobin concentrations and consequently oxygen consumption. It involves taking up to 900 mL of blood from the competitor and freezing it some weeks before the event. It is then re-infused 1 to 2 days before the event. However, it can take months for some individuals to recover after blood has been taken. The alternative is to infuse donor blood before the event, but this method introduces risks of serum sickness and transmission of blood-borne diseases (e.g. AIDS and hepatitis). There is always an increase in viscosity following blood transfusion, which carries a risk of blood-vessel blockage. Blood doping is banned by the IOC, although there are, as yet, no means of detection.

Oxygen 100% is used as an ergogenic agent in some sports because it is felt that increased oxygen in the muscles improves performance and reduces recovery time from exercise. However, studies carried out to assess its effectiveness have not conclusively demonstrated this. Oxygen is also inconvenient because it can only be administered if the activity is temporarily stopped, and the effects are short-lived. However, it is often used in American football and has not been banned by the IOC.

Partial restrictions   Some drugs (e.g. corticosteroids and local anaesthetics) have partial restrictions imposed. Certain formulations, or only specific indications may be permitted, and notification to the relevant authorities may be required in some instances.

Alcohol is a source of calories that may be used as a fuel source; it also reduces anxiety. Its use is not banned by the IOC, although breath-alcohol or blood-alcohol concentrations may be determined at the request of an International Federation. However, other sports authorities may have different rules. For example, the International Skiing Federation bans the use of alcohol by competitiors because of its disinhibiting effect. Cannabis is also not banned by the IOC Medical Commission for use in sport, although tests may be requested by an International Federation. However, UK law prohibits its possession and use.

Table 8.2 lists examples of substances included in the above categories. Details of some of the drugs that may be taken by athletes without contravening these regulations are described below.

The role of the pharmacist

For many people, participation in sport or exercise is a daunting prospect, even if they have already been convinced that it will be beneficial to their health. They may fear that exercising will be uncomfortable or painful, or they may worry about potential injuries. Many of those who have not played any sport since school are likely to be extremely lacking in confidence or too embarrassed to learn or 'relearn' a new skill. Lack of time is an important factor in many people's life-styles, and a reorganisation of other activities may be necessary. The pharmacist should, where necessary, emphasise that it is not necessary to run marathons to become fit, and explain the overload principle of training (i.e. it is only necessary to regularly increase physical activity above usual levels for a minimum of 20 minutes three times a week). The pharmacist can also suggest, for those who wish to learn a sport, that perhaps the best way is to join a beginners class so that everyone will be at a similar level of playing skill, and possibly fitness. The social advantages of participating in a sport, particularly if it involves membership of a sports club, could also be stressed.

People's goals and capabilities vary enormously, and the pharmacist's initial function is to assess what these are. There are many different ways of exercising and the pharmacist could find out what local facilities are available through the local council offices, adult education centres, or private clubs, and pass the information on to those interested. However, not everyone has the time or the inclination to take up a sport, and some people may prefer solitary exercise rather than group exercising. One of the most popular, convenient, and least obtrusive ways of exercising is walking. As long as the pace is brisk and faster than normal walking pace, and forms a regular part of an individual's normal routine, there will be a training effect. The most enjoyable way is to specifically 'go for a walk', particularly in areas of interesting scenery. However, for those truly pressed for time, there are ample opportunities throughout the course of a normal day's work to 'walk rather than ride'. Stair-climbing instead of using a lift or walking short distances instead of taking a car, bus, or train is of great benefit; the extra time taken is probably negligible compared to the time wasted in rush-hour traffic or waiting for public transport. There is the additional benefit of boosting the body's levels of vitamin D by carrying out physical activities outdoors (*see* Section 2.2.4). For those who may have difficulties in coping with sport and exercise (e.g. the elderly, or physically or mentally handicapped), specialist help is available from various organisations (*see* Section 8.6). The pharmacist can help by passing

TABLE 8.2
Examples of substances and methods banned by the Medical Commission of the International Olympic Committee (IOC)

Class A
Stimulants

Amiphenazole	Fenproporex
Amphetamine	Furfenorex
Amphetaminil	Meclofenoxate
Benzphetamine	Mefenorex
Caffeine*	Methoxyphenamine
Cathine	Methylamphetamine
Chlorphentermine	Methylphenidate
Clobenzorex	Morazone
Clorprenaline	Nikethamide
Cocaine	Pemoline
Cropropamide	Pentetrazol
Crotethamide	Phendimetrazine
Diethylpropion	Phenmetrazine
Dimethylamphetamine	Phentermine
Ephedrine	Phenylpropanolamine
Etafedrine	Pipradrol
Ethamivan	Prolintane
Ethylamphetamine	Propylhexedrine
Fencamfamin	Pyrovalerone
Fenethylline	Strychnine
	and related compounds

* The definition of a positive is a concentration in urine in excess of 12 μg/mL.

Class B
Narcotic analgesics

Anileridine	Dipipanone
Buprenorphine	Methadone
Codeine	Morphine
Dextromoramide	Pentazocine
Dextropropoxyphene	Pethidine
Diamorphine (heroin)	Phenazocine
Dihydrocodeine	Trimeperidine
	and related compounds

Class C
Anabolic steroids

Bolasterone	Methyltestosterone
Boldenone	Nandrolone
Chlordehydromethyltestosterone	Norethandrolone
Clostebol	Oxandrolone
Fluoxymesterone	Oxymesterone
Mesterolone	Oxymetholone
Methandienone	Stanozolol
Methenolone	Testosterone**
	and related compounds

** The definition of a positive is the administration of testosterone or the use of any other manipulation such that the ratio of testosterone:epitestosterone in the urine exceeds 6:1.

Class D
Beta blockers

Acebutolol	Metoprolol
Alprenolol	Nadolol
Atenolol	Oxprenolol
Labetalol	Propranolol
	Sotalol
	and related compounds

As a result of the continued misuse of beta-blockers in some sports where physical activity is of little or no importance, the right is reserved to test those sports deemed appropriate.

Table 8.2 *continued*

Class E
Diuretics

Acetazolamide	Dichlorphenamide
Amiloride	Ethacrynic acid
Bendrofluazide	Frusemide
Benzthiazide	Hydrochlorothiazide
Bumetanide	Spironolactone
Canrenone	Triamterene
Chlorthalidone	and related compounds

Class F
Peptide hormones and analogues

Chorionic gonadotrophin (HCG or human chorionic gonadotrophin)
Corticotrophin (ACTH)
Growth hormone (HGH or somatotrophin)
and all the respective releasing factors of the above-mentioned substances
Erythropoietin (EPO)

Blood doping
The practice of blood doping in sport is banned by the IOC Medical Commission.

Pharmacological, chemical, and physical manipulation
The IOC Medical Commission bans the use of substances and of methods which alter the integrity and validity of urine samples used in doping controls. Examples of banned methods are catheterisation, urine substitution and/or tampering, inhibition of renal excretion (e.g. by probenecid and related compounds).

Alcohol and marijuana
Alcohol and marijuana are not prohibited although tests may be carried out at the request of an International Federation.

Local anaesthetics
Injectable local anaesthetics are permitted under the following conditions:

- that procaine, xylocaine, carbocaine etc., are used but not cocaine
- only local or intra-articular injections may be administered; intravascular injections are not permitted
- only when medically justified (i.e. the details including diagnosis, dose, and route of administration must be submitted immediately in writing).

Corticosteroids
The use of corticosteroids is banned except for topical use (aural, ophthalmological, or dermatological), inhalation therapy (for asthma or allergic rhinitis), and by local or intra-articular injections. Any team doctor wishing to administer corticosteroids intra-articularly or locally to a competitor must give written notification to the IOC Medical Commission.

The presence in a urine sample of all listed substances (except those substances that are allowed up to a certain level) or their major metabolites, and substances belonging to the banned classes even if they are not listed, will constitute an offence.

The information contained in this table is taken from one of the booklets in the Doping Control Information series produced by the Sports Council. Copies of the booklets may be obtained from the Doping Control unit of the Sports Council (*see* Section 8.6).

Other governing bodies (both national and international) may produce their own lists of banned substances or there may be sport-specific restrictions. For example, the Modern Pentathlon bans the use of anxiolytic sedatives, hypnotics, neuroleptics, and tricyclic antidepressants, and an up-to-date copy of the list specific for a competitor's particular sport and event should always be consulted.

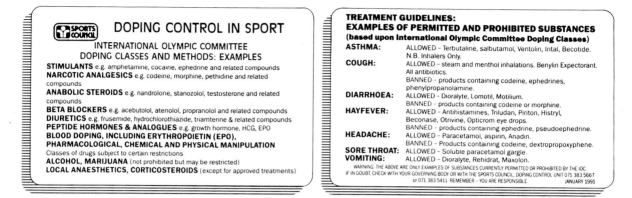

Fig. 8.3
Doping Control in Sport advice card produced by the Sports Council.

such information on and by displaying some of the many leaflets available from such organisations.

The pharmacist may become involved with amateur or professional sports clubs, and be asked for advice about items necessary to stock a medical bag to enable first-aid to be carried out on-site at a sporting event. Team doctors and physiotherapists will have their own specialist requirements (e.g. suturing equipment, drugs for emergency use, inflatable splint, infra-red lamp, and strapping) in addition to the basic items needed to cleanse and dress wounds, and carry out the **RICE** regimen (*see* Section 8.4). Many low-key events will not have professional medical help available, and it will be the responsibility of the coach to administer first-aid, followed by medical referral where necessary. For suggestions of items that may be included in a sports medical bag to cover the basic requirements of sports injury first-aid *see* Table 8.1.

A pharmacist presented with a request for advice by an athlete for the treatment of a minor ailment should first ascertain what the problem is and then check the relevant list of banned substances before counter-prescribing. The IOC produces one such list (Table 8.2), but there may be further restrictions imposed by other national or international organisations, and there may be some sport-specific restrictions. A competitor should therefore make himself fully aware of all regulations governing his specific event and present the information to the pharmacist before purchasing medicines or having a prescription dispensed. Athletes may be confused over nomenclature of substances on the banned list (e.g. trade or generic names, or metabolites), and seek guidance from a pharmacist.

In general, coughs and colds cannot be treated with any product containing sympathomimetics (e.g. ephedrine,

phenylpropanolamine, or pseudoephedrine), or codeine. However, dextromethorphan and pholcodine are not banned and antitussive preparations containing these agents may be recommended. Hay fever may be treated with antihistamines and sodium cromoglycate but not sympathomimetics, although it must be stressed that some antihistamines are currently banned in the modern pentathlon. There is no ban on the use of non-steroidal anti-inflammatory products. Aspirin and paracetamol are permitted as analgesics but codeine is not, which precludes the use of combination analgesic products. Products containing morphine or codeine may not be used to treat diarrhoea although diphenoxylate and loperamide are permitted. Hyoscine may be used as a gastro-intestinal antispasmodic and as an anti-emetic. Topical corticosteroids are permitted for the treatment of skin conditions but there are partial restrictions imposed on the use of other corticosteroid formulations.

It isalso necessary to be aware of prescription-only medicines that are banned because there may be instances where a patient has omitted to tell the prescriber that he intends to participate in a registered sporting event, and turns instead for advice to the pharmacist dispensing the prescription. Antibiotics and antihistamines are allowed, but care must be exercised when prescribing the latter when contained in multi-ingredient preparations. Oral contraceptives are usually allowed. The use of some sympathomimetics (e.g. orciprenaline, rimiterol, salbutamol, and terbutaline) is allowed in aerosol formulations for the treatment of asthma. Fenoterol is banned because it is metabolised to a stimulant, parahydroxyamphetamine. Sodium cromoglycate and nedocromil are also allowed for the treatment of asthma but isoprenaline is banned. Anticonvulsants may be used by epileptics provided that a declaration has been made beforehand. A list of drugs that may be used when competing can be obtained from the Sports Council.

Banned substances may be present in plants and hence herbal preparations. For example, Ma Huang (Chinese ephedra) contains ephedrine. At present, there is no legal requirement for ingredients to be listed on the labels of herbal products or dietary supplements. Competing athletes using such problems may inadvertently ingest banned substances.

The Sports Council has produced a 'Doping Control in Sport' advice card (Fig. 8.3). Supplies of the card may be obtained from the Doping Control Unit of the Sports Council (*see* Section 8.6).

8.6 USEFUL ADDRESSES

AMATEUR ATHLETIC ASSOCIATION
British Amateur Athletic Board
Edgbaston House
3 Duchess Place
Hagley Road
Edgbaston
Birmingham B16 8NM

ASSOCIATION OF SWIMMING THERAPY
1 Buchan Grove
Crewe
Cheshire

BRITISH OLYMPIC ASSOCIATION
1 Wandsworth Plain
London SW18 1EH
Tel: 081−871 2677

BRITISH SPORTS ASSOCIATION FOR THE DISABLED
The Mary Glen Haig Suite
34 Osnaburgh Street
LONDON NW1 3ND
Tel: 071−383 7277

THE CENTRAL COUNCIL OF PHYSICAL RECREATION
Francis House
Francis Street
London SW1P 1DE
Tel: 071−828 3163/4

CHARTERED SOCIETY OF PHYSIOTHERAPY
14 Bedford Row
London WC1R 4ED
Tel: 071−242 1941

DISABLED LIVING FOUNDATION
380/384 Harrow Road
London W9 2HU
Tel: 071−289 6111

EXTEND
1A North Street
Sheringham
Norfolk NR26 8LJ
Tel: (0263) 822479

Exercise training for the elderly and/or disabled.

THE INSTITUTE OF SPORTS MEDICINE
Burlington House
Piccadilly
London W1V 0LQ
Tel: 071−287 5269

KEEP FIT ASSOCIATION
16 Upper Woburn Place
London WC1H 0QG
Tel: 071−387 4349

LONDON SPORTS MEDICINE INSTITUTE
c/o Medical College of St Bartholomew's Hospital
Charterhouse Square
London EC1M 6BQ
Tel: 071−251 0583

THE NATIONAL COACHING FOUNDATION
4 College Close
Beckett Park
Leeds LS6 3QH
Tel: (0532) 744802

THE PHYSICAL EDUCATION ASSOCIATION OF GREAT BRITAIN AND NORTHERN IRELAND
Ling House
162 Kings Cross Road
London
WC1X 9DH
Tel: 071−278 9311

RADAR (The Royal Association for Disability and Rehabilitation)
25 Mortimer Street
London W1N 8AB
Tel: 071−637 5400

THE SCOTTISH SPORTS COUNCIL
Caledonia House
South Gyle
Edinburgh EH12 9DQ
Tel: 031−317 7200

SPECIAL OLYMPICS UNITED KINGDOM
The Management Office
Willesborough Industrial Park
Kennington Road
Ashford
Kent TN24 0TD
Tel: (0233) 639910
The aim of Special Olympics is to provide year round training and athletic competition in a variety of well coached Olympic-type sports for individuals with a mental handicap.

SPORTS COUNCIL
16 Upper Woburn Place
London WC1H 0QP
Tel: 071−388 1277

SPORTS COUNCIL FOR NORTHERN IRELAND
House of Sport
Upper Malone Road
Belfast BT9 5LA
Tel: (0232) 381222

SPORTS COUNCIL FOR WALES
National Sports Centre for Wales
Sophia Gardens
Cardiff CF1 9SW
Tel: (0222) 397571

SPORTS NUTRITION FOUNDATION
London Sports Medicine Institute
c/o Medical College of St Bartholomew's Hospital
Charterhouse Square
London EC1M 6BQ
Tel: 071–251 0583

ST JOHN AMBULANCE
1 Grosvenor Crescent
London SW1X 7EF
Tel: 071–235 5231

UNITED KINGDOM SPORTS ASSOCIATION
FOR PEOPLE WITH MENTAL HANDICAP
30 Phillip Lane
Tottenham
London N15 4JB
Tel: 081–885 1177

8.7 FURTHER READING

Fentem PH, *et al. Benefits of exercise: the evidence.* Manchester: Manchester University Press, 1990.

First aid manual. The authorised manual of St. John Ambulance, St. Andrew's Ambulance Association, and the British Red Cross Society. 5th ed. London: Dorling Kindersley, 1987.

Grisogono V, ed. *Sports injuries.* Edinburgh: Churchill Livingstone, 1989.

Jamieson RH. *Exercises for the elderly.* New York: Emerson Books, 1985.

Lamb DR. *Physiology of exercise. Responses and adaptations.* 2nd ed. New York: Macmillan, 1984.

Latto K. *Give us the chance. Sport and physical recreation with mentally handicapped people.* London: Disabled Living Foundation, 1981.

Macleod D, *et al.*, eds. *Exercise. Benefits, limits and adaptations.* London: E & FN Spon, 1987.

Marchand J. *Sport for all in Europe.* London: HMSO, 1990.

McLatchie GR, ed. *Essentials of sports medicine.* Edinburgh: Churchill Livingstone, 1986.

Mottram DR, ed. *Drugs in sport.* London: E & FN Spon, 1988.

Reilly T, *et al.*, eds. *Physiology of sports.* London: E & FN Spon, 1990.

Sperryn PN. *Sport and medicine.* London: Butterworths, 1985.

Sperryn PN. *The sports medicine handbook.* London: Medical News Tribune Group.

Thomson N, *et al.*, eds. *Sports and recreation provision for disabled people.* London: The Architectural Press, 1984.

Chapter 9

HEALTH AND TRAVEL

9.1 INTRODUCTION

The number of people travelling overseas for business or pleasure has risen steadily since the introduction of international air travel. Significant numbers also leave the UK for the continent on ferries. This steady increase has been reflected in an upsurge in requests to pharmacists for advice about health during travel. The range of destinations is varied and includes more tropical countries than ever before. The advice on prophylaxis against infectious diseases is constantly being updated, and it is essential that pharmacists keep abreast of all major developments in travel health.

The tremendous variety of infectious diseases that may befall the unwary and unprepared traveller is discussed in Section 9.3. The risk of contracting any of these diseases varies considerably and depends upon the destination, activities while abroad, standard of foreign accommodation, and numerous other factors (e.g. state of health and medical history).

This Chapter deals with some of the precautions that need to be taken before and during travel to minimise illness and discomfort, the preventive measures that need to be taken to avoid contracting infections,

management of some conditions associated with travel, and action that may be necessary on returning home. In the UK, information on recommendations for immunisation and all aspects of health abroad can be found in Department of Health (DoH) leaflets, which are updated regularly. Information is also published by the World Health Organization (WHO). Prominent display of available literature in the pharmacy helps to confirm the pharmacist as a source of information on health and overseas travel.

9.2 ACTION TO BE TAKEN BEFORE TRAVELLING

Chemoprophylaxis and immunisation

Malaria chemoprophylaxis and immunisation against infectious diseases are the most important medical considerations before setting out overseas. A clear distinction must be drawn between mandatory immunisation requirements necessary for entry to a country and recommendations for immunisation because of the potential risks to the traveller. Some vaccines are administered as courses in which doses must be separated by specified time intervals, and some vaccines may not be given at the same time as others. It is absolutely essential, therefore, that travellers start their vaccination programmes well in advance of the date of departure.

It is important that the administration of live vaccines is postponed until at least three months after stopping corticosteroids and six months after stopping cancer chemotherapy. Live virus vaccines should be given at least three weeks before or three months after an injection of normal immunoglobulin, which may interfere with the immune response. This does not apply to yellow fever vaccine since normal immunoglobulin does not contain antibody to the virus. For those about to travel, if there is insufficient time, the recommended interval may have to be ignored.

In general terms, travel to Europe, North America, Australia, and New Zealand does not warrant protection unless a stop-over is made outside these areas. The specific measures required vary according to stop-overs and final destinations. Information and details of addresses and telephone numbers of UK organisations that can be contacted for further information can be obtained from BNF 14.6; some useful addresses are also listed in Section 9.5.

Diphtheria, measles, mumps, poliomyelitis, rubella, and tetanus are all given routinely as part of the UK childhood immunisation programme and only booster doses may be required. However, full courses may be required by those who did not receive vaccines during childhood, or if courses were not completed.

Cholera   Cholera is primarily a disease resulting from poor sanitation and hygiene. Vaccination against cholera provides effective cover from six days after administration and lasts for about six months. It is not, however, completely effective, and is no substitute for stringent standards of personal hygiene, particularly when handling food (*see* Section 9.3). Cholera vaccination should only be recommended if travellers are likely to be exposed to insanitary conditions for more than a few days, or an outbreak is in progress. In recognition of the fact that vaccination against cholera cannot prevent the introduction of infection into a country, the World Health Assembly amended the International Health Regulations in 1973 so that cholera vaccination should no longer be required of any traveller.

Travellers to Lesotho, Pakistan, Pitcairn Island, Somalia, and Sudan are still required to produce a certificate of vaccination against cholera if they have arrived from endemic regions. The seventh world pandemic, which started in Indonesia in 1961 and has mainly targeted Africa and Asia, is now becoming established in parts of South America.

Hepatitis   Hepatitis A and hepatitis B occur throughout the world, particularly in warm climates where hygiene and sanitary conditions are poor. Hepatitis A is transmitted by the faecal-oral route and has no carrier state. Infection commonly arises as a result of eating raw seafood that has been contaminated by sewage or by eating vegetables grown in soil fertilised with human faeces.

The risk of contracting hepatitis B is increased by the high prevalence of asymptomatic carriers in many parts of the world. Hepatitis B is transmitted predominantly in blood and blood products, although its presence in saliva, menstrual and vaginal fluids, and seminal fluid allows the possibility of additional modes of transmission.

Passive immunisation against hepatitis A for travellers to endemic regions can be carried out by administering human normal immunoglobulin injection, which protects for 3 to 5 months. Active immunisation with hepatitis B vaccine is available for travellers considered at high risk (e.g. health-care staff, patients with malignant diseases, immunocompromised patients, and homosexual men). It should, however, be borne in mind that immunisation takes up to six months to confer adequate immunity.

Japanese B encephalitis   Japanese B encephalitis is a rare but serious insect-borne infection that occurs in most of the Far- East and South-East Asia. Vaccination is recommended for those travelling to Asia for more than one month or for those staying in rural areas.

Malaria   Travellers at particular risk from being bitten by mosquitoes infected with *Plasmodium* spp. are those going to Africa, Central and South America, and Asia. Infected mosquitoes may also occasionally be transported to non-endemic areas in luggage and aircraft, and pharmacies in the vicinity of airports should be alert to this possibility.

The potential role of pharmacists in issuing advice about malaria chemoprophylaxis is complemented by the classification of chloroquine and proguanil in the UK as pharmacy medicines for that indication. However, drug resistance varies considerably between endemic areas and the latest advice in BNF 5.4.1 or from one of the telephone advice lines listed in Section 9.5 should be given. A list of useful addresses is also given in Section 9.5. Chemoprophylaxis should ideally be started one week before departure but not later than the first day of exposure, and be taken regularly and continued for at least four weeks after return without fail, except mefloquine (*see below*); all tablets should be taken with or after food. Mefloquine is a prescription-only medicine indicated for use in areas where chloroquine-resistant falciparum malaria is endemic. It provides an alternative to the more usual chloroquine and proguanil regimen although it has been recommended that it should only be used for short stays of up to three weeks. The course is one dose a week for six weeks and should be started one week before departure. Pregnant women and immunocompromised patients should be referred for medical advice on malaria chemoprophylaxis. Chloroquine and proguanil may be used during breast-feeding, but mefloquine is contra-indicated. Chemoprophylaxis is necessary in breast-fed infants since the amounts of antimalarials excreted in breast milk are too variable to be reliable.

Poliomyelitis   Despite its disappearance from many developed countries of the western world, poliomyelitis is still prevalent in developing nations, especially in areas of poor hygiene. Poliomyelitis is contracted via the faecal-oral route or nasopharyngeal secretions.

A large proportion of the population of the UK and of other western countries is protected against poliomyelitis as a result of active immunisation programmes carried out during childhood since 1955. Nevertheless, travellers with no record of immunisation wishing to visit develop-ing countries must be immunised before setting out. Single booster doses are recommended every ten years for those who have been previously immunised.

Tetanus   The risk of contracting tetanus is rare on holidays of limited physical exertion; the risk is somewhat increased when participating in holidays of greater activity (e.g. adventure holidays, trekking, and safaris). Most people in the UK will have been vaccinated during childhood but booster doses are necessary every ten years or following injury. The DoH particularly stresses the need for travellers to regions without medical facilities to be immunised before departure.

Tick-borne encephalitis   Tick-borne encephalitis occurs in the forested areas of Scandinavia and Central Europe, particularly Austria, Czechoslovakia, West Germany, and Yugoslavia. A vaccine is available from from a limited number of centres in the UK.

Tuberculosis   BCG vaccination is recommended for travellers proposing to stay for longer than one month in Asia, Africa, or Central and South America; it should pre-ferably be given three months or more before departure.

Typhoid fever   Typhoid fever is a disease resulting from poor sanitation and hygiene. Vaccination should be recommended to all travellers to endemic regions intending to stay for longer than two weeks, and especially for travellers to the Indian subcontinent from where most of the 200 cases reported annually in England and Wales derive. However, it should be emphasised to all prospective travellers that vaccination is not a substitute for, but an adjunct to, basic hygienic measures (*see* Section 9.3). Typhoid vaccination is given in two doses separated by an interval of 4 to 6 weeks; protection from the double dose lasts up to three years. If only a single dose is administered, cover lasts for only six months. Following a completed course of two doses, a booster dose is necessary after three years for those who continue to be exposed to the risk of infection.

Yellow fever   Travellers to some parts of Africa and South America are at risk of contracting yellow fever which, like malaria, is transmitted by mosquitoes. As there is no effective treatment for the infection, the importance of prevention cannot be overemphasised (*see* Section 9.3). A yellow fever vaccine is available from a limited number of centres in the UK and, after administration, patients are issued with an International Certificate of Vaccination. The certificate becomes valid after ten days and lasts for ten years following initial vaccination; it is immediately valid on re-vaccination within the ten-year period. Certificates are required for entry into many parts of Africa and South America. Some countries (e.g. in Asia) may require a certificate of vaccination if travellers have come from an endemic region.

Travel and diabetes mellitus

Travelling can be a source of worry to diabetics, and in particular insulin-dependent diabetics, but taking adequate precautionary measures can help allay fears.

Immunisation schedules and malaria prophylaxis are the same for diabetics as non-diabetics (*see above*). It is essential that diabetics ensure that they have sufficient supplies of insulin, syringes, and urine/blood testing equipment in their luggage. Air travellers should carry insulin in hand luggage to prevent it freezing in the luggage hold at high altitudes; it is also then available for use in the event of unexpected delays before departure, while airborne, and if luggage is lost. If insulin injections are required while airborne, only half as much air should be injected into the vial to take account of the differences between cabin pressure and ground pressure (*see* Air travel below). Travellers should be reassured that although refrigeration of insulin is necessary for long-term storage in high ambient temperatures, it is not essential for short periods during a journey or in temperate climates.

A means of identification (e.g. a doctor's letter or statement of current treatment, and the name and address of the doctor or clinic) is important for diabetic travellers. It can help to smooth passage through customs if luggage is searched and the presence of needles and syringes is queried. Identification can also help first-aiders attending a solo diabetic traveller who has lost consciousness as a result of hypoglycaemia.

If diabetics are known to experience motion sickness, it is important to prevent vomiting because of the risk of dehydration, hyperglycaemia, and diabetic ketoacidosis. Drugs for motion sickness may be used by insulin-dependent diabetics. If vomiting occurs, carbohydrate intake should be maintained by sipping fluids containing glucose.

Long-distance travel across time zones can pose special problems for insulin-dependent diabetics in the timing of their injections. Flights from east to west increase the length of the first day of travel, whereas eastward flights result in a shorter length of first day. In general, changes in time zones in excess of four hours require modifications to injection schedules. However, it is recommended that diabetics should continue with their dosage schedule on home-time until arrival at their destination, or even wait until the effects of jet lag have worn off before adjusting the dose. This may be facilitated by initially leaving watches set at home-time. When making changes to the dosage schedule, the time of each injection may be altered by 2 to 3 hours until in line with the new time zone, although a dose should only be given if it can safely be assumed that a meal or snack will follow within 30 minutes. Careful and regular testing of blood and urine glucose concentrations is advised during the period of adjustment. If a urine test indicates a high concentration of sugar, which may occur when the interval between doses is increased, a supplementary injection of soluble insulin (e.g. 4 to 8 units) may be given. Conversely, when reducing the dosage interval, it may be necessary to reduce the dose by 4 to 8 units to prevent hypoglycaemia. All insulin- dependent diabetics should be advised to consult their doctor or diabetic clinic well in advance of travelling and, if necessary, have a dosage adjustment schedule worked out for them. It should also be borne in mind that the level of physical activity during a holiday may be somewhat different from that at home, and further adjustments in insulin dose, carbohydrate intake, or both, may be required. Non-insulin-dependent diabetics taking oral hypo-glycaemic agents do not need to adjust their dosage schedules on account of different time zones.

Regular dietary management may be a particular problem for diabetics. If normal eating times are delayed, additional snacks may be necessary to prevent hypoglycaemia. Diabetics should always carry a readily available form of glucose in case of insulin overdose or other cause of hypoglycaemia; this is particularly important while travelling.

Prolonged sitting in any form of transport may prevent adequate circulation in the toes and feet, which is a particular hazard for diabetics. Regular walking breaks, or determined efforts to move the toes and feet while otherwise immobile, will help to promote adequate blood flow. Legs should not be crossed while sitting for prolonged periods.

Travel and human immunodeficiency virus infection

There is no vaccine available to protect against human immunodeficiency virus (HIV) infection, and travellers must be aware of the mode of transmission of infection and means of prevention (see Section 9.3).

People who have already contracted HIV infection should consult their doctor for assessment of their fitness to travel and advice concerning any medication they may require. The WHO has advised that no restrictions should be made on entry requirements into any country for people infected with HIV because such measures are ineffective and impractical in the fight against spread of the disease. Nonetheless, many nations have taken it upon themselves to impose a variety of restrictions that travellers with HIV infection should be aware of.

Air travel

Flying can be a stressful experience, especially for those who do not fly regularly. Elements of travel that cause most stress include overcrowding, delays at airports, altered eating habits, and travel across time zones; consequences of these pressures include fatigue, indigestion, insomnia, and nausea. The predominant reasons for requests for doctors during a flight include anxiety, convulsions, mental illness, stress, and cardiovascular and gastro-intestinal disorders. Recommendations on advice for people with pre-existing medical conditions is outlined in Table 9.1.

Some drugs (e.g. antiepileptics, insulin, and oral contraceptives) require regular dosage intervals to be effective, and patients taking such medication may run into difficulties when crossing time zones. The recommendations are to remain on home-time during a long journey and to adjust carefully dosage intervals after arrival (see Travel and diabetes mellitus above). It is also strongly recommended that all essential medication is kept in hand luggage. Epileptics may need to increase

TABLE 9.1
Advice for people with pre-existing medical conditions who may be contemplating air travel

Condition	Advice	Reason
Anaemia, severe	not fit to fly	impaired oxygenation of tissues exacerbated by hypoxia
Cerebrovascular accident	do not fly for at least 3 weeks	impaired oxygenation of tissues exacerbated by hypoxia
Diabetes mellitus	*see* Section 9.2	
Epilepsy	dose of antiepileptics may need to be increased; patient should consult doctor	risk of stress-induced seizures
Fractured skull	do not fly for at least 7 days	expansion of gases may damage brain tissue
Gastro-intestinal haemorrhage, recent (e.g. as a result of peptic ulceration)	do not fly for at last 21 days	rebleeding may occur
Heart failure, uncontrolled	not fit to fly	impaired oxygenation of tissues exacerbated by hypoxia
Infectious diseases	do not fly	risk of contagion of other passengers
Myocardial infarction and severe angina	do not fly for at least 2 weeks, and preferably not before 2 months	impaired oxygenation of tissues exacerbated by hypoxia
Ostomies	carry extra bags and dressings	pressure changes may result in increased venting of gas and cause the bag to split
Otitis media, severe	do not fly	inability to vent the Eustachian tubes causes pain and discomfort, and may cause internal damage; patients with grommets may, however, be able to fly because grommets are not an airtight fit
Plaster casts	plaster may need to be split for long journeys	air trapped in the cast may expand and compress the limb
Pneumothorax (collapsed lung)	do not fly until lung has re-expanded	expansion of gases may impair lung function
Psychiatric disorders	trained escort and sedation may be required	stress and excitement of flying may exacerbate some psychiatric conditions
Respiratory disorders that cause breathlessnes at rest	flying permissible if fit to walk 50 m and climb 10 to 12 steps	impaired oxygenation of tissues exacerbated by hypoxia
Sinusitis, severe	do not fly	inability to vent the Eustachian tubes causes pain and discomfort, and may cause internal damage
Skin diseases, repulsive	do not fly	carriers feel that offence may be caused to other passengers and air crew, who must handle food, and cannot provide nursing assistance
Surgery, recent		
abdominal	do not fly for at last 10 days	expansion of gas may weaken the wound
air introduced into a body cavity (e.g. laparoscopy)	do not fly until the condition has resolved	expansion of gas may compress and damage surrounding tissue
chest	do not fly for at least 21 days	expansion of gases may impair lung function
intracranial	do not fly for at least 7 days	expansion of gases may damage brain tissue
ear (e.g. stapedectomy)	do not fly for at least 2 weeks, preferably not before 2 months	expansion of gases may cause severe damage
facial	must be accompanied by someone trained to release the wires holding the jaws together in the event of vomiting	if the jaws are wired, vomiting as a result of motion sickness may asphyxiate
Terminal illness	at the discretion of the airline, provided that death is not likely to occur on board	death on board presents difficult legal problems and is distressing to other passengers

their dose of antiepileptic drugs to avoid seizures induced by the stresses of flying and should consult their doctor well in advance of the flight.

The environment within an aircraft is pressurised to counteract the low atmospheric pressure and decreased temperature at high altitudes. At all altitudes, the conditions within the aircraft are maintained so as to be equivalent to those at 2000 metres above sea level. The partial pressure of oxygen at 2000 metres is about 80% of that at sea level, which may have adverse effects on some individuals as a result of hypoxia. Heavy smokers are at risk because carbon monoxide in cigarette smoke reduces the oxygen-carrying capacity of the blood. Similarly, people who consume excessive quantities of alcohol are at risk because alcohol enhances the effects of hypoxia. Smoking and alcohol should, therefore, be avoided during flight. Hypoxia may also affect those with acute upper respiratory-tract infections who should, where possible, avoid flying.

The air in the cabin is very dry and all passengers on long flights are at risk of dehydration; regular drinks should be taken, avoiding tea, coffee, or alcohol, which cause dehydration. Elderly people are particularly at risk of myocardial infarction or cerebrovascular accident if they become dehydrated. Contact lens wearers should be warned that both hard and soft contact lenses may appear to feel dry.

Reduction in pressure and prolonged sitting during a flight results in postural oedema, which causes swollen legs and feet; difficulty may be experienced in replacing shoes at the end of a flight. Oedema and venous stasis may produce serious problems for anyone predisposed to, or already suffering from, deep vein thrombosis. It is strongly recommended that air passengers should walk about the cabin as often as is practicable. When sitting down, leg exercises involving isometric contractions of the large muscles (see Section 8.2) may help reduce venous pooling.

The reduction in total pressure in the aircraft causes expansion of gases within body cavities, which can also produce adverse effects. Expansion of gases in healthy individuals may be felt as tightness of clothes around the waistline. This is exacerbated by carbonated drinks, alcohol, and foods that produce a lot of intestinal gas (e.g. cabbage, beans, and turnips), which should be avoided before and during flight. Wearing loose-fitting clothes may help to minimise the feelings of discomfort.

Air in the sinuses and middle-ear cavities expands during ascent and escapes passively via the Eustachian tubes producing the familiar feeling of 'popping'. As the aircraft descends, gas in the sinuses and middle-ear cavities contracts, and air must pass in from outside the body via the Eustachian tubes to equalise the pressure.

Venting may be assisted by various techniques including swallowing, yawning, moving the jaw from side to side, or opening the mouth wide; some people find that chewing or sucking sweets is helpful. Valsalva's manoeuvre involves holding the nose and venting the oesophagus into the postnasal space. If this does not clear the Eustachian tube, Toynbee's manoeuvre should be tried instead, which involves holding the nose and swallowing with the mouth closed. Sleeping should be avoided during descent so that Eustachian tubes can be vented. If the air passages are blocked (e.g. if they are swollen and inflamed as a result of infection), it is difficult to equalise the pressure and this may cause mild deafness, discomfort, pain, and a feeling of fullness. Babies and young children are less likely to be affected by pressure changes because of anatomical differences in the middle ear.

SCUBA divers must be aware that decompression sickness (the 'bends') may occur during high altitude air travel if a flight is taken too soon after a deep dive, because reduction in pressure allows nitrogen to be released too rapidly from body tissues. Divers should check with their diving clubs for the exact rules to be observed when flying after diving, but a general rule is that the maximum depth of any dive in the 24 hours before a flight should be 9 metres, and diving should cease at least 2 to 3 hours immediately before the flight (deep diving should cease much longer before).

Almost all airlines have imposed a ban on carrying pregnant women on long-haul flights if they are more than 34 to 35 weeks into confinement, and after 36 weeks on short-haul flights because of the risk of early labour and foetal hypoxia; flying is also contra-indicated until seven days after delivery. Neonates under 48 hours of age should not be subjected to the pressure changes within aircraft because of the poor development of the alveoli and the associated risk of hypoxia.

Hypoxia and expansion of gases in body cavities may produce additional problems for those with specific medical conditions. People most at risk from experiencing adverse effects are those suffering from cardiac and respiratory illnesses. Any weakened tissue (e.g. recent surgical incisions or blood-vessel damage) may be further weakened by distension, particularly in the abdominal region. Flying should be avoided if there is a recent history of gastro-intestinal haemorrhage (e.g. as a result of peptic ulceration) as this may be exacerbated; there is also a danger of hypoxia if haemorrhage has been sufficient to produce anaemia. Air travel should be avoided during the period following introduction of gas into the body for whatever reason (e.g. fractured skull or intracranial surgery, laparoscopy, pneumothorax, or surgical emphysema). Air entrapped within a plaster cast may expand and cause compression damage to enclosed tissues, which is exacerbated by the effects of postural oedema (*see above*). Recent dental work may produce pain during a flight as a result of expansion of air trapped beneath fillings.

MEDIF (Medical Information) forms are available from travel agents for patients who are not sure if they are fit to fly. The first part is filled in by the patient wishing to travel and the second by his or her doctor; the final decision is, however, the carrier's. The settings on body scanning security checks used in some countries may induce changes in the electrical components of pacemakers, and patients fitted with a pacemaker should notify the airline at the time of booking. If a patient with a pulmonary disorder is likely to require oxygen during a flight, the airline must be notified in advance as there is a limit as to how much oxygen may be carried on board; for safety reasons patients may not take their own cylinders.

First-aid kits for travel

There is an almost never-ending list of preparations and materials that could be recommended to prospective travellers to local and foreign destinations. Indeed, many international companies issue their own special medical packs to travelling employees, although these comprehensive products are not usually necessary for short-term travel. A selection of some of the items that may be recommended for inclusion in first-aid kits for travel is listed in Table 9.2. There may be additional specific requirements for those with pre-existing medical conditions, and travellers must ensure that they take sufficient supplies. Travellers should be aware of the legal status of any drugs that they wish to carry in the countries they intend to visit. It may be necessary to carry a doctor's note or certificate covering essential drugs, or choose suitable alternatives for non-essential drugs likely to pose problems at customs.

The risk of contracting HIV infection and hepatitis B from injection of contaminated blood products and use of contaminated injection equipment has led to the availability of kits containing sterile needles, syringes, disposable gloves, giving sets, cannulae, and plasma substitutes (e.g. modified gelatin preparations). Certain kits contain prescription-only preparations and can only be supplied against a doctor's prescription.

All airliners should carry a medical emergency kit in order that sick passengers may be assisted. Ideally, medical kits should contain diagnostic equipment, first-aid supplies, and a range of drugs; some of which can be given by the crew and others that are for use only by a travelling doctor.

TABLE 9.2
General items that may be considered for inclusion in a traveller's first-aid kit

Analgesics, non-opioid
Antacids
Antibiotics, broad-spectrum (for emergency use in remote regions)
Antidiarrhoeal drugs
Antihistamines, oral
Antifungal preparations
Antiseptic preprations
Calamine lotion
Condoms
Forceps or tweezers (fine-pointed)
Hydrocortisone 1% cream or ointment
Insect repellents
Laxatives
Magnesium sulphate paste
Malaria prophylactics (where appropriate)
Motion sickness prophylactics
Needles and syringes, sterile
Oral rehydration salts
Scissors
Sunscreens
Water purification products
Wound cleansing products
Wound dressings (including bandages and self-adhesive plasters)

Travellers should check the legal status of drugs that they wish to carry in the countries they intend to visit from the embassy, and if necessary obtain a doctor's note or substitute with another product.

9.3 PREVENTION AND MANAGEMENT OF CONDITIONS ASSOCIATED WITH TRAVEL

Motion sickness

Anyone who has experienced the trauma of sickness while travelling is understandably keen to prevent its recurrence. Motion sickness can occur on land, in the air, or at sea. It is thought to be caused by excessive stimulation of the vestibular apparatus by motion but treatment is merely palliative, and the condition can be severe enough to devastate holidays or business trips.

Symptoms of motion sickness follow a characteristic cascade pattern. Stomach discomfort, facial pallor, and cold sweating of the hands and face are common early symptoms. Increased salivation, lightheadedness, and lethargy may also precede vomiting and, in the event of continued exposure to the motion, the cycle of symptoms may be repeated. Vestibular stimulation can be severe enough to produce symptoms for hours or sometimes days after the journey.

Airsickness commonly occurs when an aircraft cannot rise above turbulent weather or while ascending to, or descending from, cruising altitudes. People's susceptibility to seasickness varies tremendously; some may experience symptoms on the calmest of seas whereas others are not affected by seas whisked up by force ten gales. The introduction of stabilisers, especially on cruise liners, has reduced the incidence of symptoms although roll-on roll-off ferries may not be similarly equipped. Passengers aboard ships should be advised to stay on deck whenever the weather conditions allow this. In aircraft, and in sea conditions that preclude decktop travel, travellers should sit with their eyes closed and their heads fixed in one position. Occupying the mind may assist in the prevention of symptoms.

Drug prevention of motion sickness requires dosage at least half an hour before travel (two hours for cinnarizine). Doses may be repeated according to the regimen of individual drugs. Hyoscine is the most effective drug in preventing motion sickness, but antihistamines (e.g cinnarizine, cyclizine, and dimenhydrinate) are better tolerated; cyclizine and cinnarizine are the least sedating. Antihistamine preparations are, however, best avoided during pregnancy. Care must be taken in the administration of sedating drugs if driving is to be undertaken immediately after a flight or sea-crossing. Once the symptoms of motion sickness have started, further treatment is ineffective, and the importance of strict adherence to the recommended prophylactic dosage schedule must therefore be stressed; this is particularly important in the event of flight or ferry delays. Children under two years of age do not generally suffer from motion sickness and are, therefore, unlikely to require prophylactic treatment.

Jet lag

Long-distance air travel in an easterly or westerly direction can result in passage across several time zones. Disturbances to physiological systems, and in particular to sleeping, waking, and mental activity, occur as a result of disruption of normal circadian rhythms, which are governed by the periods of light and dark, temperature, and time. Symptoms of jet lag, which are often worse when travelling from west to east, include decreased mental and physical performance, disturbances to appetite and bowel function, disrupted sleep, and lightheadedness. Excessive alcohol consumption and dehydration can aggravate symptoms.

Jet lag can be minimised by a combination of the following measures: sleeping for as long or as frequently as is practicable during the flight and on arrival; adopting local sleeping patterns as quickly as possible; and avoiding food at times when sleep should be taken.

Infectious diseases

There are many ways that infectious diseases may be contracted, and it is essential to be familiar with the different modes of transmission in order to give advice to travellers about effective means of prevention. Immunisation and chemoprophylaxis have already been discussed (see Section 9.2) but, in some cases, these measures are not completely effective and travellers should be advised of extra precautions. Additional precautions are strongly recommended, and are essential to prevent those infections for which no vaccine is available. A knowledge of infections endemic in the areas to be visited is necessary, and it is important not to assume that all infectious diseases are confined to tropical countries.

All of the infections discussed in this Section require medical attention, and any untoward, chronic, or recurrent symptoms should not be ignored. Some of these diseases are life-threatening emergencies whereas others are generally debilitating and only fatal in vulnerable groups (e.g. infants, immunocompromised patients, and the elderly). Some are insidious in onset or have long incubation periods and may not present until some time after the traveller has returned home (see Section 9.4). Traveller's diarrhoea (see below) may be caused by micro-organisms present in food or water, but it is generally a self-limiting condition and does not necessarily require medical referral.

Food and water-borne infections   A common mode of transmission for many infections is via food or drinking water. Many micro-organisms are excreted in faeces, and in areas where poor sanitation exists or human faeces is used to fertilise crops, pathogenic species may enter the food chain. Faecal contamination of food or water may also deposit the eggs of some species of helminth. Direct contamination of food by foodhandlers may occur if strict standards of hygiene are not observed, and flies may also be responsible for transporting micro-organisms from faeces to food. Examples of infections contracted via the faecal-oral route include:

- amoebiasis (amoebic dysentery)
- ascariasis
- cholera
- dwarf tapeworm infection
- giardiasis
- hepatitis A
- hookworm infection
- hydatid disease
- intestinal fluke disease

- paratyphoid fever
- poliomyelitis
- shigellosis (bacillary dysentery)
- trichuriasis
- typhoid fever.

Contaminated food may also be derived from an infected animal: unpasteurised milk, or dairy products made from it, may contain the bacteria that cause brucellosis and tuberculosis; and transmission of some helminthic infections may be effected by consumption of meat or fish containing the larval stages of the parasite. Examples of the latter include:

- fish tapeworm infection (freshwater fish)
- liver fluke disease (freshwater fish)
- lung fluke disease (freshwater crustaceans)
- taeniasis (beef or pork)
- trichiniasis (any meat).

Dracontiasis is a helminthic infection contracted via drinking water that has been contaminated by adult worms discharging embryos directly into environmental water through the skin of the host's leg.

The general principles relating to food hygiene and safety have been discussed in Section 2.4, and these also apply to travellers. However, in view of the low standards of sanitation and hygiene prevalent in some countries, travellers to such destinations may need to take additional action.

Food and water-borne infections may be prevented by ensuring that all food is thoroughly cooked before eating. It should be freshly prepared and not reheated; pre-cooked food should only be eaten if it has been properly refrigerated. All raw food should be avoided unless in the form of fruits and vegetables that can be peeled. Food should be personally prepared where possible, or eaten only in restaurants and hotels where a high standard of hygiene may be safely assumed; the temptation to purchase food from roadside vendors or other dubious outlets should be resisted. Strict rules of personal hygiene must be observed before handling or eating food, and anyone suffering with diarrhoea should not prepare food for others. Food and drink should be kept covered at all times before consumption to prevent flies from gaining access to it; this is particularly important when eating in the open air. All unpasteurised milk and dairy products made from it should be avoided.

Drinking water is a major source of pathogenic organisms but contaminated water may also be ingested from unexpected sources (e.g. ice cubes, when brushing teeth, during a shower, or when swimming in polluted water). Water should be boiled or treated with chemicals before drinking, and treated water should be used to wash all food before cooking. Boiling is practicable only for small quantities, and it should be stressed that the water must be maintained at 100°C for at least five minutes. Once boiled, the water can be stored for up to two hours if covered and kept in the vessel it was boiled in.

Chemical treatment of water by chlorine liberated from chlorine-based disinfectants (e.g. chloramine), is an alternative means of disinfecting water in the absence of facilities for boiling. However, the vessel used for disinfection must be free from organic matter to prevent inactivation of the disinfectant. The water itself should also be free of organic matter and should, where possible, be filtered before disinfection. The manufacturers' recommendations on rate of use and standing time must be followed. Some manufacturers recommend a higher concentration of disinfectant for water used to wash food than for drinking. However, it is necessary to ensure that washed food is subsequently rinsed in water containing a lower concentration of disinfectant. Iodine is an alternative to chlorine for disinfection. Five drops of the 2% tincture are added to one litre of clear water and allowed to stand for 20 to 30 minutes; if the water is cloudy, ten drops are necessary.

Infections transmitted by insect vectors   Many pathogenic micro-organisms have a complex life-cycle that involves insects and man. In some cases, there are several possible mammalian hosts, and man becomes an incidental host when entering areas where the infection exists in animals. Examples of insect-borne infections include:

- African trypanosomiasis (tsetse flies)
- American trypanosomiasis (bugs)
- dengue haemorrhagic fever
- filariasis (mosquitoes, black-flies, deerflies)
- leishmaniasis (sandflies)
- Lyme disease (ticks from deer and other forest animals)
- malaria (mosquitoes)
- plague, bubonic (fleas from rats)
- typhus fevers (human body louse, fleas from rats)
- yellow fever (mosquitoes).

Mosquitoes are active between dusk and dawn, and the preventive measures to be undertaken need only be applied during these hours; however, this may not be true for all insects and the general principles outlined may need to be applied at all times. Clothes that cover as much of the body as possible should be worn, choosing fabrics with a close weave and light colour; wet clothing should be replaced immediately as insects may bite through it.

Topical insect repellents interfere with the sensory apparatus of insects, and may be mixed with synthetic pheromones that confuse the insect. Some products are a combination of repellents and insecticides. The most commonly used insect repellents are butopyronoxyl, dibutyl phthalate, diethyltoluamide (DEET), and dimethyl phthalate; butylethylpropanediol may be used to impregnate clothing. Preparations should be applied to all exposed parts and reapplied according to manufacturer's instructions (usually every four hours) and after swimming, washing, or if sweating profusely; eyes and mucous membranes should be avoided. Travellers should be warned that some insect repellents soften plastics.

Netting (which may be impregnated with an insect repellent) should be used around beds, and it should be inspected regularly for holes. It should completely cover the bed and be tucked in all around; there should be no point of contact with the skin. A knock-down insecticide should be sprayed in the bedroom before retiring for the night, and the netting examined to make sure that there are no insects inside it.

Infections acquired directly from the environment
Some infections (e.g. hookworm infection and strongyloidiasis) may be acquired directly from the soil as a result of walking barefoot, and footwear should be worn at all times in endemic regions. Soil is also contaminated with tetanus spores, and penetrating wounds pose a risk for non-immunised individuals. All wounds should be cleansed thoroughly and medical attention sought as soon as possible.

Anthrax is still endemic in some parts of the world, and spores present in the environment are a potential risk for travellers. Anthrax is also transmitted from spores present in the products derived from infected animals (e.g. bones, hair, hide, wool, and meat), which should be handled with extreme care in endemic regions.

Schistosomiasis (bilharziasis) is contracted by swimming or washing in fresh water harbouring certain species of snail that are intermediate hosts in the life-cycle of *Schistosoma* spp., and such activities should be avoided in endemic regions. It occurs in Africa, Asia, and South America. In general, to avoid contracting any water-borne infection, bathing should be confined to chlorinated swimming pools or the sea.

Lassa fever is acquired by contact with urine from infected rats (who represent the reservoir of infection) although the exact mode of transmission is unknown.

Infections acquired directly from animals   The most notable example is rabies and contact with domestic and wild animals should be avoided in endemic regions. The virus is present in the saliva of an infected animal, and is transmitted to man during a bite. Rabies may also be acquired by inhalation of infected secretions in bat caves. Any animal bite should be thoroughly washed with detergent and running water, and any residual debris removed. The application of 40 to 70% alcohol (e.g. in an emergency, whisky or gin is acceptable) or povidone- iodine may help to inactivate the virus, but urgent medical attention is essential. If the animal can be safely captured, it should be handed over to the local authorities for examination. The potential seriousness of animal bites is emphasised by the invariably fatal outcome of rabies once symptoms are seen. Post-exposure vaccination may be successful if the treatment course is started as soon as possible after a bite.

Infections transmitted directly from person to person   Some infections are contracted directly from other people via airborne droplets or by contact with body fluids and secretions (e.g. blood and blood products, seminal fluid, breast milk, or nasopharyngeal secretions). This may represent the only form of transmission for some infections, or it may be a secondary mode for those that were primarily acquired from other sources.

Examples of infections that may be transmitted directly between people include:

- Ebola fever
- hepatitis B
- HIV infection
- Lassa fever
- leprosy (from untreated persons)
- Marburg disease
- meningococcal infections
- plague, pneumonic
- poliomyelitis
- sexually transmitted diseases
- tuberculosis.

It is absolutely essential to avoid unnecessary surgery, dental treatment, acupuncture, tattooing, ear piercing, or any other invasive technique in developing countries. First-aid kits for travel containing sterile syringes and needles (*see* Section 9.2) are available, and should be carried by travellers to countries where the standards of medical hygiene are questionable. In some countries, screening of blood and blood products is not routinely carried out; however, blood transfusion may be essential in emergencies. Travellers should not indulge in casual sex (especially with prostitutes), or at least use condoms (*see* Section 4.4). The only means of preventing transmission of airborne micro-organisms is by isolation of infected cases. However, there is no guarantee that all cases will be isolated, particularly in remote rural areas, and for many infections a patient is infectious during the incubation period, which is often asymptomatic. An unsuspecting traveller may therefore unwittingly come into contact with infected individuals. The only means of protection is by immunisation where possible, and immediately reporting to a doctor, symptoms of any sort or general feelings of malaise.

Traveller's diarrhoea

Traveller's diarrhoea affects between 25 and 50% of all those travelling abroad, and may be sufficiently severe in one-third of sufferers to result in confinement to bed. However, reassurance can be gained from the knowledge that most episodes last less than 72 hours. Although diarrhoea is a common symptom of gastro-intestinal infections, many cases of traveller's diarrhoea are caused by a sudden change in diet and eating habits, and not necessarily the result of ingestion of contaminated food or water. Food poisoning does account for some cases, and pathogenic micro-organisms commonly implicated include *Escherichia coli*, *Campylobacter* spp., *Salmonella* spp., *Staphylococcus aureus*, and *Vibrio parahaemolyticus*. Food poisoning may be prevented by observing stringent standards of personal hygiene, particularly when handling food (*see* Food and water-borne infections above).

Traveller's diarrhoea may be treated by the administration of oral rehydration salts, ensuring that only boiled or treated water is used to make up the solution. Antidiarrhoeal drugs may be used if necessary, but it must be emphasised that they are of secondary value, and must not detract from oral rehydration therapy. This is particularly important in infants because of the serious adverse effects of dehydration. Medical assistance should be sought if diarrhoea lasts longer than five days, is recurrent, or is associated with the passage of blood or mucus.

Bites and stings

The unwary traveller may be prone to a wide variety of bites and stings that will, in most cases, be no more than a source of minor irritation. However, pharmacists, should be particularly aware of the potential hazards in hypersensitive individuals.

Bites
Some infectious diseases are transmitted to man during an animal or insect bite (e.g. rabies, malaria, or yellow fever). There is an additional hazard, even if bitten by a non-rabid animal, of contamination of a penetrating wound by micro-organisms present in the animal's saliva. Insect bites may also result in infection if scratched excessively.

Insect bites   Insect bites may be caused by flies, gnats, midges, or mosquitoes, which suck up blood from below the skin surface. Simultaneously, insect saliva, which contains substances that are pharmacologically active and capable of provoking allergic reactions of varying degrees, is deposited. Insect bites should be treated by cleansing the area followed by application of a cooling lotion (e.g. calamine lotion). Administration of topical antihistamine preparations is not recommended because of the occasional risk of allergic contact dermatitis in sensitive individuals. Topical hydrocortisone (*see* Fig. 9.1) or oral antihistamines may be beneficial. For preventive measures to avoid insect bites *see* Infections transmitted by insect vectors above.

Snake bites   Snake bites occur more commonly in remote regions of travel, although it should not be forgotten that a venomous snake, the adder (*Vipera berus*), inhabits some regions of Great Britain. Snakes only attack humans as a means of defence, and it is therefore prudent to avoid deliberately provoking a snake. Bites as a result of accidental contact with a snake may be avoided by:

- wearing boots, socks, and trousers in areas known to be inhabited by snakes
- carrying a torch when walking at night (when snakes are most active)
- inspecting bedding when sleeping on open ground
- not disturbing boulders, brushwood, burrows, or other similar places where snakes may be resting, without first checking the area carefully and protecting the arms, hands, and face.

Almost all venomous snakes secrete their poison through fangs located on the upper jaw. Venoms are mixtures of enzymes, peptides, and metalloproteins, and produce a wide variety of effects including haemolysis, haemorrhage, neurotoxic signs, oedema, shock, myonecrosis, pituitary failure, and renal failure. However, about 25% of snake bites fail to envenomate. The most common immediate reaction on having been bitten is fear and panic, and there may be breathlessness, dizziness, and chest pain. Tenderness and pain may develop at the site of the bite, indicating envenomation, and may be followed by lymphadenopathy and swelling of the distal limb.

Proprietary brands of hydrocortisone cream (0.1 and 1.0%) and ointment (1.0%) may be sold to the public for the treatment of:

- allergic contact dermatitis
- irritant dermatitis
- insect bite reactions.

It is unlawful to sell any hydrocortisone preparation if it is to be used:

- on the eyes or face
- on broken or infected skin (including cold sores, acne, athlete's foot)
- around the anogenital region
- on children under 10 years of age
- in pregnancy.

Preparations should be applied sparingly over a small area once or twice daily, for a maximum of one week.
    The label must include 'If the condition is not improved, consult your doctor'.

Fig. 9.1
Sale of over-the-counter hydrocortisone preparations in the UK.

The most appropriate action after a snake bite is to calm the patient and immobilise the limb. The age-old remedy of applying a tourniquet is not recommended because, in inexperienced hands, it may lead to gangrene; however, a tight crepe bandage may be of value. Leaching blood by cutting tissue from an area around the wound is also no longer advocated because haemorrhage may occur, the site may become infected, and further damage may be caused to surrounding tissues. Aspirin should not be given as it may exacerbate gastro-intestinal haemorrhage. First-aiders should ensure that an adequate airway is maintained, and regularly check that the patient is still breathing. Signs of systemic poisoning, which may appear within 30 minutes or up to 24 hours later, include loss of consciousness, spontaneous bleeding from the gums, and muscle paralysis. Because of the wide variety of clinical syndromes produced by the venom of different snake species, the dead snake (held by the tail) should, whenever possible, be transported with the patient to a local hospital to aid identification of the venom; attempts should not be made to capture live snakes. Gloves must be worn at all times when carrying a dead snake because venom can ooze from the body, especially if the head has been severed.

Spider bites   Almost all spiders are venomous, but only a few species are dangerous to man. They possess a small pair of fangs attached directly to venom glands. Spider bites are particularly common in Australia, South America, USA, Israel, North Africa, and Mediterranean areas. Spider venoms may be neurotoxic (e.g. black widow spider), or produce local necrosis and haemolysis (e.g. brown recluse spider). As with snake bites, first-aid measures include immobilisation of the limb and immediate transportation to hospital; neurotoxic symptoms may develop rapidly.

Ticks   Ticks are commonly carried by domestic pets, especially in North America and Australia, and usually bite in hairy crevices or orifices and on the scalp. The tick embeds itself in the skin by a barbed protrusion (the hypostome), which injects saliva containing a neurotoxin.

Stings

Many creatures have developed highly specialised stings. Most social insects (e.g. honeybees, wasps, hornets, and ants) will only sting if they perceive a threat to themselves or their colony; accidental disturbance of a nest or of a feeding insect may provoke attack. Insect venom contains a variety of pharmacologically active substances (e.g. dopamine, histamine, acetylcholine, serotonin, formic acid, and noradrenaline).

Bee and wasp stings   Having delivered its sting, a honeybee may remain attached to the victim's skin by its barbed sting. Brushing the insect away invariably leaves the sting with its venom and appendages embedded in the skin and these must be carefully extracted. The location of the pocket of venom at the distal end of the barb demands that only tweezers with fine tips should be used for extraction; it is important that the venom sac is not squeezed, injecting further venom into the wound. Scraping away the sting with a blade or fingernail may be a more effective means of removal. By comparison, wasp stings are smooth and are usually extracted from the skin by the insect itself after attack.

Symptoms include immediate local pain followed by erythema and oedema. In most cases, the swelling lasts for a few hours only, although more severe reactions may result from stings on the face; gross oedema resulting from stings in the mouth may cause respiratory distress and asphyxiation. One in 200 people appear to develop hypersensitivity to bee and wasp stings, and fatal anaphylactic responses may occur in a small minority of cases on subsequent exposure to the allergen. An initial symptom of a hypersensitive reaction after stinging is bronchoconstriction, which may be followed by generalised erythema, nausea and vomiting, oedema, hypotension, and shock. Serious systemic reactions generally occur within the first 30 minutes after a sting, and most fatalities occur in the middle-aged or elderly, presumably as a result of associated conditions (e.g. ischaemic heart disease).

The affected area should be cleansed and a cooling lotion (e.g. calamine lotion) applied. Administration of topical antihistamine preparations is not recommended because of the risk of allergic contact dermatitis in some individuals. Topical hydrocortisone (*see* Fig. 9.1) or oral antihistamines may be beneficial. If stung within the mouth, ice should be used to reduce the swelling, and medical attention sought as soon as possible.

Atopic individuals may be particularly susceptible to developing hypersensitivity reactions and should, where possible, avoid contact with stinging insects. Anyone known to have experienced hypersensitivity to a previous insect sting may benefit from carrying oral anti-histamines, and an adrenaline inhalation or pre-filled adrenaline syringe to relieve bronchoconstriction, which is the primary cause of anaphylactic death. Carrying identification that can alert others to a known history of hypersensitivity (e.g. in the form of a medallion or bracelet) can also be life-saving. Full measures for the treatment of allergic emergencies are described in BNF 3.4.3.

Ant stings   Ant stings contain a high concentration of formic acid, the effects of which can be neutralised by the application of alkaline solutions containing sodium bicarbonate or 1% ammonia.

Scorpion stings   Travellers to the Americas, the Middle East, India, South Africa, and North Africa are liable to scorpion stings. Different species produce different venoms with varying clinical symptoms, and stings from some species may be fatal, especially to young children. A scorpion sting may cause intense local pain, oedema, and lymphadenopathy. Symptoms of systemic distribution of the venom may be produced almost immediately or up to 24 hours later. Overactivity of the autonomic nervous system produces a wide range of symptoms, including dilated pupils, excessive salivation and sweating, diarrhoea, and vomiting. Increased release of catecholamines produces cardio-vascular hyperactivity, hypertension, and arrhythmias. Urgent medical attention is essential, although the onset of systemic effects may be delayed by immobilisation of the affected part.

Stinging fish   Some fish (e.g. scorpion-fish, sting-rays, stone-fish, and weeverfish) have bony spines that are covered in venom-secreting tissues. Weeverfish may be found in waters around the UK although most other species inhabit tropical waters. Swimming should be avoided in infested waters and attempts to handle fish (either dead or alive) should only be made by swimmers who are confident in their identification. The venom causes intense local pain, but may be inactivated by heat. The affected area should first be irrigated with cold salt-water, and then immersed for a few seconds in the hottest water that is bearable (but not so hot as to scald and blister). The process should be repeated until the pain no longer recurs, which usually takes about 30 minutes. If it is not practicable to immerse the wound, hot compresses should be applied. Stone-fish stings may require the administration of an antivenom to prevent potentially life-threatening systemic reactions.

Jellyfish   Jellyfish are equipped with stinging capsules (nematocysts) which release vasoactive substances (e.g. histamine and kinins) that cause erythema, wheals, and local pain. Most jellyfish are harmless, but death has occurred following stings from a Portuguese man-of-war; the most dangerous of all is the box jellyfish (sea wasp) found in seas off north-east Australia. Underwater clothing can act as a barrier to the dermal penetration of nematocysts. Tentacle remains should be removed, although great care must be taken not to discharge more of the venom in doing so. Application of vinegar, dilute acetic acid, or calamine lotion may also be beneficial. Intensive supportive therapy may be necessary for serious cases.

Sunburn

The most harmful component of sunlight that reaches the earth's surface is ultraviolet (UV) radiation, which has a wavelength between 200 and 400 nm. UV radiation is made up of three components: UVA radiation (wave-length 320 to 400 nm), which represents about 80% of the UV radiation that reaches the earth's surface; UVB radiation (wavelength 290 to 320 nm), which is partially absorbed by the earth's atmosphere and only constitutes about 20% of the total UV radiation reaching the earth's surface; and UVC (wavelength 100 to 290 nm), which is totally absorbed by the earth's atmosphere, particularly by the ozone layer. UVB is more energetic than UVA but is less capable of penetrating human epidermis.

Melanocytes in the basal layer of the epidermis are responsible for the formation of a pigment, melanin, which develops as a protective response to exposure to UV radiation. The number of melanocytes is constant, and the varying rates at which different people tan is a function of the rate of production of melanin, which is genetically determined. UVA radiation causes oxidation of melanin already present in the skin, producing an immediate but transient tan. UVB radiation stimulates the melanocytes to produce melanin granules, which move to the surface layers of the skin. This process takes 24 to 48 hours and accounts for the delay in tanning after exposure. UVA radiation is less effective than UVB in producing a tan by this mechanism. A further protective mechanism is skin thickening, which is only initiated by UVB radiation. Sunbeds utilise UVA radiation and do not, therefore, offer protection against subsequent exposure to UVB radiation. The tanning and thickening mechanisms are a response to an adverse stimulus, and only occur after the skin has already been damaged (i.e. sunburn). A tan does not completely protect the skin from further damage.

Sunburn is an inflammatory reaction and is not immediately apparent during exposure; the first symptoms may not be felt until 2 to 8 hours later. The most common symptom is erythema, which usually fades within 36 to 72 hours. Severe sunburn may result in bullae, oedema, pain, and tenderness, which generally reach a peak on the second day. Peeling starts after about 72 hours and lasts for up to five days. Extensive areas of sunburnt skin may produce constitutional symptoms (e.g. fever, chills, malaise, and headache). The symptoms of sunburn can be severe enough to ruin part or all of a holiday or trip. If preventive measures (*see below*) have not been adopted or have been unsuccessful, sunburn may be relieved by cooling the skin with cold-water compresses or by sponging. A cooling lotion (e.g. calamine lotion) may be of value, but administration of topical antihistamine preparations is not recommended because of the risk of allergic contact dermatitis in sensitive individuals. Non-opioid analgesics may be used for pain relief. Further exposure to UV radiation should be avoided until all symptoms have subsided.

Sunburn can be caused by both UVA and UVB radiation, although the dose of UVA radiation required is 1000 times that of UVB; however, more UVA radiation reaches the earth's surface than UVB (*see above*). Prolonged and repeated exposure to UV radiation may, in time, cause premature ageing of the skin and the development of malignant skin diseases (e.g. melanoma or rodent ulcer). People most susceptible to the harmful effects of UV radiation are fair skinned, and tend to have red hair, freckles, or both. Infants and children are particularly vulnerable to the damaging effects of UV radiation. To prevent the long-term consequences of damage by UV radiation, children should be protected from overexposure and should be educated about the dangers. People at risk should examine their skin regularly for any sudden appearances of sinister skin lesions, or changes in existing moles, freckles, or birthmarks.

Photosensitivity reactions may occur in those taking some medicines (e.g. griseofulvin, immunosuppressants, nalidixic acid, non-steroidal anti-inflammatory drugs, sulphonamides, tetracyclines, or thiazide diuretics) or using topical preparations containing coal tar; contact with some plants or use of perfumes may also have the same effect. Photodermatoses may also occur in individuals suffering from some medical conditions (e.g. systemic lupus erythematosus, porphyrias, or chronic actinic dermatitis). These adverse reactions are caused predominantly by UVA radiation and can develop from exposure to normal amounts of sunlight. All those at risk should be advised to avoid any exposure to UV radiation, or to cover exposed areas; use of sunscreens (*see below*) that absorb both UVA and UVB radiation or total sunblocks may be necessary.

Throughout most of the year, the majority of people living north of the tropic of Cancer and south of the tropic of Capricorn are exposed to only limited quantities of sunlight. Sunlight received at these latitudes is generally of low intensity because of the relatively low angle at which the rays impinge on the earth's surface. Holidays in sunnier regions mean that for 2 or 3 weeks each year people are exposed to increased amounts of high intensity UV radiation. There is also an increased risk of sunburn at high altitude, even during the winter, because the atmosphere is less capable of filtering UV radiation than at ground level.

The skin-damaging effects of UV radiation may be minimised by observing the following simple rules:

- keep out of the sun as much as possible, and wear a hat and clothes that offer adequate protection
- if tanning, increase exposure times gradually (*see below*)
- always use a sunscreen (*see below*) on exposed parts.

Unless the sun is completely blocked, sunburn can occur on cloudy days because clouds scatter radiation over a wide area. There is the additional danger that as clouds absorb infra-red radiation (the heat-producing rays), people may stay out of doors for longer periods increasing the time of exposure to UV radiation. It is also important to recognise that sitting in the shade may afford little protection because ultraviolet rays may be deflected by sand, snow, or concrete; the sun's rays can also penetrate water and thin or wet clothing.

It is recommended that the maximum time of exposure during periods of high intensity UV radiation (i.e. between 10.00 and 15.00 h) should not exceed 15 minutes on the first day. This may be increased to 30 minutes on the next day, and to one hour on the third day; thereafter, exposure may be increased by one hour per day.

Sunscreens

Sunscreens protect the skin from receiving high doses of UV radiation by either a physical or chemical mechanism. In total sunblocks, the active ingredient (e.g. finely divided calamine, talc, titanium dioxide, or zinc oxide) completely blocks skin absorption of UV radiation (both UVA and UVB) by scattering and reflecting the rays. These compounds are thick and opaque, and cosmetically too conspicuous for general use. They may, however, be useful in areas that are more prone to sunburn than others.

The most commonly used sunscreen preparations contain agents that act by a chemical mechanism and absorb UVB radiation (e.g. aminobenzoates and salicylates); some also absorb UVA radiation (e.g. benzophenones and cinnamates).

The rational selection of sunscreens has been assisted by the development of the Sun Protection Factor (SPF), which is the ratio of the minimal dose of UVB radiation necessary to produce delayed erythema in skin protected by the sunscreen to that in unprotected skin. The higher the SPF value, the greater protection afforded by the sunscreen (i.e. the longer the period of exposure necessary to cause a similar degree of erythema). For example, if delayed erythema occurs in unprotected skin following 15 minutes exposure to UV radiation, then applying a sunscreen with a SPF of 4 would allow 60 minutes exposure to elicit the same reaction. There are two main test methods determining SPFs *in vivo* used in Europe and USA. The methods differ in the details of procedure but give similar results for UVB radiation. However, the actual exposure time required to produce delayed erythema is an individual variable and also depends on the intensity of UV radiation. It is also difficult in practice to control the amount of sunscreen applied. A guide to the selection of appropriate products for different skin types is given in Table 9.3. It should be remembered that SPFs generally refer to protection against UVB, not UVA radiation. Until there is a recognised factor system for denoting UVA protection, a sunscreen that offers good protection against both UVB and UVA radiation should be chosen (e.g. one containing a combination of either a benzophenone, mexenone, or padimate O with a cinnamate). It may be necessary to choose a sunscreen with a high SPF for particularly vulnerable areas of the body (e.g. breasts, buttocks, lips, nose, ears, or a bald head); people susceptible to cold sores, which may be triggered by sunlight, should use lipsalves with a high SPF. It should be noted that benzophenones may cause photoallergic contact dermatitis in sensitive individuals. Choosing a product with protection against UVB radiation only, effectively increases the exposure time to UVA radiation, which is

TABLE 9.3
Classification of skin types and recommended sun protection factors

Skin type category	Recommended sun protection factor (SPF)
I – Always burns; never tans	10 to 15
II – Always burns; minimal tan	8 to 9
III – Burns moderately easily; gradually tans	6 to 7
IV – Never burns; tans well	4 to 5
V – Asian and Mongoloid skin	2 to 3
VI – Afro-Caribbean skin	none

It may be necessary to use a higher SPF than recommended above at high altitudes and for travel to sunny regions from a winter climate.

particularly hazardous to those at risk of hypersensitivity reactions (*see above*).

Sunscreens should be applied evenly and thickly to be effective; studies have shown that in many cases, too little is applied and the actual SPF value may be reduced by up to 50%. For maximum effect they should be applied at least 30 minutes before exposure to allow time for absorption into the skin, and in the case of preparations containing para-aminobenzoic acid (PABA), two hours beforehand. Sunscreens must be reapplied after swimming or during profuse sweating; reapplication does not, however, prolong the protective time (i.e. it does not increase the SPF value). PABA penetrates the skin and binds with keratin, and is therefore less easily removed by water than other sunscreens. However, it only protects against UVB radiation.

Sunscreens are generally available throughout the year because of the demand generated by winter holidays, either in the sun or snow. Travellers to sunny regions from a winter climate should initially select products with a higher SPF value than they would for a summer holiday, to allow for the fact that their skin is unlikely to have had any exposure to UV radiation for several months. The reflectant property of snow is strong, and skiers should likewise select a sunscreen with a high SPF value. The choice of sunscreen product for those at higher altitudes and in colder regions should also be determined by the vehicle containing the active ingredient. Many water-based sunscreens will freeze at low temperatures, and this has prompted the manufacture of a range of products specifically for use in colder temperatures.

A limited range of sunscreening preparations (BNF 13.8.1) is prescribable for a range of dermatoses, and for patients at risk of photosensitivity reactions (*see above*). Items cannot be prescribed for any other groups, but the choice for the majority of holidaymakers and business travellers is considerably wider, and pharmacists are often asked to advise on the selection of appropriate products.

9.4 ADVISING TRAVELLERS ON RETURN

Travellers who have experienced illness while away will, in all likelihood, be prompted to seek medical attention on returning home if symptoms persist or recur. The greatest danger lies with those who felt perfectly fit while away but develop symptoms on return; the patient may not realise that the symptoms could be related to an infection contracted abroad, and fail to alert the doctor to this possibility, or not seek medical attention at all.

A change in temperature and humidity on returning home may provoke symptoms of the common cold and nasal congestion. However, the presence of a cough or other respiratory symptoms may suggest that a viral or bacterial infection has been contracted, and such patients should be referred to their general practitioner. Feverish, 'flu'-like symptoms may be early signs of malaria in travellers returning from tropical or subtropical regions. Fever or chills may also be the presenting symptom of many other infectious diseases, and returning travellers reporting such symptoms to a pharmacist should always be referred. Some infectious diseases, particularly helminthic infections, may remain silent for years before symptoms present.

Pharmacists should, as a matter of routine, ask all patients with gastro-intestinal symptoms or fever, or any unusual symptoms if they have recently travelled; if the answer is in the affirmative, referral is strongly recommended and the patient should be asked to tell the doctor where they have travelled. Some authorities recommend routine tropical screening for travellers returning from high-risk areas if they have been away a long time or if their life-style put them at risk of contracting endemic infections.

9.5 USEFUL ADDRESSES

AIR TRANSPORT USERS COMMITTEE (AUC)
2nd Floor
Kingsway House
103 Kingsway
London WC2B 6QX
Tel: 071–242 3882

BRITISH DIABETIC ASSOCIATION (BDA)
10 Queen Anne Street
London W1M 0BD
Tel: 071–323 1531
Provides advice and information about travel for diabetics among other services.

COMMUNICABLE DISEASES (SCOTLAND) UNIT
Ruchill Hospital
Glasgow G20 9NB
Tel: 041–946 7120

DEPARTMENT OF COMMUNICABLE AND TROPICAL DISEASES
East Birmingham Hospital
Birmingham B9 5ST
Tel: 021–772 4311

INTERNATIONAL AIR TRANSPORT ASSOCIATION (IATA)
Imperial House
15–19 Kingsway
London WC2B 6EN
Tel: 071–497 1048

LIVERPOOL SCHOOL OF TROPICAL MEDICINE
Pembroke Place
Liverpool L3 5QA
Tel: 051–708 9393

MEDICAL ADVISORY SERVICES FOR TRAVELLERS ABROAD (MASTA)
London School of Hygiene and Tropical Medicine
Keppel Street
London WC1E 7HT
Tel: 071–631 4408

PHLS MALARIA REFERENCE LABORATORY AND ROSS INSTITUTE ADVISORY SERVICE
London School of Hygiene and Tropical Medicine
Keppel Street
London WC1E 7HT
Tel: 071–636 7921; 071–927 2212/2435
These telephone numbers give recorded messages, and may be given to patients.
Tel: 071–636 8636
This telephone number is for use by physicians and pharmacists only, and not the general public.

RADAR (The Royal Association for Disability and Rehabilitation)
25 Mortimer Street
London W1N 8AB
Tel: 071–637 5400
Provides advice for the disabled traveller among other services.

TRAVEL CLINIC
Hospital for Tropical Diseases
4 St Pancras Way
London NW1 0PE
Tel: 071–388 8989/9600
(0898) 345081 (Telephone Healthline)

9.6 FURTHER READING

Dawood R, ed. *Travellers' health. How to stay healthy abroad.* 2nd ed. Oxford: Oxford University Press, 1989.

DoH, Central Office of Information. *Health advice for travellers inside the European Community.* London: HMSO, 1991.

DoH, Central Office Of Information. *Health advice for travellers outside the European Community.* London: HMSO, 1991.

Walker E, Williams G. *ABC of healthy travel.* 3rd ed. London: British Medical Journal, 1989.

Walker E, Williams G. *Well away. A health guide for travellers.* London: British Medical Journal, 1988.

WHO. *International travel and health. Vaccination requirements and health advice.* Geneva: WHO, 1991.

Chapter 10

CONTACT LENS CARE

10.1   INTRODUCTION

Contact lenses were first designed more than 100 years ago and consisted of large corneoscleral glass shells. In the 1940s, hard lenses made of Perspex became available and were followed 20 years later by the introduction of soft hydrogel lenses. Further developments have included gas permeable hard lenses, which allow the movement of oxygen through the lens to the cornea, soft lenses for extended wear, and most recently disposable lenses.

In 1988, it was estimated that about 2.32 million people in the UK between 16 and 60 years of age were regular contact lens wearers. Contact lenses are worn primarily by adults, although a baby can be fitted with lenses if clinically necessary. Lenses are obtained from an optometrist (ophthalmic optician), who will advise on the type of lens that will be suitable after considering the individual's visual requirements, daily environment, leisure activities, and personal choice. Some optometrists have an additional qualification in contact lens management.

Contact lenses are often preferred to spectacles for cosmetic reasons, and may also provide better peripheral vision. Visual defects that can be corrected by contact lenses include myopia (short sight), hyperopia (long sight), and corneal astigmatism (irregularly-shaped cornea). Contact lenses are not available on the NHS unless they are indicated for a serious eye disorder as determined by a hospital ophthalmologist.

Contact lenses may be used following removal of the lens of the eye in cataract surgery, and can also be fitted to protect the eye in diseases affecting the cornea including bullous keratopathy (a severe form of corneal oedema), dry eye, and recurrent corneal ulceration. Cosmetic contact lenses are sometimes used to disguise eyes that have developed unacceptable appearances, usually following injury or surgery. Contact lenses are also indicated for severe refractive errors where suitable spectacles cannot be made or are impractical; in these cases, contact lenses provide effective correction of vision and are cosmetically acceptable.

Contact lenses are contra-indicated in certain conditions, particularly active eye diseases. People unable to wear contact lenses include those with a history of allergy, or disease presenting with eye symptoms. Patients with hay fever may not be able to wear contact lenses during the period in which they are affected. Manual dexterity is important in insertion and removal of contact lenses, and for effective care. Consequently, patients with arthritis, stroke victims, young children, and the elderly may not be able to use contact lenses.

Tolerance to contact lenses tends to become reduced during pregnancy, but should not necessarily mean that women have to stop wearing their lenses; all that may be required is a reduction in wearing time or allowing an hour or two during the day without lenses. People who are diabetic or immunocompromised are at greater risk of developing eye infections, and should be advised of this if contact lenses are considered.

10.2 CONTACT LENSES AND CARE REGIMENS

Contact lenses are broadly classified as either hard lenses, which include gas permeable hard lenses, or soft lenses. Special lenses may be required in certain circumstances, and include scleral lenses (*see below*). Soft lenses are less durable and need to be replaced every 6 to 18 months, whereas hard lenses and gas permeable hard lenses tend to last for a number of years.

At the time of fitting, contact lens wearers are instructed how to take care of their lenses. This includes the correct techniques for insertion and removal of lenses, and appropriate methods for cleaning and storing them. Meticulous care with a strong commitment is essential in order to obtain the maximum benefit from contact lenses, ensure maximum life of the lenses, and prevent eye infection. These objectives are primarily achieved by using an effective care regimen designed for the particular lens type.

Solutions labelled for use with one type of contact lens are not usually intended to be used with another lens type, although there are exceptions. Solutions for hard lenses and gas permeable hard lenses contain preservatives that may be absorbed by soft lenses and slowly released onto the eye; these solutions should not therefore be used for soft lenses.

In addition to caring for the contact lenses, lens storage cases need to be thoroughly cleaned and air dried between use to remove contaminants. At weekly intervals, lens cases should be cleaned using hot water and a small brush. Soap and detergents should not be used. The case should be shaken to remove surplus water and be left to air dry before its next use.

When contact lenses are first fitted, there is a period of time during which the eyes adapt to the presence of lenses; this is called the adaptation time. Initially, the lenses are worn for short periods and the wear time gradually increased in increments until lenses can be worn comfortably for the desired duration. The adaptation time is generally shorter with soft lenses than with hard or gas permeable hard lenses, and is often associated with transient symptoms, which include:

- awareness of the lenses in the eyes
- blurred vision (momentary episodes)
- discomfort from exerting extreme eye movements (to the left or the right) and when looking upwards
- discomfort in a smoky or dry atmosphere
- excessive blinking
- excessive lachrymation
- reflections from light (prominent at night)
- temporary blurred spectacle vision after lens removal.

Hard contact lenses and gas permeable hard contact lenses

Hard contact lenses and gas permeable hard contact lenses are both rigid in nature. Hard contact lenses are made of polymethylmethacrylate (PMMA, Perspex). They are inert, hydrophobic, and have a very low water content; they are also impermeable to oxygen. Gas exchange with the corneal epithelium is therefore dependent on tears flowing behind the lens. The initial tolerance to hard lenses is poor, with a failure rate of about 30%. Hard lenses have now been almost completely replaced by gas permeable hard lenses, although in some cases they may be the most appropriate type of lens for large refractive errors (high prescription lenses).

Gas permeable hard lenses were developed to try and overcome the disadvantages of hard lenses, and to include some of the advantages of soft lenses. The lenses are hard, hydrophobic, and have a low water content. They allow the transmission of oxygen through the lens to the cornea, facilitating more normal metabolism. All gas permeable hard lenses are smaller than the diameter of the cornea, and float freely in the tear film. Generally, gas permeable hard lenses are made from one of the following polymer materials:

- CAB; cellulose acetate butyrate (low gas permeability)
- siloxane/methylmethacrylate copolymers (medium gas permeability)
- fluorocarbons/siloxane copolymers (high gas permeability).

The oxygen permeability of the lens, which ranges from low to high, is dependent on the silicone content.

Compared to hard lenses, gas permeable hard lenses tend to scratch more easily and the accumulation of lipid deposits is also more of a problem, although they are more comfortable to wear. Visual acuity is good with gas permeable hard lenses, but compared to soft lenses, the fitting is more complex.

Preparations used in the care of hard lenses and gas permeable hard lenses include:

- daily cleaning solutions
- rinsing and soaking (disinfecting) solutions
- wetting solutions
- rewetting and comfort solutions
- protein removal preparations.

The solutions available to perform these tasks may be single-function (e.g. cleaning only) or multi-function (e.g. for wetting, cleaning, and soaking). Multi-function solutions may be less effective because some properties may be compromised in their formulation. Therefore, it may be advisable to reserve the use of multi-function solutions for situations when convenience is required (e.g. during travel).

Essentially, the solutions used for the care of gas permeable hard lenses are the same as those used for hard lenses. However, in some instances, solutions for use with hard lenses may not be compatible with gas permeable hard lenses. For this reason, the optometrist's instructions must be followed, and only those solutions labelled for use with the particular lens type should be used.

Cleaning   Hard lenses and gas permeable hard lenses need to be cleaned daily to remove accumulated deposits. The type and amount of deposit varies with the type of lens material. Lipids tend to accumulate on PMMA and CAB lenses whereas both proteins and lipids are attracted to silicone acrylates.

A preserved, enzyme-free cleaning solution for use on hard and gas permeable hard lenses should be used at the end of the day to remove environment-derived and tear-related deposits from the lens surface and break down the microbial biofilm that collects during wear. The cleaning solution should be applied to both surfaces of the lens and gentle digital pressure used in a rotating manner in the palm of the hand.

Solutions for daily cleaning are isotonic, and usually consist of a nonionic or amphoteric surfactant, and a preservative. Some cleaning solutions contain a chelating agent (e.g. disodium edetate), which is present to remove calcium deposits. Disodium edetate also acts as an antimicrobial synergist.

A preservative-free preparation containing isopropyl alcohol 20% is available for cleaning both rigid and soft lenses and is reported to be effective against *Acanthamoeba* spp. (*see* Section 10.3).

Rinsing and disinfection   In general, following cleaning, contact lenses are disinfected by overnight storage in fresh soaking solution. Before soaking, the cleaning solution should be rinsed off each lens, in order to reduce contamination of the soaking solution. Soaking solutions are normally used for rinsing lenses after cleaning as well as disinfecting them. Soaking solutions are isotonic and consist of wetting agents, disinfectants, and a chelating agent. Soaking solutions for rigid lenses usually contain the same preservatives that are used in solutions for soft lenses, with the exception of benzalkonium chloride. The compatibility of benzalkonium chloride with gas permeable hard lens is controversial. It has been suggested that the preservative binds to the silicone acrylate lens material, and may also increase the hydrophobicity of the lens surface. Some authorities consider that it is probably expedient to rinse cleaning fluid off rigid lenses with tap water as the lenses will subsequently be placed in a soaking solution. However, tap water should not be applied to lenses after they have been disinfected. Mineral water and distilled water are not sterile and the former contains minerals which can accumulate and discolour lenses, especially soft contact lenses.

Disinfection of hard lenses and gas permeable hard lenses between periods of use is essential, and is accomplished by storing them in a soaking solution. After daily cleaning and subsequent rinsing, the lenses are placed in their storage case containing fresh soaking solution, and ideally left overnight. Daily replacement of the soaking solution is essential to prevent micro-organisms from proliferating in the storage case.

Among the alternative methods of disinfection for contact lenses, the use of hydrogen peroxide 3% is probably the most effective. However, contrary to some manufacturers' recommendations, it is necessary to clean the lenses before disinfection. In addition, although a ten minute disinfection cycle may be specified in the instructions, a soaking time of at least two hours has been reported to be necessary to eliminate acanthamoeba trophozoites and cysts, and overnight soaking is therefore recommended. Only hydrogen peroxide solutions that are specifically formulated for contact lenses should be used. Contact lenses must be neutralised after soaking in the hydrogen peroxide solution. This neutralisation process is usually achieved using a preparation of the enzyme catalase, or of sodium pyruvate. The advantage of using this system is the fact that no residual preservatives are present when the lenses are inserted into the eyes.

Heat disinfection (*see below*) is not a suitable method for disinfecting hard or gas permeable hard lenses.

Wetting   Wetting solutions are used for hard lenses and gas permeable hard lenses to reduce the contact angle of tears with the contact lens. They are formulated to be slightly viscous so as to cushion the lens on the eye for greater comfort. Wetting solutions are isotonic, and consist of wetting agents, viscosity increasing agents, and preservatives. Polyvinyl alcohol, or cellulose derivatives, or both, are commonly used in the formulation of wetting solutions. Generally, wetting solutions increase the comfort of contact lens wear and prevent the accumulation of deposits.

Saliva should not be used as a wetting substance on contact lenses because serious eye infections may be caused by micro-organisms that are present in saliva.

Rewetting and comfort solutions   The purpose of these solutions is to improve comfort when lenses are being worn, reduce lens irritation, and augment tear flow. They are administered directly onto the eye with the contact lens in place. These solutions are formulated on similar principles to wetting solutions (*see above*). Hypertonic solutions may be used in some cases to reduce lens irritation caused by slight corneal oedema associated with lens wear.

Protein removal   Periodic cleaning with protein removing preparations is necessary for all types of contact lenses. Protein removal is carried out as an extra stage after cleaning the lenses (*see above*) and before disinfection. Protein removing preparations containing proteolytic enzymes (e.g. papain or subtilisin A) are capable of removing stubborn deposits from the lenses. Pancreatin, a preparation containing enzymes having protease, lipase, and amylase activity, is included in some periodic cleaning products. Periodic cleaning preparations are usually presented as tablets for reconstitution. The tablets are generally dissolved in sterile sodium chloride 0.9% solution, and the lenses are soaked for a period which varies according to the type of lens and the particular preparation. It is advisable to clean and rinse the lenses again afterwards, before disinfecting them, as the enzymes may only loosen the deposits and a mechanical action is necessary to complete their removal. The frequency of periodic cleaning varies according to the instructions of the product manufacturer. These preparations are usually suitable for both soft lenses and gas permeable hard lenses. The use of protein removal preparations is not an alternative to daily cleaning; the two processes are complementary.

Soft contact lenses

Soft lenses are made of materials based on polyhydroxyethylmethacrylate (poly-HEMA), and are the most popular types of contact lens in use. Soft lenses are hydrophilic and have a water content of 30 to 80%. They allow the transfer of oxygen to the cornea through the lens, with the oxygen dissolving in the liquid in the lens and diffusing through. The higher the water content, the better the oxygen transmission of the lens, although this is usually accompanied by problems of greater fragility and accumulation of dirt in and on the lens. Silicone rubber soft lenses have a higher water content and oxygen permeability, and are used in patients with dry eye and where there is a high corneal oxygen demand. However, they are more difficult to fit and have a tendency to form deposits despite attempts to reduce this by surface coating.

There are two main types of soft lens: daily wear soft lenses, which are designed to be removed for cleaning each night; and extended-wear lenses, which are thinner, have a higher water content than daily wear lenses, and are designed to be worn for a minimum of 24 hours and usually several weeks. However, it is generally recommended that extended-wear soft lenses should be removed for cleaning and disinfection at least once a week, and the eyes allowed to rest for a night. Disposable extended-wear soft lenses are also available and are usually discarded after 1 to 2 weeks of continuous wear. This is intended to avoid the complications associated with the accumulation of deposits. However, disposable extended-wear lenses are expensive and reports indicate that they do not eliminate all the potential problems of contact lenses (*see* Section 10.3).

Compared with hard lenses and gas permeable hard lenses, soft lenses are well tolerated and more comfortable, and because the adaptation time is short they are suitable for occasional use. Soft lenses are larger than hard lenses, and cover the cornea and part of the sclera; this makes them less likely to dislodge, and hence more suitable for use during sport and exercise. However, soft lenses are more expensive, less resilient to damage, and readily accumulate deposits. In addition, they require greater care and are not able to provide the same degree of visual acuity.

The care of soft lenses involves cleaning, rinsing, and disinfection. It is time-consuming and requires a much greater degree of commitment compared with hard lenses and gas permeable hard lenses. Contaminated soft lenses are considered to be primarily responsible for the complications associated with the use of soft lenses.

Cleaning   The routine for cleaning soft contact lenses is similar to that described for hard lenses (*see above*). Cleaning is one of the most important aspects in the effective care of soft lenses; it is also one of the most neglected. Daily cleaning is necessary to remove fresh deposits of lipids, proteins, and other contaminants. Daily use cleaning solutions are isotonic, and usually contain surfactants, preservatives, and a chelating agent.

Rinsing and disinfection   Sterile sodium chloride 0.9% solution is commonly used to rinse soft lenses after cleaning. Sodium chloride 0.9% solutions may contain preservatives, but unpreserved solutions are available in unit-dose packs and aerosol formulations are available. The use of homemade saline solutions is strongly discouraged because of the likelihood of contamination, which may cause serious eye disorders (*see* Section 10.3). Soaking solutions are also commonly used for rinsing lenses. Soft contact lenses should never be rinsed or soaked in water, as changes to the structure of the lens may occur. Soaking solutions for soft lenses usually contain the same preservatives that are used in solutions for hard lenses, with the exception of benzalkonium chloride.

Soft lenses can be disinfected by one of two methods: chemical disinfection or heat disinfection. Chemical disinfection is the more popular method. Such solutions contain disinfectants and a chelating agent. Following cleaning, the lenses are rinsed and placed in fresh soaking solution, ideally for overnight storage. Subsequently, the lenses can be inserted into the eyes without further rinsing, although it is commonly recommended that the lenses are rinsed before insertion.

An alternative method of disinfection using hydrogen peroxide 3% is described above under Hard contact lenses.

A chlorine-based method for disinfection of soft contact lenses using sodium dichloroisocyanurate is also available. It acts by releasing available chlorine when it is dissolved in chloride 0.9% solution. The lenses should be rinsed thoroughly with unpreserved sodium chloride 0.9% solution before they are worn.

A preservative-free preparation containing isopropyl alcohol 20% is available for cleaning both rigid and soft lenses and is reported to be effective against *Acanthamoeba* spp. (*see* Section 10.3).

Heat disinfection requires the use of units designed specifically for the purpose. It is a technique suitable for use with low water content soft lenses, and is the method of choice for patients who are sensitive to the preservatives used in some contact lens solutions. Preserved sodium chloride 0.9% or non-preserved sterile sodium chloride 0.9% solutions may be used to store the lenses during the heating process. It is essential to follow the method of disinfection outlined by the manufacturer of the disinfection unit. Heat disinfection is more detrimental to the lenses than chemical disinfection and can reduce the lens-life considerably. Soft contact lenses that are subjected to heat disinfection may last as little as six months.

Heat disinfection is not a suitable method for disinfecting hard or gas permeable hard lenses.

Comfort solutions   These solutions are formulated for instillation directly into the eye with the lens in place. They provide fluid to maintain adequate lens hydration and improve the comfort of soft lenses. The regular use of these solutions is important with extended-wear and disposable soft lenses.

Protein removal   Periodic cleaning with the use of protein removal preparations is required (*see above*). Protein removal preparations are usually suitable for both soft lenses and gas permeable hard lenses, and should be used according to the manufacturer's instructions.

Special contact lenses

Special contact lenses are used to correct particular problems affecting the eye. Scleral lenses cover the cornea and the sclera, and are used to mask damaged eyes. They can also be used in certain sports (e.g. water skiing) because they are less easily dislodged.

Toric lenses can be made with most materials and are used to correct astigmatism. They have an uneven surface curvature and correct irregular astigmatism and keratoconus (protrusion of the cornea) more effectively than spectacles.

Bifocal lenses can also be fitted for age-related changes to the eye, although the success rate is not very high.

Tinted contact lenses can be used to alter cosmetically the colour of the eyes, or they can be used instead of sunglasses, but the degree of protection from ultraviolet light is lower since the lens does not cover the entire eye.

10.3 COMPLICATIONS RELATED TO CONTACT LENS WEAR

Most complications associated with the wearing of contact lenses are self-limiting if the lens is removed at the first sign of trouble. The problems encountered are usually caused by the reaction of the eye to deposits on the lens or to chemicals absorbed by the lens. In addition, complications may be a result of poor lens care, inadequate hygiene, corneal hypoxia, overwear, or poor fitting.

Daily contact lens wear is associated with accumulation of deposits on the lens surface, which are responsible for many of the complications. Deposits on contact lenses may consist of:

- abraded corneal materials
- cosmetics
- divalent and trivalent cations
- dust
- lysozyme
- mucoproteins
- oils and lipids
- pollutants
- tear proteins.

The type and extent of lens deposits are influenced by tear consistency, flow rate, and volume. Increased lens deposits are seen in hot, dry environments as a result of evaporation of tears and increased concentration of constituents. The extent of deposit formation appears to be proportional to the water content of the lens. Accumulated lens deposits are relatively easy to remove from hard lenses by routine cleaning, they are less easily removed from gas permeable hard lenses, and may become chemically bound to soft lenses. The consequences of contact lens deposits include:

- allergy caused by denatured protein accumulation
- irritation as a result of poor wetting
- lens discoloration
- ocular irritation caused by binding of cationic preservatives to lens deposits
- pitting in surface of lens upon removal of calcium deposits
- reduced visual acuity
- reduction of antimicrobial activity of contact lens solutions caused by binding of preservatives to deposits on lens.

Daily wear gas permeable lenses are associated with the lowest incidence of complications and extended-wear soft lenses appear to cause most problems. Soft contact lenses are slightly larger than hard lenses and the long circumference tends to irritate the conjunctival membrane of the eyelid; the high surface area of the contact lens maximises the deposition of potentially antigenic deposits. The most common and potentially serious complication associated with daily wear soft contact lenses is corneal ulceration. Extended-wear soft lenses have been associated with a high incidence of suppurative keratitis, the risk of which appears to be related to the number of nights that the lenses are worn.

Contact lenses may cause chronic conjunctival problems. Purulent conjunctivitis is probably more common in contact lens wearers than in the general population. Contact lens associated papillary conjunctivitis may be caused by antigenic deposits on contact lenses. It occurs in approximately 3% of hard lens wearers and 8% of soft lens wearers. Symptoms include red eye, itching, and mucous discharge that causes smeared lenses and blurred vision. The condition is similar to allergic conjunctivitis and is thought to be an immune system-mediated reaction to the lens deposits. In the late stages, the condition may be associated with the appearance of giant papillae on the underside of the eyelid.

High water content soft lenses may become tight during wear, particularly if worn overnight. Immediate lens removal is essential to prevent corneal ulceration. A small degree of corneal oedema is inevitable with contact lens wear, but more extensive oedema may increase the risk of other complications. Contact lens removal and refitting with new lenses may resolve the problem, but some people have to stop using contact lenses. Prolonged wear of soft lenses may cause corneal opacities, which only infrequently occur with hard lenses and almost never with gas permeable hard lenses.

Toric lenses may have a thick inferior edge to prevent excessive rotation. The lower portion of the cornea may then become oxygen starved which could lead to the formation of new blood vessels (neovascularisation).

Ulcerative keratitis is a rare, but serious, complication of contact lens wear; it is more common with soft lenses because of increased microbial adherence to the lens and lens deposits. Other predisposing factors include overnight wear of daily wear lenses and long intervals between cleaning. The risk of keratitis is further increased with extended-wear soft lenses and disposable lenses. Infecting organisms are commonly bacterial (e.g. *Pseudomonas aeruginosa*), although fungal keratitis is occasionally encountered.

Acanthamoeba keratitis is a protozoal infection that is being increasingly encountered, particularly in soft lens wearers. It is a serious, sight-threatening condition, which is also difficult to diagnose since it mimics the symptoms of herpes virus infection. Symptoms include red eye, a purulent discharge, visual impairment, and pain. *Acanthamoeba* spp. can cause corneal scarring with partial or complete loss of sight. Homemade saline solutions have been implicated as a source of *Acanthamoeba* infection.

Red eye is a symptom of many complications associated with the use of contact lenses. It can also be caused by accumulated deposits and scratches on the lenses. Treatment involves stopping lens wear until the red eye has subsided and refitting with new lenses. Wearing lenses for longer than the recommended period of time may result in corneal oedema, which causes blurred vision and epithelial necrosis. Symptoms of overwear are common with hard lenses, but infrequently seen with gas permeable hard lenses and soft lenses; they resolve within a few hours of lens removal, although some people may require active treatment.

Allergic reactions to the preservatives and disinfectants included in contact lens solutions may occur. Chemicals used for cleaning and disinfection may be taken up by the lenses and released onto the eye. Symptoms may include itching, stinging, and, in more serious cases, severe discomfort and visual impairment. Patients may be advised to use alternative formulations to avoid a particular allergen. Heat disinfection is the method of choice for soft contact lens wearers who are sensitive to components of the solutions.

10.4 THE ROLE OF THE PHARMACIST

Contact lens wear demands motivation, commitment, and meticulous care to prevent problems. Wearers must realise that it is essential to conform to the recommended regimens of maintenance and use for their particular type of lens. The regimen that is necessary will have been explained to wearers by the optometrist; however, it has been demonstrated that compliance is commonly poor. The complexity of care regimens and the correct use of lens care products requires effective education to ensure compliance and problem-free wear.

The pharmacist should emphasise to contact lens wearers that they should visit the optometrist regularly for contact lens after-care. New contact lens wearers will usually be required to visit the optometrist at frequent intervals in the period immediately after fitting. There-after, regular visits at six-monthly intervals for soft lens wearers and yearly intervals for those with rigid lenses are recommended. Symptom-free wear does not nec-essarily mean that the contact lenses are not causing undesirable effects. These visits are important to keep the contact lens prescription updated and identify insidious complications at an early stage. All contact lens wearers should also have their spectacle prescription kept updated, and have a pair of spectacles to use in place of their contact lenses, either in an emergency or on an occasional basis to rest the eyes.

Advice on the prevention of complications associated with the use of contact lenses is essential because inadequate lens care is one of the many causes of eye infections. Lenses should only be worn for the recommended length of time, and should not be worn during sleep, unless they are extended-wear or disposable lenses designed for the purpose. It is important to refer wearers immediately if any of the following are apparent:

- discomfort
- excessive lachrymation
- frequent eye infections
- itching
- pain
- photophobia
- recurrent red eye problems
- visual impairment.

The pharmacist is ideally placed to advise contact lens wearers on contact lens products and effective care regimens. The type or brand of contact lens solutions should not be changed by wearers without first obtaining guidance from the optometrist or pharmacist. Lens care products are intended to be used in clean surroundings, and hands should be washed and dried before attempting to remove or insert lenses. If working over a sink, it is essential to put in the drainage plug to stop the accidental loss of a lens.

Awareness of circumstances and situations that can adversely affect contact lens wearers will assist pharmacists to advise on achieving comfortable and problem-free wear. Adverse environmental conditions (e.g. dry heat, air-conditioning, and windy days) may cause burning, stinging, and blurred vision; comfort solutions can be used to alleviate discomfort if the stimulus cannot be avoided. The use of cosmetics with contact lenses is acceptable provided simple guidelines are followed. Generally, contact lenses should be inserted before applying cosmetics; however, hairspray and other aerosol applications should be used before contact lenses are inserted. It is preferable to use water-based, fragrance-free cosmetics because oily cosmetics tend to stain lenses or bind with lens material. Cosmetics should not be applied to the edge of the eyelids, and mascara should be water-resistant and applied only to the tips of the eyelashes. Contact lenses are fragile, and sharp objects (e.g. fingernails) can scratch hard lenses and gas permeable hard lenses and tear soft lenses.

Contact lens wearers should be advised that lenses cannot disappear behind the eye; they may need to be recentred if they slip out of position and the techniques, which vary with different lenses, will have been explained to them by the optometrist. Lenses should not be worn when swimming unless advised to do so by the optometrist. During illness, the duration of contact lens wear should be shortened and built up after recovery.

The pharmacist should be aware of the effects of systemic and topical eye medication in contact lens wearers (Table 10.1).

Systemic medication   Systemic medication can have adverse effects on the wearing of contact lenses, or on the lens material itself. Reduced tolerance to contact lenses has been reported with the use of oral contraceptives, particularly those containing higher doses of oestrogen. Reported effects have included corneal and eyelid oedema, reduced visual acuity, photophobia, allergic conjunctivitis, and altered tear composition. Corneal oedema appears to be less of a problem with the present low-dose oral contraceptives and modern lenses. Preg-nancy can produce the same effects on contact lens wear.

Anxiolytics, hypnotics, antihistamines, and muscle relaxants can reduce the blink rate. Adequate blinking is necessary to maintain proper hydration of lenses, par-ticularly with soft lenses. Blinking also removes stale tears and provides a fresh supply.

Atropine, antihistamines, antimuscarinic drugs, chlorpromazine, some beta blockers, diuretics, and tricyclic antidepressants can all decrease tear volume, which may lead to corneal drying and irritation. Reserpine, ephedrine, or hydralazine may cause an increase in lachrymation and can adversely affect contact lens wear by impairing the fit.

Conjunctivitis can occur with isotretinoin and it is wise to avoid wearing contact lenses during treatment. Primidone and chlorthalidone may produce ocular or eyelid oedema causing interference with lens wear. After taking aspirin, salicylic acid appears in tears and may be absorbed by soft lenses resulting in ocular irritation and redness. Rifampicin and sulphasalazine both cause discoloration of soft contact lenses.

Topical medication Generally, topical eye medication should not be used while lenses are being worn. Eye drops should be administered 30 minutes before the insertion of lenses. Topical treatment of an eye infection necessitates the removal of contact lenses for the duration of treatment, as the lenses may harbour the micro-organisms. The lenses may need professional cleaning and sterilisation, services which are available from the optometrist.

The effect of topically applied drugs on soft contact lenses may be exaggerated due to the following effects:

- absorption and consequent concentration of drug can occur with gradual release over a period of time
- increased drug absorption due to compromised cornea in contact lens wearers
- lenses can increase contact time of drug medication.

Dark discoloration of soft lenses with repeated use of phenylephrine and adrenaline has been observed. At after-care visits, diagnostic stains (e.g. fluorescein sodium) may be used to detect corneal abrasions. Fluorescein is capable of staining contact lenses, and spectacles should be worn following its use in an examination, for a period specified by the optometrist. Acne medications containing benzoyl peroxide can fade tinted soft lenses.

Smokers have a higher incidence of stained soft lenses than non-smokers. This may be due to stimulation of melanin products in tears by nicotine and other aromatic compounds in cigarette smoke. Patients should be counselled about the potential for lens spoilage and the importance of disinfection. Nicotine transferred to lenses by smoke or fingers can reduce their clarity.

TABLE 10.1

Reported drug interactions with contact lenses

Drug	Hard	Soft	Interaction mechanism
Adrenaline, topical		.	discoloration
Anxiolytics	.	.	decreased blink rate
Aspirin		.	absorption by lens causing irritation and redness
Antihistamines	.	.	decreased tear volume; blink rate
Antimuscarinics	.	.	decreased tear volume
Benzoyl peroxide, topical		.	fading of lens tint
Diuretics		.	decreased tear volume; ocular and eyelid oedema with chlorthalidone
Fluorescein, topical		.	concentration by lens and subsequent discoloration
Hypnotics	.	.	decreased blink rate
Muscle relaxants	.	.	decreased blink rate
Oral contraceptives		.	ocular and eyelid oedema; altered tear composition
Phenylephrine, topical		.	discoloration
Primidone	.	.	ocular and eyelid oedema
Reserpine	.	.	increased lachrymation
Rifampicin		.	orange discoloration of the lens
Rose bengal, topical		.	concentration by lens and subsequent discoloration
Sedatives	.	.	decreased blink rate
Sodium sulphacetamide 10%, topical		.	lens dehydration due to hypertonicity of solution
Sulphasalazine		.	yellow discoloration of the lens
Tricyclic antidepressants	.	.	decreased tear volume

INDEX